Gastrointestinal Tract Imaging

Commissioning Editor: Claire Wilson
Development Editor: Catherine Jackson
Project Manager: Sukanthi Sukumar
Designer: Stewart Larking
Illustration Manager: Merlyn Harvey
Illustrator: Robert Britton

Gastrointestinal Tract Imaging

An evidence-based practice guide

Edited by

Julie M. Nightingale, MSc DCR(R)
Director of Radiography/Chair of the GI Radiographers'
Special Interest Group (GIRSIG), University of Salford, Salford, UK

Robert L. Law, DCR(R) MRCR(Hon)
Consultant Gastrointestinal Radiographer,
North Bristol NHS Trust; Visiting Research Fellow,
University of the West of England, Bristol, UK

Foreword by

Giles Maskell, FRCP FRCR
Consultant Radiologist,
Royal Cornwall Hospital, Truro, Cornwall, UK

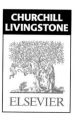

Edinburgh   London   New York   Oxford   Philadelphia   St Louis   Sydney   Toronto   2010

CHURCHILL LIVINGSTONE
ELSEVIER

First published 2010, © Elsevier Limited. All rights reserved.

ISBN 978 0 443 06789 1

British Library Cataloguing in Publication Data
A catalogue record for this book is available from the British Library

Library of Congress Cataloging in Publication Data
A catalog record for this book is available from the Library of Congress

Notice
Knowledge and best practice in this field are constantly changing. As new research and experience broaden our knowledge, changes in practice, treatment and drug therapy may become necessary or appropriate. Readers are advised to check the most current information provided (i) on procedures featured or (ii) by the manufacturer of each product to be administered, to verify the recommended dose or formula, the method and duration of administration, and contraindications. It is the responsibility of the practitioner, relying on their own experience and knowledge of the patient, to make diagnoses, to determine dosages and the best treatment for each individual patient, and to take all appropriate safety precautions. To the fullest extent of the law, neither the Publisher nor the Editors assume any liability for any injury and/or damage to persons or property arising out of or related to any use of the material contained in this book.

The Publisher

Printed in China

Contents

List of Contributors

Jessie Aw, MBChB MRCP FRCR
Radiology Fellow, Austin Health,
Melbourne, Australia

Neil Bayman, MBChB MRCP FRCR
Consultant Clinical Oncologist,
Clinical Oncology, Christie
Hospital, Manchester, UK

Christine Bloor, BSc (Hons) MSc Cert Ed
Consultant Radiographer, Department
of Clinical Imaging, Royal Cornwall
Hospital, Cornwall, UK

Alison Booth, DCR(R) MSc
Research Fellow, Centre for Reviews
and Dissemination, University of
York, York, UK

Helen Carter
North Bristol NHS Trust, Radiology
Department, Frenchay Hospital,
Bristol, UK

David Gary Culpan, DCR(R) PgCHSM
PgCHEP MSc
Lecturer in Radiography, Course
Leader PgC GI Reporting, University
of Bradford, Division of Radiography,
School of Health Studies, Bradford, UK

S. Gandhi
Consultant Radiologist, Department
of Radiology, Frenchay Hospital,
Bristol, UK

Najib Haboubi, MBChB FRCPath
Professor of Health Sciences, Liver
and Gastrointestinal Pathology,
Consultant Histopathologist,
Trafford Healthcare NHS Trust,
Manchester, UK

Peter Hogg
Professor of Radiography,
Department of Radiography,
University of Salford, Salford, UK

Myke Kudlas, MEd RT(R)(QM)
Assistant Professor of Radiology
and Director, Radiography
Program, Mayo Clinic College of
Medicine, Jacksonville, Florida, USA

Robert L. Law, DCR MRCR(Hon)
Consultant Gastrointestinal
Radiographer, North Bristol NHS
Trust; Visiting Research Fellow,
University of the West of England,
Bristol, UK

Derrick Martin, FRCR FRCP.Mb CHb
Professor of Gastrointestinal
Radiology, Department of
Radiology, Wythenshawe Hospital,
Manchester, UK

Nyla Nasir, MBBS FRCPath
Consultant Histopathologist,
Department of Histopathology,
Trafford Health Care NHS Trust,
Urmston, Manchester, UK

Roger D. Newman, BSc(Hons) MRCSLT
Senior Specialist Speech and
Language Therapist, NHS Central
Lancashire, Preston, UK

Julie M. Nightingale, MSc DCR(R)
Director of Radiography/Chair
of the GI Radiographers' Special
Interest Group (GIRSIG), University
of Salford, Salford, UK

Anne M. Pullyblank, MBBS BSc FRCS (gen surg) MD
Consultant Coloproctologist, Department of Surgery, Frenchay Hospital, Bristol, UK

Liza Ricote, DCR PostGradDip
Senior Radiographer, Emergency Department

Vivian E. Rushton, PhD MDS BDS FRCR DDRRCR MFGDP PgCertEd
Senior Lecturer and Honorary Consultant in Dental and Maxillofacial Radiology, School of Dentistry, University of Manchester, Manchester, UK

Emil Salmo, FRCPath
Consultant Pathologist, Trafford Healthcare NHS Trust, Manchester, UK

Mark P. Saunders, MBBS MRCP FRCR PhD
Consultant Clinical Oncologist (Radiotherapy), Radiotherapy Department, Christie Hospital, Manchester, UK

Ian S. Shaw, MBChB MSc FRCP
Consultant Gastroenterologist, Department of Gastroenterology, Gloucestershire Royal Hospital, Gloucester, UK

Charlotte Thompson
Department of Radiography, University of Salford, Salford, UK

Christopher Wong, MB BCH PhD FRCS
Consultant Upper GI and Endocrine Surgeon, Department of Surgery, Frenchay Hospital, Bristol, UK

Foreword

The advances in medical imaging in recent decades are well recognized, and nowhere is their impact better exemplified than in the field of gastrointestinal disease. From fluoroscopy to ultrasound, endoscopy, multidetector CT, and MRI, the range of tools that are available to examine the GI tract has continued to grow. At the same time, the pattern of gastrointestinal disease has changed with the virtual disappearance of peptic ulceration from Western populations and the rise of diseases of affluence and old age. Medical imaging should never be seen in isolation and any professional seeking expertise in this area must pay as much attention to the epidemiology and pathophysiology of gastrointestinal tract disease as to the imaging techniques available for its investigation. A sound knowledge of anatomy, physiology and the other basic building blocks of clinical medicine is required before the increasingly sophisticated imaging tools can be employed for the benefit of patients.

For this book, the editors, acknowledged leaders in radiography education and clinical radiographic practice, have assembled a group of expert contributors from a wide range of clinical and professional backgrounds. There are chapters by surgeons, physicians, pathologists, therapists, radiologists and radiographers and in fact almost the whole multidisciplinary team involved in the care of patients with GI tract conditions. Contributions cover the full range of gastrointestinal disease and its investigation from mouth to anus and from barium to CT colonography and PET-CT. There is a consistent focus on the essential clinical background and on the evidence base for each type of investigation. The underpinning ethos of the book is multiprofessional and multidisciplinary. The editors have skilfully melded the contributions into a book which has a consistent and coherent style and message. The message, in essence, is that patients with gastrointestinal problems are best served by a clinical team which makes full use of the talents and skills of all involved, regardless of their professional background.

This is much more than a textbook of gastrointestinal tract imaging. Whilst it stands as a comprehensive account of the role of imaging in gastrointestinal disease, it goes beyond that to form a chronicle of the progress made by a dedicated group of clinical radiographer leaders in expanding not only their own horizons but also those of the whole profession of radiography. This book is testament to their achievements and will serve to inform and inspire future generations of radiographers and radiographic technologists.

Dr. Giles Maskell FRCP FRCR

Preface

Over the last two decades, radiology departments around the world have witnessed significant changes in the way their services are delivered. Rapid technological advancements, coupled with an increasing emphasis on patient outcomes and experience, have resulted in a changing professional landscape within the radiology department. Within the United Kingdom and America, radiographers have been successfully delegated a number of roles formerly undertaken by consultant radiologists. In the Gastrointestinal Imaging (GI), branch of radiology in particular, radiographers have developed a wide spectrum of advanced practice, and these role changes have promoted a renewed enthusiasm for critical evaluation of the GI imaging service.

Numerous text books focus upon individual aspects of the GI patient pathway, such as radiology image interpretation, surgery or pathology. This textbook, however, offers a unique collaboration between expert clinicians and health care professionals involved with different stages of the patient pathway, from initial consultation, through imaging procedures, to eventual treatment. It is hoped that this collaboration, and the resultant textbook, reflect the multi-disciplinary way in which services are now delivered. Through discussions of the evidence base at each stage of this pathway, we have attempted to provide a concise, single volume guide or handbook for all professionals involved in either referring patients for GI procedures, or performing and interpreting GI imaging studies.

We hope that this book will be of particular value for radiographers and radiologic technologists who are involved in performing GI imaging procedures or managing a GI radiology service, or those who wish to aspire to advanced and consultant practice roles. Detailed chapters spanning the range of diagnostic and therapeutic GI procedures will be of value not only to radiographers, but also to radiologists in training student radiographers and nurses with a GI interest. Whilst we did not aim to create a 'radiology image interpretation' textbook (many excellent resources are already available), we do attempt to refer to commonly encountered pathologies within each imaging chapter. Complementary to the 'imaging' chapters are a number of 'fundamental knowledge' chapters which span all related aspects of the GI service. These include detailed discussions on medico-legal and ethical issues, pharmacology, image interpretation and report writing, and applied anatomy and physiology.

It is hoped that this text will be a valuable addition to the bookshelves of referring clinicians (General practitioners, surgeons and gastroenterologists), medical students, gastroenterology nurses and any health professional who is interested in developing a role associated with the gastrointestinal tract.

We would like to express our appreciation to the many individuals who have contributed chapters for this book. As leaders and pioneers within their field we are indebted to them for sharing their knowledge and enthusiasm. We appreciate how much work is involved in producing chapters to this standard, and thank them for their dedication.

Whilst the majority of contributors are from the UK, we sincerely hope that the book offers an international perspective of GI radiology in the 21st century, and will be welcomed by professionals in other countries who wish to ensure that they offer an effective GI imaging service. If any reader would like to contact us for further information, discussion or debate, please do not hesitate to do so.

Julie M. Nightingale MSc DCR(R)
J.Nightingale@salford.ac.uk

Robert L. Law DCR(R) MRCR (Hon)
Robert.Law@nbt.nhs.uk

Acknowledgments

Instrumental to the development of my interest in gastrointestinal (GI) fluoroscopy have been a number of people. In the early 1980s, during his time at Frenchay Hospital, GI radiologist Dr. David Mackenzie-Crooks willingly offered the enthusiastic teaching and practical training that initiated my interest in GI fluoroscopy. Over the following 25 years, GI radiologists, Drs Nicky Slack and Andrew Longstaff had the faith to allow me to develop and expand my interest, and the friendship, clinical and editorial mentorship and red pen guidance of gastroenterologist, Dr. Richard Harvey has been an inspiration. Lastly, but most particularly I want to thank Sally, my wife, who has put up with my love affair with my work from the beginning.

Robert L. Law

I would first like to offer my sincere thanks for the dedication and hard work shown by all the contributors of this book. It has been a privilege to work with a number of health professionals who, over the last few years, have inspired and encouraged me to develop my knowledge, and that of others, within the gastrointestinal imaging field. In particular, I would like to acknowledge Andrea Owen and Christine Bloor (Consultant Radiographers), Sue Conroy and Ian Sutton (GI Advanced Practitioners) and Alison Booth (research fellow and former GI practitioner), who have shared my enthusiasm for educating our future GI advanced practitioners and promoting research within the specialty. Similarly, I would also like to acknowledge the essential support for skills mix projects within the GI radiology field shown by Consultant Radiologists Professor Nigel Thomas, Dr. Hans-Ulrich Laasch, Professor Derrick Martin and Dr. Rob Bisset.

As a result of the encouragement, direction and vision shown by all of these radiographers and radiologists, I developed a range of Gastrointestinal Imaging programs, which ultimately provided the impetus for this text book.

Most of all, however, I would like to thank my husband Graham and my children Christopher and Jonathan, who have provided endless support throughout this long-term project.

Julie M. Nightingale

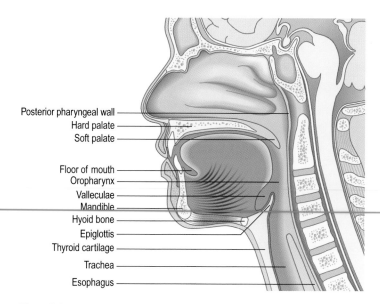

Posterior pharyngeal wall
Hard palate
Soft palate

Floor of mouth
Oropharynx
Valleculae
Mandible
Hyoid bone
Epiglottis
Thyroid cartilage
Trachea
Esophagus

Figure 7.1 Lateral view of the oral cavity and oropharynx.

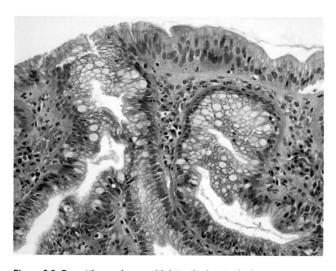

Figure 9.2 Barrett's esophagus with intestinal metaplasia.

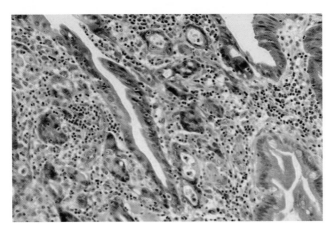

Figure 9.3 Barrett's esophagus with intramural carcinoma.

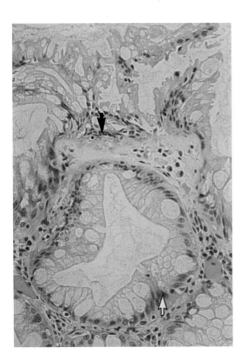

Figure 9.6 Microscopic appearance of hyperplastic/regenerative polyp.

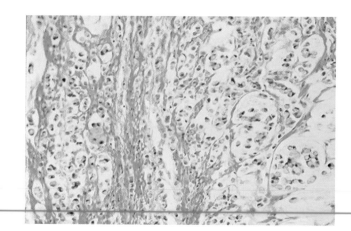

Figure 9.8 Signet ring cell adenocarcinoma infiltrating the gastric wall.

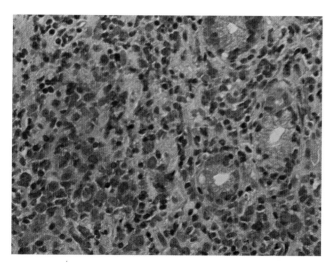

Figure 9.11 Gastric lymphoma: heavy population of lymphocytes infiltrates diffusely into the mucosa, invading gastric glands to form lymphoepithelial lesions with florid destruction of gastric glands.

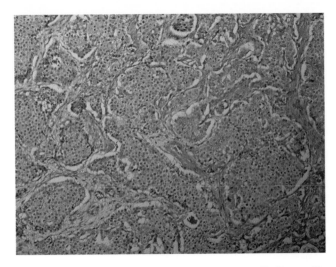

Figure 9.12 Carcinoid tumor composed of monotonous cells dispersed in an organoid pattern.

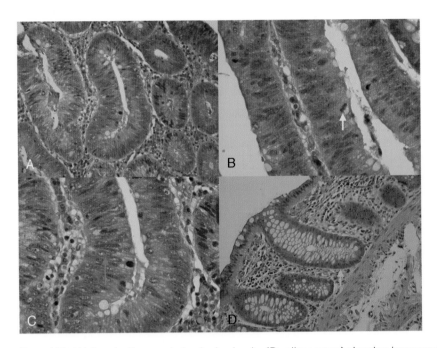

Figure 14.3 (A) Dysplastic crowded colonic glands, (B yellow arrow) showing increased mitotic figures and (C red arrow) epithelial nuclear stratification, multilayering and hyperchromasia. (D) Normal colonic glands lined by a single layered epithelium (blue arrow).

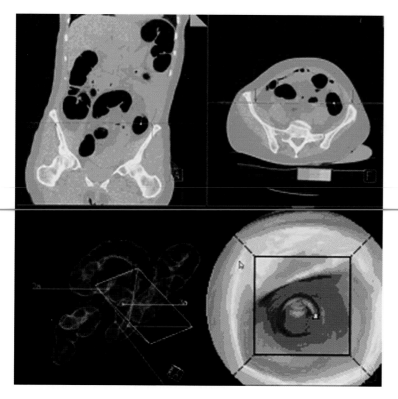

Figure 17.15 Shows the workstation display for CT colonographic assessment.

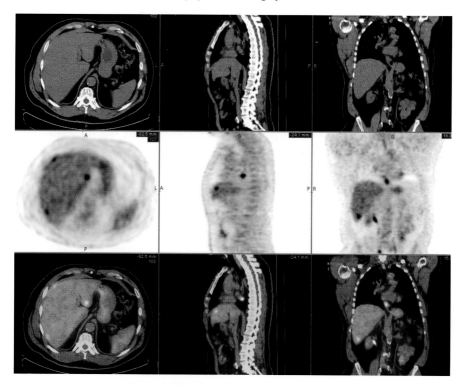

Figure 17.17 PET-CT: esophageal primary with liver metastases. (Courtesy of Dr Julie Searle.)

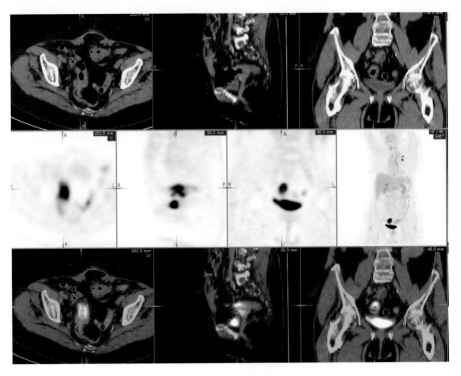

Figure 17.18 **PET-CT: sigmoid primary with lung metastases.** (Courtesy of Dr Julie Searle.)

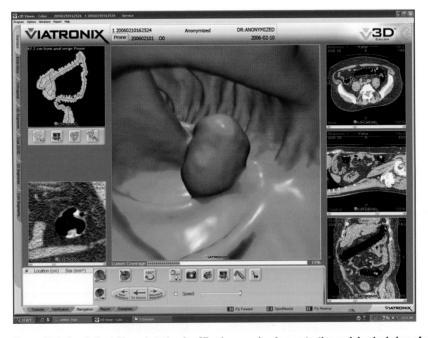

Figure 18.4 **Specialized 3D workstation for CT colonography, demonstrating endoluminal view of a polyp alongside corresponding 2D slices** (Courtesy of Viatronix, Inc).

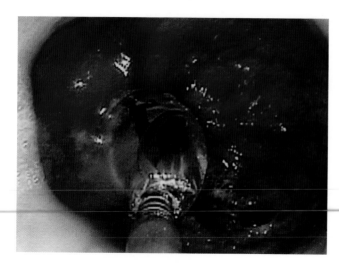

Figure 20.1 Esophageal balloon dilatation.

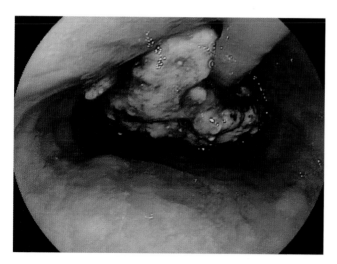

Figure 20.2 Esophageal carcinoma.

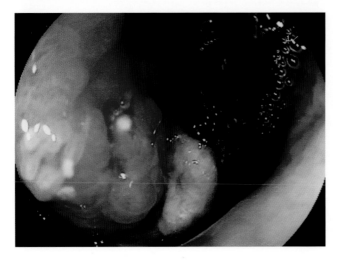

Figure 20.3 Esophageal carcinoma, retroflex view from gastroscopy.

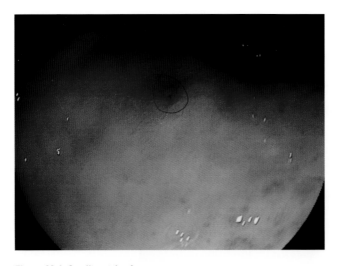

Figure 20.4 Small gastric ulcer.

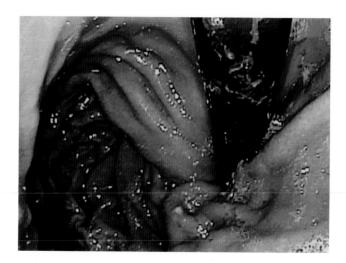

Figure 20.5 Nissen wrap, retroflex view.

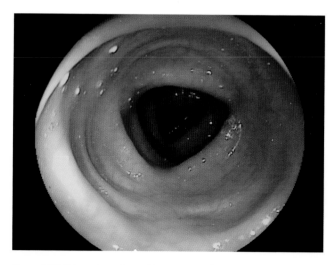

Figure 20.6 Triangular nature of transverse colon.

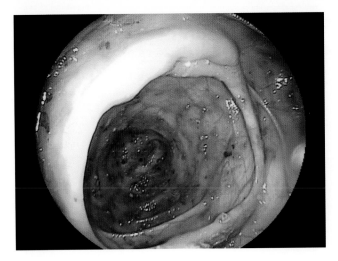

Figure 20.7   Cecum, shows ileocecal valve and appendix orifice.

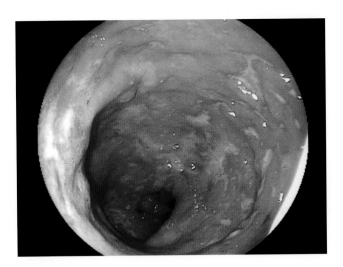

Figure 20.8   Colitis.

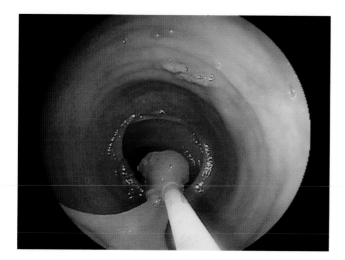

Figure 20.9 Polyp being snared.

Evolving practice and shifting boundaries in gastrointestinal tract imaging

Julie M. Nightingale, Myke Kudlas, Liza Ricote

Contents ||||||||||||||||||||||||||||||||||||||||||||||||||||||||||||||||||||||||||||

Advances in GI imaging

Fluoroscopic techniques to image the gastrointestinal (GI) tract have been available since the early 20th century, although it was not until the 1970s (with the introduction of image intensification and double contrast techniques) that their effectiveness as a diagnostic tool was firmly established. While some fluoroscopic procedures have remained dominant as the method of choice for investigation of particular pathologies, a number have been replaced by alternative procedures, or are experiencing challenges to their position as a first line investigation. The barium meal, for example, has largely been replaced by endoscopy, with the double contrast barium enema (DCBE) being challenged by colonoscopy and computed tomography (CT) colonography. While fluoroscopic investigations have always been the examination of choice for investigating the small intestine (being difficult to access endoscopically), they also are being challenged by CT and MR enteroclysis techniques, as well as direct visualization by capsule endoscopy.

CT has been the mainstay of staging for most GI cancers, although we are seeing an increasing role for ultrasound and magnetic resonance (MR) imaging, particularly in peri-rectal imaging. PET (positron emission tomography) and hybrid scanning methods are also likely to have an expanding role in the assessment of more complex cases, particularly in the investigation of cancer recurrence or identification of an unknown primary cancer.

Many radiology departments have also introduced an increasing array of interventional and therapeutic GI procedures, especially for palliation of cancer. These have included esophageal and colonic stenting and balloon dilatations for different types of stricture. More recently, fluoroscopic guidance and radiological expertise for gastric banding is being used to assist in the management of patients with obesity, demand for such involvement being likely to increase in developed nations. While being time consuming and resource intensive for the radiology department, such procedures provide hospitals with the ability to support effectively those unsuitable for major surgery.

Throughout the 20th century, the GI radiology service has involved a multiprofessional team of radiologists, radiographers, radiology nurses and health care assistants. During the 1980s, the skills mix within the fluoroscopy department began to change and the following section will consider how this affected radiology departments within the UK.

Shifting professional boundaries

The gradual refinement of fluoroscopic techniques, coupled with the progressive exploration of new imaging modalities, has resulted in a much wider contribution of radiology to the gastrointestinal (GI) patient care pathway. Over the last three decades, there has been a huge shift in the role of the professions that are involved in providing the GI radiology service, particularly in the UK (Nightingale and Hogg, 2003a, 2007). However, the UK is not alone in this, with gradually shifting professional boundaries being seen within other English-speaking countries, including the USA, Australia, New Zealand and Canada.

The health services of the world are highly complex organizations, often being among the largest national employers. Introducing radical change into such organizations is challenging, as they often have many stakeholders with different needs to satisfy. Analysis of a number of historical role developments, both within and outside radiology, suggests that a range of overlapping drivers is necessary to implement the changes effectively (Box 1.1) (Nightingale and Hogg, 2003b). In the early 1990s, a major shift in professional roles began to take place within UK radiology departments. One of the

---

BOX 1.1 Drivers promoting successful introduction of new roles

- A perceived deficiency in the service
- A proposed solution
- A legal framework within which to introduce the change
- A 'champion' of the change, at national and local level
- Evidence (research) that the change will be effective
- A benefit to stakeholders (interested parties)

most rapid to be adopted was the introduction of radiographer-performed double contrast barium enema (DCBE) examinations (known as the air contrast barium enema examination in the USA). The introduction of this role will be explored further, considering the relevant drivers that came together to result in successful implementation on a national scale.

A perceived deficiency in the service

According to the UK professional body, The College of Radiographers (2006), diagnostic imaging and interventional services have increased by 2.5–5% per annum over the last 10 to 12 years. This continuing rise in demand for imaging services, coupled with a shortage of radiologists, led to UK radiology services being severely over-stretched. The shortfall in radiologists was estimated by the Royal College of Radiologists in 2002 to:

> Need to double just to match existing workloads, let alone take into account future service pressures.

Not surprisingly, perceived deficiencies were noted within the service. These included excessively long waiting times for complex examinations (including the DCBE) and radiological reports turned around too slowly to affect patient management, or not reported at all (Audit Commission, 1995). The DCBE examinations were often single reported, even when double reporting was considered to be best practice (Markus et al., 1990; Leslie and Virjee, 2002; Halligan et al., 2003). This raised serious concerns for patient care and the impact upon their prognoses, particularly where cancer was suspected. The shortage of radiologists also inevitably held back the further development of the service at that time, with less time available for audit, research and the introduction of new services.

A possible solution

Radiographers had expanded their pre-registration education to degree level (from a 2-year diploma course) and experienced radiographers had begun to explore postgraduate master's level opportunities. Radiographers have long been perceived to be working below their potential (Swinburne, 1971), often moving into managerial or education positions due to a lack of challenging opportunities in clinical practice. One solution, to train radiographers to undertake DCBE examinations, as these had unacceptably long waiting lists in many hospitals, offered an important new challenge and yet could be 'easily described within a protocol' (Somers et al., 1981).

A legal framework within which to introduce the change

A number of changes to legislation and professional body guidance was introduced within the 1990s, some acting as a catalyst to encourage role development and some, inevitably, being brought about in response to what was already happening at a local level. These included the introduction of the Ionising Radiation (Medical Exposure) Regulations (Department of Health, 2000a) and Department of Health publications such as the NHS Cancer Plan (2000b). The professional body and trade union for radiographers (the Society and College of Radiographers) was very supportive to radiographers wishing to develop their roles, issuing a series of guidance documents between 1996 and the present day (e.g. The College of Radiographers 1996, 1997, 2006). In essence, these documents suggested a framework in which radiographers could potentially develop any role, as long as they were appropriately trained, worked within agreed protocols, audited their practice and maintained their competence through continuing professional development (CPD). Protocols have been found to be appropriate frameworks within which radiographers can safely and effectively practice advanced roles (Nightingale, 2008). The Royal College of Radiologists (RCR; the UK radiologists' professional body) has also been supportive towards radiographer role development, although with a slightly more cautious approach (RCR 1996, 1999, 2007). This is understandable when their members are delegating existing tasks and may still bear the ultimate responsibility for the delegated role.

A 'champion' of the change, at national and local level

There has to date been no direct professional body steer to introduce a particular role development across the UK. However, as with most new roles, there is often a champion at national level. For the introduction of radiographer-performed DCBE, this champion has arguably been the national gastrointestinal radiographers' special interest group (GIRSIG), which has both promoted and supported radiographers involved in these roles for several years (Nightingale and Hogg, 2000). However, it is not clear if the role would have been introduced so successfully across the UK if it had not been for the presence of radiologist champions, promoting radiographer role development both within and beyond radiology (e.g. Chapman, 1997; Robinson et al., 1999; Thomas, 2005b). The radiologists appeared at that time to be the 'gatekeepers' to service development and this largely appears to be the case today. The radiologists provided clinical training and supervision for the radiographers, who had access to a short course or Master's level module for theoretical underpinning.

National drivers for role development have also emerged in the wake of a series of government targets, most notably the introduction of a maximum waiting target of 2 weeks from referral to diagnosis for suspected cancer (NHS Executive, 2000) and, more recently, the 18 week maximum from referral to treatment (Department of Health, 2006). With medical imaging being heralded by the Government as the primary bottleneck resulting in failure of hospitals to meet these targets (Department of Health, 2005), it is little wonder that modernizing services and new ways of working are being championed in political circles.

Evidence (research) that the change will be effective

Published evidence that the role change is effective is vital to promote the widespread introduction of a new service. While UK radiographers have been rather reticent to engage in research, where the DCBE examination has been concerned, one finds a wealth of literature supporting the new role. This has included a number of studies comparing radiographer performance in performing and/or reporting DCBE examinations with trainee radiologists (Mannion et al., 1995; Schreiber et al., 1996; Davidson et al., 2000) or with consultant radiologists (McKenzie et al., 1998; Culpan et al., 2002; Murphy et al., 2002; Vora and Chapman, 2004). It also includes performance against pathology databases (Law et al., 1999, 2008) and national surveys of practice (Bewell and Chapman, 1996). While most of these studies have concentrated on small numbers of individuals in single-center studies, they nevertheless provide very useful and plausible performance data across large numbers of patients.

A benefit to stakeholders (interested parties)

However, without there being a clear benefit to the relevant stakeholders, it is unlikely that a new role will be introduced. The benefits to radiology departments have been clear, with vastly reduced waiting lists for DCBE and, where radiographer reporting has been introduced, quicker turn-around for report writing. There are potential cost savings, with the hourly rate of a radiographer being considerably less than that of a consultant radiologist (Brown and Desai, 2002). Surprisingly little published literature is focused upon patient acceptability, although in practice many unpublished patient surveys have suggested that patients are happy to be cared for by a radiographer without recourse to a radiologist. The patient benefits directly from these improvements, reducing anxiety with shorter waits and having a potentially better prognosis associated with a shortened referral to diagnosis timeframe. The benefits to the radiologist are clear, in that they have more time to fulfil their other duties or to introduce new services. Anecdotal evidence would suggest that, for most radiologists, the rather unglamorous aspects of the DCBE procedure have not been missed from their portfolio of duties!

So what about the radiographers? Again anecdotal evidence would suggest that performing these complex procedures has given them a great deal of satisfaction, in particular in relation to improved patient care and team working. For many who have continued their training to include reporting on the images and the performing of other GI procedures, they have increased their confidence and esteem, becoming highly valued members of the multidisciplinary team. This has led to re-grading and increased salaries for many radiographers within the new career framework.

Beyond the DCBE

The radiographer-performed DCBE role has been so well received that radiographer-led services are now the norm across the UK National Health Service (NHS), with recent estimates suggesting that over 1200 radiographers have been trained to perform DCBE (Nightingale and Hogg, 2007); 82% of hospitals surveyed by Price and Le Masurier (2007) had implemented a radiographer-led DCBE service. Many such radiographers have gone on to undertake postgraduate training to enable them to write an official report on the DCBEs, with published data supporting this practice (Law et al., 1999; Murphy et al., 2002). While most of the available courses prepare and assess radiographers to report independently, in practice, many will report as part of a double reporting system, whereby two people view the images independently and then compare reports. Double reporting is recommended in the

UK for the DCBE procedure, as it is associated with a high level of potential perception errors (Markus et al., 1990; Leslie and Virjee, 2002).

Some radiographers have further expanded their role to perform and report barium swallows and meals, videofluoroscopy swallowing assessments, small bowel studies, proctograms and other non-GI fluoroscopy (e.g. hysterosalpingography) (Law et al., 2005; Nightingale and Mackay, 2009). While most DCBE radiographers have further developed their role within the confines of the fluoroscopy room, increasingly GI radiographers are crossing traditional imaging modalities to run a CT colonography service, often in conjunction with a CT radiographer. Some are not only working across imaging modalities, but have also crossed professional boundaries to work with teams outside radiology. Although nurse-performed endoscopy is far more common (Maruthachalam et al., 2006, Kelly et al., 2007), a handful of UK radiographers have trained to undertake sigmoidoscopy or colonoscopy, with the potential advantage over nurses of being able to offer continuity of care with combined DCBE and direct visualization on one day.

However, despite the exciting opportunities presented, relatively few UK radiographers have developed their role beyond the DCBE examination (Price and Le Masurier, 2007). This may be because the required drivers for effective role changes (see Box 1.1.) are not firmly in place. In Table 1.1, we present possible reasons, based upon both published and anecdotal evidence, regarding the apparent stalemate in the adoption of further role developments and advanced practices.

Clearly from Table 1.1, a number of drivers for effective implementation of widespread role changes are not currently in place. While a clear service need for other GI advanced practices may exist within any given hospital, the role is unlikely to be adopted as national standard practice without there being a perceived service deficiency, coupled with a champion at national level.

At the time of writing, it appears that we are once again on the threshold of a new role change for radiographers, which may well be implemented on a national basis. CT colonography (CTC) (alternatively known as virtual colonoscopy), a relatively new technique to examine the bowel, has been extensively researched around the world. Advocates of this procedure are proposing that it will eventually replace the barium enema for symptomatic work and may have an important role to play in bowel screening. For this reason, the government and professional bodies have also taken a keen interest, with a national working party currently developing a framework for implementation. A UK wide study (SIGGAR 1 trial) comparing CTC to barium enema and colonoscopy for bowel cancer in older symptomatic patients is soon to report its findings (Halligan et al., 2007). Nevertheless, hospitals around the UK have already introduced this procedure to varying degrees, with many proposing that radiographers play an important part in both performing the procedure, managing the scanning protocols and, in some way, contributing to the reporting process. Table 1.2 considers the presence or absence of drivers for implementation of radiographer involvement in CTC.

While CTC presents an exciting opportunity for radiographers (and possibly radiology nurses) to expand their role beyond the DCBE, a number of radiographers have already developed a 'package' of expertise that has enabled them to attain the highest level of clinical speciality in the UK – that of consultant radiographer status. At the time of writing, there are 26 consultant

Table 1.1 Criteria for effective implementation of role changes beyond the DCBE examination since 2000

Driver for change	Evidence for the presence of the driver
A perceived deficiency in the service	The waiting lists for other GI examinations and their report turnaround times are reasonably short The shortage of radiologists is no longer as acute as in the 1990s Additional funded radiology training places results in competition for training sessions in some hospitals
A proposed solution	Radiographers could take on new roles
A legal framework within which to introduce the change	There are concerns about the greater risks involved in some procedures (e.g. endoscopy)
A 'champion' of the change, at national and local level	Some examinations are not attracting interest from the government, compared to others which are seen as high priority (e.g. examinations for colon cancer screening) While special interest groups and professional bodies still support role development, there is a lack of appropriate education and training for new roles
Evidence (research) that the change will be effective	There is a lack of published evidence that radiographer-performed studies other than the DCBE are safe or effective
A benefit to stakeholders (interested parties)	Radiologists do not want to give up these procedures Radiographers already rewarded within the career structure for doing an advanced role (advanced practitioner level) are unlikely to receive any additional payment for taking on a new role (and new responsibility)

radiographers in the UK, five being GI sub-specialists. While the ethos of the consultant practitioner role should be applauded, 5 years since their introduction the actual numbers achieving this accolade are still woefully low (Price and Le Masurier, 2007). Their roles vary depending upon local needs, but predominantly their post is concerned with service development, including aspects of expert clinical practice, research and involvement in education (College of Radiographers, 2005). They often work alongside GI advanced practitioners, radiographer practitioners, assistant practitioners and radiology nurses within the GI service (see Table 1.3), with several crossing professional boundaries to work within the gastroenterology or endoscopy departments. It is likely that the numbers of advanced and consultant GI practitioners will grow in the next few years, although funding such posts will always be a major issue.

Inevitably, the role of the radiologist will also continue to evolve, with medical imaging always being central to clinical medicine. However, it is

Table 1.2 Criteria for effective implementation of radiographer role development in CTC, as of 2008

Driver for change	Evidence for the presence of the driver
A perceived deficiency in the service	Insufficient capacity on CT scanners New 18-week targets from referral to treatment in force and difficult to meet Expensive procedure in terms of radiologist involvement to perform and report examinations Possible need to double report, yet limited radiologist time to do so
A proposed solution	Radiographers who currently perform DCBE examinations already have many transferable skills for performing the procedure (e.g. rectal catheterization and IV cannulation) Radiographers skilled in CT have the expertise to manage the CT examination, and may be skilled in IV cannulation DCBE radiographers who report on their examinations may have transferable skills to report the intraluminal findings of the CTC examination Both CT and GI radiographers can be trained to interpret the extraluminal findings Radiographers will be cheaper to employ than radiologists, could work extended days to offer additional lists, and could contribute to a double reporting system
A legal framework within which to introduce the change	Supportive to role developments
A 'champion' of the change, at national and local level	Attracting interest from the government and professional bodies for radiology and radiography, for both screening and symptomatic groups National working parties set up to consider nature of any implementation A number of training courses offered, with several master's level courses under development
Evidence (research) that the change will be effective	Whilst there is a lot of evidence to support CTC, limited data is found regarding the radiographer role
A benefit to stakeholders (interested parties)	Radiologists have more time to concentrate on reporting CTC, or have additional 'back-up' from a double report by a radiographer GI radiographers have an opportunity to diversify their role beyond fluoroscopy CT radiographers have an opportunity to develop their role in an advanced practice area Radiographers already rewarded within the career structure for doing an advanced role (Advanced Practitioner level) are unlikely to receive any additional payment for taking on a new role (and new responsibility)

Table 1.3 The career framework for radiographers within the UK

Career level	Band	Education	Descriptors
Assistant practitioner	4	NVQ level III or equivalent	Specific task related skills supervised by registered practitioners An assistant practitioner performs non-complex, protocol-limited clinical tasks under the direction and supervision of a registered radiographer
Practitioner	5–6	BSc(hons)	A practitioner in radiography autonomously performs a wide-ranging and complex clinical role, is accountable for his or her own actions and for the actions of those they direct They undertake a wide range of both simple and complex imaging examinations or radiotherapy and oncology treatments on the full range of patient types and conditions and in a variety of settings
Advanced practitioner	7	Master's level education	An advanced practitioner, autonomous in clinical practice, defines the scope of practice of others and continuously develops clinical practice within a defined field Advanced practitioners work in a specific area of expert clinical practice and are involved in delivering specialist care to patients. They also contribute to the evidence base and the development of other staff, act as an expert resource for their particular field of practice and demonstrate team leadership
Consultant practitioner	8	Master's and working/studying at doctorate level	A consultant practitioner provides clinical leadership within a specialism or area of service, bringing strategic direction, innovation and influence through practice, research and education, based on specialized knowledge and skills Such roles will nominally comprise at least 50% clinical work and significant work on research and development, audit, education and training of others, and policy and practice development

From The College of Radiographers, Implementing Radiography Career Progression: Guidance for Managers, May 2005.

Beyond the DCBE

CHAPTER 1

likely that, similar to the situation within radiography, radiologists will continue to specialize to ensure they can provide the best care for their patients and will need to introduce innovative solutions to respond to changing patterns of care, including a move towards a 24/7 department and increasing opportunities in molecular imaging (Thomas, 2005a).

International perspectives

Having outlined the historical and current situation in the UK, we will now consider how these compare to shifting professional boundaries within selected other countries, and will attempt to ascertain why any differences exist. Cowling (2008) offered a global overview of the changing roles of radiographers, suggesting that the UK has led the way in widening their scope of practice and is unquestionably the world leader in advanced practice. She outlines four different levels of role advancement, with the UK and the USA being in the first tier, having implemented an effective system of role advancement. In the second level lie countries such as Australia and New Zealand, Canada, South Africa and Japan, where the driving forces are the same but implementation has not yet happened to any great degree. The third level countries have made moves towards having formal recognition for their profession, with role development being their next step, and the fourth group have yet to achieve formal acceptance of radiography as a distinct profession. The situation in the USA, Australia and New Zealand will now be explored further in terms of gastrointestinal imaging role advancements and will be compared to that of the UK.

The United States of America

In the USA, the practice of GI radiography varies widely from state to state. In some states, radiographers are able to perform many examinations independently, while in other parts of the country radiographers are limited to more of an assistant's role. There are few national statutes regulating the practice of GI radiography, however, the American Society of Radiologic Technologists (ASRT) has developed practice standards and the American Registry of Radiologic Technologists (ARRT) designed a task inventory that provides general guidance to radiographers in the performance of GI exams (ASRT, 2007a; ARRT, 2004). These principles would be further defined by the individual states, whose law supersedes those of the national Societies.

According to the practice standards and task inventory mentioned above, radiographers in the USA are able to obtain a patient history, confirm a proper preparation for an exam, take a lead role in radiation safety during the GI exam and set the technical factors on the radiographic and fluoroscopic equipment. In addition, the radiographer may perform particular non-fluoroscopic (over-couch) projections, including individual images of the esophagus and upper GI series and abdominal images as part of a small bowel series and barium enema.

The radiographer's role in a majority of these studies is to assist the radiologist during the fluoroscopic portion of the exam and perform any additional over-couch follow-on images independently. The most notable exception to the role of the radiographer compared to the situation in the UK is results reporting. Fluoroscopy can be performed by a radiographer, as long as there is no reporting connected to the procedure (ASRT, 2007a).

Within the last several years, however, the role of the radiographer in GI imaging has been evolving, in large part due to the developing role of the radiologist assistant (RA). The RA is a relatively new role for radiographers in the USA that can actually trace its development back to the 1970s. The idea of an additional rung on the career ladder for radiographers in the USA has gained a great deal of support recently when, in 2002, the ASRT began to explore an expanded role for radiographers. The RA concept was approved by the American College of Radiology (ACR) in 2003 and the ARRT began offering a certification exam to radiologist assistant graduates in June of 2007.

The additional role of the RA was developed for several reasons: to provide a career ladder for radiographers; to increase the job satisfaction of radiographers; to reduce radiographer attrition; to address the radiologist shortage; to increase efficiency; and to reduce expenses (Smith and Applegate, 2004; McLeod and Montane, 2006; Carlos and Keast, 2006). These drivers for change are not dissimilar to those culminating in role developments within the UK. The concept of a radiologist assistant was also developed because there was a wide acceptance that properly trained radiographers could perform specific examinations independently. Arguably, the area of imaging identified where RAs could make the greatest impact was in GI imaging. Several studies performed in the USA indicate that properly trained radiographers can perform fluoroscopic GI examinations to a level comparable to radiology residents (Schreiber et al., 1996; Davidson et al., 2000) and, in some cases, even practicing radiologists (Van Valkenburg et al., 2000; Thompson et al., 2006).

In their new roles, radiologist assistants are able to perform an expanded array of procedures in GI radiology and the ASRT and ARRT have consequently expanded the guidelines for RAs, allowing them to perform many examinations with some degree of independence. According to the ARRT's (2005) Registered Radiologist Role Delineation, RAs may perform the following GI procedures without the physical presence of the radiologist in the room (although they must be immediately available for consultation if necessary):

Upper GI
Esophagus
Small bowel series
Barium enema
Nasogastric or oroenteric feeding tube placement.

Although the exam can be performed by the RA and preliminary findings can be reported to the radiologist, the RA is still prevented from rendering a final diagnostic reading of the images (ASRT, 2007b). Similar to the 'Red Dot' system utilized in other countries, the RA may strictly point out areas of concern for the radiologist but the final report is approved by a board certified radiologist. This limitation imposed upon radiographers is perhaps understandable while these new roles are in their infancy, particularly in the absence of published literature supporting radiographer reporting in the GI field.

However, one approach strongly advocates that the person undertaking a dynamic, real-time examination is in the best position to write a diagnostic report on the findings, as they have been party to the fluoroscopic findings which may not have all been captured on static images (Halligan et al., 2003). Perhaps the fact that the USA operates a fee per service system (including the report) may influence the professional latitude awarded to the radiographers. Within the UK National Health Service, a fee per service system does not affect the pay and awards of an individual radiologist. However, over time, it may be possible to develop the radiographers' reporting skills to enable them to contribute fully to a double reporting system, where they write the report, which is then verified by the radiologist.

By November 2007, there were 59 radiologist assistants who had graduated from 10 educational programmes (May et al., 2008). Early evaluations showed that there was the potential to save radiologists an average of 100 minutes per day, with a resultant cost saving, even though RA salaries are some 62% higher than radiographers (Wright et al 2008). Based on evidence such as this, radiologist support for the RA program is growing (May et al., 2008).

Regardless of the degree of performance in GI radiography, all radiographers in the USA must understand the general principles behind GI radiography, GI anatomy and how the examination is performed. This knowledge is vital whether the radiographer is performing the examination or assisting the radiologist. The ability to anticipate the needs of the radiologist and to act as a second pair of eyes during the GI examination can sometimes make all the difference in providing a quality examination for the patient.

Australia and New Zealand

At the time of writing, Australia and New Zealand has no formalized system of either role extension or expansion. In a national system where private healthcare and fee for service is well entrenched and has dominated the greater percentage of not only imaging services, but healthcare provision generally for many years, the incentive for change and the change itself is made considerably more difficult.

It may be considered that Australia is perhaps somewhere in the order of 20 years behind the UK in the area of radiographer role development. In comparison to the UK, Australia is a very large country with a number of states that act as their own governors; thus regulations vary from state to state. Most imaging services are delivered within private radiology groups, some operating in very remote places. While a limited extension of the scope of practice is occurring in small pockets around Australia (e.g. IV cannulation, contrast injections and Red Dot flagging), it has normally come about through approval at hospital level as a result of local need, rather than as part of a coordinated national approach (Smith et al., 2008). In Australia, there is currently little radiographer involvement in GI procedures beyond acting in an 'assistant to the radiologist' capacity, although in New Zealand, two radiographers are currently performing DCBE examinations.

The topic of radiographer role development is gathering momentum, however, with a continuing shortfall of radiologist numbers required for timely service delivery, coupled with an increase in the demand for imaging services in light of technological evolution and the aging population (Smith and Baird, 2007). Journal and press articles raising awareness and concern are increasing in number, detailing reporting backlogs, unmet service demands and associated risks regarding patient welfare and diagnostic outcomes (Patty, 2007). In New Zealand, a high rate of colorectal cancer, coupled with difficulties in providing a responsive service in some of the more remote areas, would seem to be potential catalysts for future radiographer-led GI services. However, the current fee for service system seems to work against radiologists delegating the examinations and, in particular, the reporting aspects, to radiographers. As has been evident in both the UK and the USA, the radiologists continue to be the gatekeepers to the role development of radiographers.

The Productivity Commission's Health Workforce Report of 2005 (Productivity Commission, 2005) examined the impact on healthcare services taking into account the supply and demand of trained health practitioners, and the current workforce's ability to meet service demands. As has already been established in other countries, the question of limited task transfer in some professions within Australia has been identified as holding the key to alleviating some of the current stress (Smith and Baird, 2007). To date, an advanced practice model has been developed and implemented within the Australian Nursing Profession.

The Australian Institute of Radiography (AIR) is Australia's leading national body representing radiographers, radiation therapists and sonographers. In anticipation of the escalation of this mis-match of supply, demand and increased patient risk, AIR is actively working towards implementation of an advanced practice model to suit the Australian workforce environment. The AIR is simultaneously negotiating with the Australian government and with the Royal Australian and New Zealand College of Radiologists (RANZCR) to propose a new hierarchical structure that includes an advanced practitioner tier. RANZCR's position, in a similar stance to that of the USA professional organizations, is that a radiological report cannot at this time be provided by anyone who is not a trained medical practitioner and who has not subsequently undergone training as an imaging specialist (Kenny and Andrews, 2007).

In 2005, the AIR, committed to this initiative, commissioned the Professional Advancement Working Party (PAWP). The aim of PAWP was to identify a pathway of role evolution for radiographers and radiation therapists that would ultimately improve the healthcare status of the patient, the functioning of the healthcare team and add value to the role of the radiographer (PAWP report 2006). Subsequently, the AIR has commissioned the Advanced Practitioners' Working Group (APWG) which is currently working to further the recommendations of the PAWP report and will be active until April 2009.

In New Zealand, however, the previously 'ad hoc' role developments have gained national interest, culminating in working groups specifically set up to look at the future skills mix in radiology departments. Reports from both the New Zealand Institute of Medical Radiation Technology (NZIMRT) and the District Health Boards of New Zealand were due to be published in 2008. The NZIMRT has approved a recommendation to introduce a three-tier career framework, including assistant practitioners, practitioners and advanced practitioners. It is anticipated that the first advanced practice roles will be introduced before the end of 2008 (Smith et al., 2008).

Change takes time, but it is hoped that, in the future, workforce restructuring in the delivery of Australian and New Zealand medical imaging and radiation therapy services will allow for an improved patient focused care and delivery.

Summary

While radiographers in the UK have embraced role developments, particularly within the GI field, the pace of change has been slower in other countries. The USA, in particular, has implemented education and training for the new RA roles on a national scale, albeit limited to performing GI exams and not contributing fully to the report. However, in Australia and New Zealand, also largely dominated by private radiology practice, there has been much resistance to change, even in remote regions where it could potentially improve the patient experience. Nevertheless, in the light of published evidence of the success of role changes, the weight of public and professional opinion will shift and this may, ultimately, effect change.

While the scope of practice of the radiographer has gradually expanded, the practice of GI imaging has evolved rapidly at the same time. Conventional radiography and fluoroscopy, once the foundation of GI imaging, are quickly being replaced by other imaging modalities. Computed tomography (CT) imaging of the GI tract and flexible sigmoidoscopy have become commonplace in the USA and the UK. Even magnetic resonance imaging (MRI) is beginning to compete for GI patients (Goldberg and Margulis, 2000; Tait and Allison 2001). Although there will probably always be a need for fluoroscopic imaging where function is a concern, the acquisition of cross-sectional images via CT, MR, ultrasound and hybrid imaging (such as PET-CT) will be likely to reduce the number of conventional fluoroscopic procedures being performed in the future. It is therefore even more critical that radiographers strive to develop and maintain their competence in GI imaging so that when they are involved in GI examinations they are up to the challenge.

References

American Registry of Radiologic Technologists, 2005. Registered radiologist assistant role delineation. <http://www.arrt.org/radasst/finalraroledelineation.pdf> Accessed 10 Nov 2007.

American Registry of Radiologic Technologists, 2004. Task inventory for radiography. <http://www.arrt.org/examinations/practiceanalysis/radti2005.pdf> Accessed 10 Nov 2007.

American Society of Radiologic Technologists, 2007a. The practice standards for medical imaging and radiation therapy. <http://www.asrt.org/media/pdf/standards_rad.pdf> Accessed 10 Nov 2007.

American Society of Radiologic Technologists, 2007b. Radiologist Assistant Practice Standards. <http://www.asrt.org/media/pdf/practicestds/GR06_OPI_RA_Stnds_Adpd.pdf> Accessed 10 Nov 2007.

Audit Commission, 1995. Improving your image – how to manage radiology services more effectively. HMSO, London.

Australian Institute of Radiography, 2006. Professional advancement working party report. <http://www.ar.com.au/documents/PAWP_Report_Final_April06.pdf> Accessed 4 Dec 2007.

Bewell, J., Chapman, A.H., 1996. Radiographer-performed barium enemas – results of a survey to assess progress. Radiography 2, 199–205.

Brown, L., Desai, S., 2002. Cost-effectiveness of barium enemas performed by radiographers. Clin. Radiol. 57 (2), 129–131.

Carlos, R.C., Keast, K.C., 2006. Radiology physician extenders and their perspective in their own words. J. Am. Coll. Radiol. 3, 190–193.

Chapman, A.H., 1997. Changing work patterns. Lancet 350, 581–583.

Cowling, C., 2008. A global overview of the changing roles of radiographers. Radiography 14 (Supplement 1) e28–e32.

Culpan, D.G., Mitchell, A.J., Hughes, S., et al., 2002. Double contrast barium enema sensitivity: a comparison of studies by radiographers and radiologists. Clin. Radiol. 57, 604–607.

Davidson, J.C., Einstein, D.M., Baker, M.E., et al., 2000. Feasibility of instructing radiology technologists in the performance of gastrointestinal fluoroscopy. Am. J. Roentgenol. 175 (5), 1449–1452.

Department of Health, 2006. NHS takes next step in tackling hidden waiting lists, Press release, reference no. 2006/0072, 21 February 2006. <www.dh.gov.uk/PublicationsAndStatistics/PressReleases.htm> Accessed 06.05.06.

Department of Health, 2005. Quicker scans, endoscopies and imaging for NHS patients. £1 billion to tackle hidden diagnostic waits – Reid, Press releases. Saturday 19 February 2005 Reference number: 2005/0064.

Department of Health, 2000a. Ionising radiation (medical exposure) regulations, The Stationery Office, London.

Department of Health, 2000b. The National Health Service Cancer Plan, Department of Health, London. <http://www.doh.gov.uk/cancer/cancerplan.htm>

Goldberg, H.I., Margulis, A.R., 2000. Gastrointestinal radiology in the United States: an overview of the past 50 years. Radiology 216, 1–7.

Halligan, S., Lilford, R.J., Wardle, J., et al., 2007. Design of a multicentre randomized trial to evaluate CT colonography versus colonoscopy or barium enema for diagnosis of colonic cancer in older symptomatic patients: the SIGGAR study. Trials 8, 32. Published online, 2007. October 27. doi: 10.1186/1745-6215-8-32.

Halligan, S., Marshall, M., Taylor, S., et al., 2003. Observer variation in detection of colorectal neoplasia on barium enema: implications for colorectal cancer screening and training. Clin. Radiol. 58, 948–954.

Kelly, S.B., Murphy, J., Smith, A., et al., 2007. Nurse specialist led flexible sigmoidoscopy in an outpatient setting. Colorectal Dis. 2007 May 17; [Epub ahead of print] PMID: 17509042 [PubMed – as supplied by publisher].

Kenny, L.M., Andrews, M.W., 2007. Addressing radiology workforce issues. Med. J. Aust. 186, 615–616.

Law, R.L., Longstaff, A.J., Slack, N., 1999. A retrospective 5-year study on the accuracy of the barium enema examination performed by radiographers. Clin. Radiol. 54 (2), 80–83, discussion 83–84.

Law, R.L., Slack, N., Harvey, R.F., 2008. An evaluation of a radiographer-led barium enema service in the diagnosis of colorectal cancer. Radiography 14 (2), 105–110.

CHAPTER 1

Law, R.L., Slack, N., Harvey, R.F., 2005. Radiographer performed single contrast small bowel enteroclysis. Radiography 11 (1), 11–15.

Leslie, A., Virjee, J.P., 2002. Detection of colorectal carcinoma on double contrast barium enema when double reporting is routinely performed: an audit of current practice. Clin. Radiol. 57, 184–187.

Mannion, R.A., Bewell, J., Langan, C., 1995. A barium enema training programme for radiographers: a pilot study. Clin. Radiol. 50 (10), 715–718, discussion 718–719.

Markus, J.B., Somers, S., O'Malley, B.P., et al., 1990. Double-contrast barium enema studies: effect of multiple reading on perception error. Radiology 175, 155–156.

Maruthachalam, K., Stoker, E., Nicholson, G., et al., 2006. Nurse led flexible sigmoidoscopy in primary care – the first thousand patients. Colorectal Dis. 8 (7), 557–562.

May, L., Martino, S., McElveny, C., 2008. The establishment of an advanced clinical role for radiographers in the United States. Radiography 14 (Supplement 1), e24–e27.

McLeod, D., Montane, G., 2006. The radiologist assistant: the solution to radiology workforce needs. Emerg. Radiol. Online. http://www.springerlink.com/content/7746t77h73133215 10 Nov 2007

McKenzie, G.A., Mathers, S., Graham, D.T., et al., 1998. An investigation into radiographer-performed barium enemas. Radiography 4, 17–22.

Murphy, M., Loughran, C.F., Birchenough, H., et al., 2002. A comparison of radiographer and radiologist reports on radiographer conducted barium enemas. Radiography 8, 215–221.

NHS Executive, 2000. Cancer Referral Guidelines, Health Service Circular, HSC 2000/013. <www.doh.gov.uk/coinh.htm> Accessed 06/05/06.

Nightingale, J., 2008. Developing protocols for advanced and consultant practice. Radiography 14 (Supplement 1), e55–e60.

Nightingale, J., Hogg, P., 2007. The role of the GI radiographer: a UK perspective. Radiol. Technol. March/April 2007, 78 (4), 1–7.

Nightingale, J., Hogg, P., 2003a. The gastrointestinal advanced practitioner: an emerging role for the modern radiology service. Radiography 9, 151–160.

Nightingale, J., Hogg, P., 2003b. Clinical practice at an advanced level: an introduction. Radiography 9, 77–83.

Nightingale, J., Hogg, P., 2000. Gastro-intestinal imaging for radiographers: current practice and future possibilities. Synergy, 16–19.

Nightingale, J., Mackay, S., 2009. An analysis of changes in practice introduced during an educational programme for practitioner-led swallowing investigations. Radiography 15 (1), 63–69.

Patty, A., 2007. X-ray backlog: patients at risk, Sydney Morning Herald 6 Oct 2007. <http://www.smh.com.au> Accessed 2 Dec 2007.

Price, R.C., Le Masurier, S.B., 2007. Longitudinal changes in extended roles in radiography: a new perspective. Radiography 13 (1), 18–29.

Productivity Commission Research Report, 2005. Australia's Health Workforce. Canberra. <http://www.pc.gov.au> Accessed 5 Dec 2007.

Robinson, P.J.A., Culpan, G., Wiggins, M., 1999. Interpretation of selected accident and emergency radiographic examinations by radiographers: a review of 11 000 cases. Br. J. Radiol. 72, 546–551.

Schreiber, M.H., van Sonnenberg, E., Wittich, G.R., 1996. Technical adequacy of fluoroscopic spot films of the gastrointestinal tract: comparison of residents and technologists. Am. J. Roentgenol. 166 (4), 795–797.

Smith, T., Yielder, J., Ajibulu, et al., 2008. Progress towards advanced practice roles in Australia, New Zealand and the Western Pacific. Radiography 14 (Supplement 1), e20–e23.

Smith, T.N., Baird, M., 2007. Radiographers' role in radiological reporting: a model to support future demand. Med. J. Aust. 186, 629–631.

Smith, W.L., Applegate, K.E., 2004. The likely effects of radiologist extenders on radiology training. J. Am. Coll. Radiol. 1, 402–404.

Somers, S., Stevenson, G.W., Laufer, I., et al., 1981. Evaluation of double contrast barium enemas performed by radiographic technologists. J. Can. Assoc. Radiol. 32 (4), 227–228.

Swinburne, K., 1971. Pattern recognition for radiographers. Lancet 589–590.

Tait, P., Allison, D., 2001. Imaging of the gastrointestinal tract. Drugs Today 37 (8), 533–557.

The College of Radiographers, 2006. Medical image interpretation and clinical reporting by non-radiologists: the role of the radiographer. COR, London.

The College of Radiographers, 1997. Reporting by radiographers: a vision paper. The College of Radiographers, London.

The College of Radiographers, 1996. Role development in radiography. The College of Radiographers, London.

The Royal College of Radiologists/The Society and College of Radiographers, 2007. Team working within clinical imaging – a contemporary view of skills mix. Joint guidance from the Royal College of Radiologists and the Society and College of Radiographers, London.

The Royal College of Radiologists, 2002. Clinical radiology: a workforce in crisis, BFCR (02) 01. The Royal College of Radiologists, London.

The Royal College of Radiologists, 1999. Skills mix in clinical radiology. BFCR (99)3. The Royal College of Radiologists, London.

The Royal College of Radiologists, 1996. Advice on delegation of tasks in departments of clinical radiology. The Royal College of Radiologists, London.

The Society and College of Radiographers, 2005. Implementing radiography career progression: guidance for managers. The Royal College of Radiologists, London.

Thomas, A., 2005a. The role of the radiologist in 2010. Imaging and oncology 2005. The College of Radiographers, London.

Thomas, N., 2005b. A radiologist's perspective. In: McConnell, J., Eyres, R., Nightingale, J. (Eds.), Interpreting trauma radiographs. Blackwell Publications, Oxford, pp. 7–18.

Thompson, W.M., Foster, W.L., Paulson, E.K., et al., 2006. Comparison of radiologists and technologists in the performance of air-contrast barium enemas. Am. J. Radiol. 187, 706–709.

Van Valkenburg, J., Ralph, B., Lopatofsky, L., et al., 2000. The role of the physician extender in radiology. Radiol. Technol. 72 (1), 45–50.

Vora, P., Chapman, A., 2004. Complications from radiographer-performed double contrast barium enemas. Clin. Radiol. 59, 364–368.

Wright, D.L., Killion, J.B., Johnston, J., et al., 2008. RAs increase productivity. Radiol. Technol. 79 (4), 365–370.

Medico-legal aspects of gastrointestinal imaging practice

Peter Hogg, Charlotte Thompson

Contents ||||||||||||||||||||||||||||||||||||||||||||||||||||||||||||||||||||||||||||||||||

Introduction

The past two decades have witnessed significant advances in clinical care; alongside this, national standards of care have been implemented. The availability and quality of information to inform care has also increased and various vehicles for sharing information and practice have been improved. To enhance services further, many non-medical health professionals such as gastrointestinal radiographers and gastroenterology nurses have engaged with a wide range of diagnostic and interventional/therapeutic advanced clinical roles. Not surprisingly, the potential to deliver a good standard of healthcare is high. In the past two decades, the rights of patients have also improved significantly; this includes the patient's ability to: contribute to healthcare policy formation; receive information about their health and care; exercise choice on where and when they receive their care; exercise their right to complain about the standard of care they receive and, associated with this, their ability to initiate a [legal] negligence claim.

Negligence on the part of the healthcare team, or their employer, can result in a legal claim. Such claims are on the increase (Berlin, 1999; Alderson and Hogg, 2003), possibly because of a greater awareness about compensation being sought from a suboptimal outcome – where the fault lies with another, or possibly because there is a greater awareness of the claims process itself – particularly notable on local radio stations through advertising. Some argue that public expectations of healthcare have been raised to an unrealistic level (Butt, 1998) requiring an increasing emphasis to be placed upon educating the public about realistic expectations. This might be worth considering during your contact with patients during the explanatory and consenting phases.

Within this chapter, we shall explore aspects of clinical negligence associated with imaging and therapy of the GI tract. The general principles outlined are likely to apply to most countries; however, it is important that you familiarize yourself with the legal processes in the country in which you practice, because conceptual and procedural differences will exist. We will not consider the detail of the legal claims process; however, if this interests you we would recommend the article by Alderson and Hogg (2003) which explains the process of a legal claim in English law.

Negligence – a definition

Negligence is a legal concept in which there is failure to act with the prudence that a reasonable person would exercise under the same circumstances, resulting in an unintended injury to another party. Negligence is the most common form of Tort, and Tort is a civil wrong committed against a person for which compensation will be sought through a Civil Court.

Where might negligence claims arise in GI imaging and therapy?

A claim can arise whenever a patient in your care is exposed to a risk that has not been explained adequately, minimized appropriately or contingency planned for. If your patient feels aggrieved by their standard of care, they may seek legal advice on what might be done to help them. Important points for you to consider about your clinical practice are:

- have you identified, adequately, risks that patients in your care will be exposed to and,
- after identifying the risks have they been addressed adequately to deal with actual or potential consequences?

Table 2.1 offers a number of circumstances where claims might arise.

On examining the list in Table 2.1, it becomes clear that the points are representative of unreasonable/poor clinical practice. Alternatively, engaging in reasonable clinical practice (the converse of the above) would improve the patient experience and outcome and also minimize the chance of a legal claim. Reasonable clinical practice, therefore, does not need to have a purely litigious basis; its basis would build on reasonable standards of care and management that are expected of highly skilled and educated practitioners.

Table 2.1 Circumstances in which claims could arise

Category of claims	Examples
Inadequate patient care	Not identifying your patient adequately Failure to identify that the examination requested is inappropriate for the related clinical history, (for example) if a barium enema has been requested for a patient with bloody diarrhea Harming your patient because of a basic failure to care for them Causing the death of your patient Not adapting technique in accordance with any pre-existing patient conditions Gaining inadequate consent from your patient Failing to maintain confidentiality
Poor medicines management for the prescription, supply and administration (including x-ray contrast media)	Administering the wrong medicine/drug such as the inappropriate use of Buscopan or Glucagen or not ascertaining whether a patient had renal impairment before administering magnesium citrate (e.g. Citramag) as a bowel preparation Administering the wrong dose of medicine/drug Failing to check the medicine/drug for technical matters (e.g. contamination, expiry date, concentration) Administering the medicine/drug by the incorrect route Failing to check whether your patient would react adversely to the medicine/drug; this would include allergies, sensitivities and drug incompatibilities
Poor radiation protection measures	Not observing radiation protection measures, particularly for females of child-bearing potential Failing to plan, adequately, radiation therapy fields (under- or over-irradiation)
A lack of competence to perform the task	You are not competent Junior qualified staff are not competent and have inadequate supervision Staff 'in training' are not competent and have inadequate supervision
Failure to articulate significant known risks about the procedure to your patient	Failure to advise on treatment of side effects to radiotherapy, initially and on follow up Failure to indicate that a diagnostic or interventional procedure has associated side effects and/or complication rates

(Continued)

Where might negligence claims arise in GI imaging and therapy?

CHAPTER 2

Table 2.1 Circumstances in which claims could arise—cont'd

Category of claims	Examples
Failure to interpret and articulate the result of a diagnostic procedure	Writing a report that is misleading or open to misinterpretation (ambiguous)
	Failing to detect an abnormality/pathology when one is present
	Failing to inform the referring clinician that you have found an abnormality/pathology
	Identifying an abnormality/pathology on the incorrect side of your patient
Inadequate communication of bad news to patients	

How does your patient succeed with a (legal) negligence claim?

Duty of care

Following a prescribed legal format, the claimant (e.g. your patient) alleges there has been personal injury (or even death). To be successful the claimant needs to establish that:

1 You (the defendant) owed them a duty of care
2 You were in breach of that duty
3 Your breach of duty caused (predictable) harm to the patient (claimant).

Let us consider the duty of care. It is fair to assume that healthcare workers have a duty of care towards their patients and typically this is made explicit by professional and regulatory bodies such as the UK Society and College of Radiographers. Statement 3 for professional conduct from the Society and College of Radiographers (2002) indicates:

> Radiographers have a duty of care towards patients they accept for imaging/treatment procedures and must act in a manner appropriate to the standards of care imposed by law on a responsible body of radiographers.

Adding weight to this, the radiographers' regulatory body indicates that radiographers must…

> …exercise a professional duty of care (Health Professions Council, 2007).

In the case of a radiographer, duty of care is easy for the claimant to establish – the only exception is where the fetus is involved. In English law, the fetus does not have a duty of care associated with it. However, if it is born alive and has sustained harm as a result of a breach of duty owed to its mother then it will be able to make a claim (Alderson and Hogg, 2003).

Breach of duty

Having understood how duty of care is established, we shall now determine how a decision is made about a breach of duty. Deciding whether there has been a breach of duty necessitates an understanding of the standard of care to be expected. This is achieved in the UK by applying the principles of Bolam v Friern Hospital Management Committee (1957), with due regard to Bolitho v City of Hackney Health Authority (1997). Invariably this is often described as 'the Bolam test'. Here, for any given clinical situation, the healthcare worker would be expected to act in a fashion as accepted by other healthcare workers (i.e. in line with peer practice) and that their actions would be responsible (i.e. based upon evidence). There is an expectation that other healthcare workers, with comparable responsibilities (and competencies), would act similarly when presented with a similar clinical situation and that the way in which they act would be positively influenced by formal evidence (e.g. journal articles). As such, patients should expect the same level of care and management for a particular examination or procedure – irrespective of which professional group conducted it.

National standards, where they exist, should be adopted into practice. There would be an expectation that clinical effectiveness research and professional and scientific body guidance would form a basis from which practice would develop. Tawn et al. (2005), for example, conducted a national audit for the Royal College of Radiologists to review the standards of sensitivity provided by the double contrast barium enema. National audits such as this provide practitioners with a baseline against which to assess their own standards. Where national standards do not exist, a literature search of published data in peer review journals can provide legitimate support as to whether an individual's standard of competence is 'reasonable'. If a Trust/hospital fails to meet national standards and a patient proves they have suffered harm as a consequence, then this could be used as evidence in a claim to support a breach of duty. Similarly, for competence of professionals to practice, national occupational standards could be used as a benchmark 'within the Bolam test'. Having said this, it is important to recognize that there is no intention to assess clinical performance against levels of excellence; rather the intention would be to assess clinical performance against what would be considered to be 'reasonable'. Additionally, even with the existence of evidence and guidelines, there is a need to recognize that patients are individual and professional latitude can be exercised when justified.

Did the breach cause harm to your patient?

Let us now consider the third component of the claims process – whether the breach of duty caused [predictable] harm to the claimant. Establishing causation (i.e. that harm was caused as a result of the breach of duty) is often the main and most complicated issue to be considered in a legal claim and it is the responsibility of the claimant to do this.

For this to be established, the claimant must prove that the harm, on balance of probabilities, was caused by the breach. This can be quite complicated for the claimant to do, as illustrated by this fictitious scenario:

The radiographer interpreted the barium enema images in accordance with approved hospital practice. However, the radiographer failed to articulate, in writing or otherwise, the result to the referring clinician.

For this scenario we will assume the barium enema images demonstrated colon cancer at a very advanced stage and this was the first presentation of this patient to determine if they had colon cancer.

The radiographer clearly owes this patient a duty of care and they have breached that duty. However, for a legal claim to be successful, the claimant must establish that they have suffered harm as a result of the breach (the third component of the claim process). In this case, it could be argued that the cancer was 'so advanced' that the report of the barium enema images would have made no difference to the long-term patient outcome, in that irrespective of any treatment they would be likely to have only months to live. As such, articulating or not articulating the enema report to the referring clinician would have the same ultimate end – the patient would die. The only claim that might be advanced would be along the lines of palliative therapy, in which the barium report might have played a role in the planning of the appropriate palliative therapy – to minimize unpleasant symptoms related to the colon cancer. In this case, damages might be sought for increased suffering, among other things.

By contrast, if the cancer in the scenario was at a very early stage and the enema report had not been articulated to this effect to the referring clinician and the patient had ultimately died as a consequence then there may be a basis for a substantial legal claim.

Regulatory body investigations

With the above scenario in mind, it is worth introducing the role of the regulatory body; for UK radiographers this would be the Health Professions Council (HPC). The purpose of regulatory bodies is to protect patients from harm. As such, whether a claim is successful or not, the regulatory body may take an interest and conduct its own investigation. The central question the regulatory body will ask is whether you are fit to practice and procedures exist for teams acting on behalf of the regulatory body to follow in such cases. Within the HPC website (located in the public domain) are investigations of 'fitness to practice'. Some of these are cases where patients could have lodged a legal negligence claim and whether the claim is successful or not may not impact particularly on the HPC investigation. For instance, a patient may lose their claim but the healthcare worker may be investigated and consequently be struck off the professional register because of malpractice. Box 2.1

BOX 2.1 Published reasons for Health Professions Council investigation into 'fitness to practice'

The healthcare worker:

- failed to follow instructions which put the patient at risk
- failed to maintain accurate records
- failed to respond to patient needs in an appropriate and timely manner
- failed to work within their legal and ethical boundaries, including not exercising a professional duty of care and not knowing the limits of their practice and when to seek advice
- imaged the wrong body part

demonstrates the range of published reasons why the HPC have investigated healthcare workers for fitness to practice.

If the regulatory body chooses to investigate your practice then you are unlikely to receive support from your Trust/hospital. By contrast, your professional body is highly likely to provide you with support and professional representation and this heightens the value of being a member of a professional body, such as the Society and College of Radiographers.

It is important to note that, in regard of competence of practice, healthcare workers should keep up to date with the advancing body to professional knowledge and make changes to their own practice, as required.

Where will the financial liability lie?

Returning to legal claims to consider who will be sued, it is unlikely that you would be sued personally if you are employed by an organization. Employers are [usually] vicariously liable for their employees, assuming certain conditions are met. For instance, where radiographers engage in advanced clinical practices, their employer should formally approve what the radiographer does with patients before they actually do it. Approval processes vary from Trust to Trust/hospital to hospital; do be mindful that local (departmental) approval may not be adequate. Typically, written procedures would be required for this (these are often referred to as protocols) and these will be discussed shortly.

If you are doing private/independent work then you would have to accept personal liability for your actions and inactions; as such, personal indemnity would be required.

Time limits for claims

Normally this is 3 years from the point at which the claimant realized that they had been [allegedly] harmed by the defendant. There are exceptions, including mental disability and children. For children, the clock starts at 18, with an additional 3 years included. Children therefore have up to 21 years, in normal circumstances.

Consent

Consent is worthy of special mention as it is a critical communication point between the patient and healthcare worker. It is here that information is shared and decisions by both parties are made and patient expectations are set as a consequence. You should be mindful that patient consent should include: purpose of examination; what it involves; its benefits; its risks. It is critical that consent is given by your patient, as this can act as a defense to an action of trespass or even assault. The healthcare worker must give adequate information to the patient when obtaining consent. Failure to provide adequate information to the patient could result in a legal claim. Consent should be sought in a non-threatening fashion and the patient giving consent must be in a position to do so (e.g. of sufficient mental capacity, of sufficient age).

There are various ways in which consent is given, including verbal, written and implied (i.e. the patient simply willingly complies with your professional requests). Consent for most GI examinations is initially implied by a patient attending the appointment having read the description of the procedure despatched with the appointment letter, at which time there is the option for the patient to discuss any queries over the telephone. The level of intervention and associated risk and the potential for patients to feel embarrassment or a loss of personal dignity associated with a procedure would determine how consent is given. A formal written response from your patient might be advised for a highly risky intervention such as surgery. The nature of consent as applied to gastrointestinal radiographers and the procedures they may perform covers a varying range of associated interventional risk, be it the double contrast barium enema, problematic intubations or the performance of upper or lower gastrointestinal endoscopy. A simple minimally invasive imaging procedure may only require implied consent. However, gastrointestinal examinations can be personally invasive; these also require consent. A good example is defecating proctography during which the patient is not only required to be imaged during defecation but may also require vaginal contrast.

Generally speaking, it is incumbent upon the healthcare worker to inform the patient of the nature of the examination and any 'significant risks' that the examination may carry. While general risks exist across the whole patient population, there may be added risks specific to a particular patient. An example of the latter could be related to age and/or a co-existing medical condition complicating the proposed procedure. Patients will be individual and the healthcare worker should assess the risks on a patient-by-patient basis and decide what information needs to be articulated in order to reach informed consent. If potential harm is not explained to the patient and the patient suffers harm subsequently then the patient may proceed to a legal claim.

Protocols

Protocols, typically comprising of written instructions, are valuable in healthcare for many reasons. Protocols: provide a detailed framework within which patients can be managed; allow for variations in care to be minimized; enable a reasonable level of care to be given; are a way to prove what was done to a particular patient. All these factors are evidence of good clinical practice and such information can help in defending a claim. For the last example (providing written evidence of what was done to a particular patient), protocols can have particular value in legal claims, especially when the 'alleged incident' happened several years ago – when the memory of the incident has faded in the healthcare worker's mind.

Protocols apply to a specific category of patients (e.g. those having a barium enema examination) and they can be used by the range of professionals who would undertake the task. Protocols should be developed by involving the appropriate people and typically a team of stakeholders would be required. A good protocol should include the information/characteristics listed in Box 2.2.

> **BOX 2.2** Essential information contained within a protocol
>
> - The names of those responsible for creating it
> - The date it came into force
> - Definitions of terms and concepts
> - The working practices should be detailed
> - When the working practices should be done
> - Who is allowed to do the working practices (professional groups and names of people)
> - Evidence should be used to inform the advocated practices
> - Peer practice should be indicated, if possible
> - Audit of practice should be indicated, including: method; audit standard; frequency; what to do with the results; and remedial action as appropriate
> - Staff training requirements/competencies should be indicated for those who will work within the protocol
> - 'What to do next' should be indicated for when the healthcare worker reaches the limit of their ability

The protocol must be authorized for use and the local approval process must be followed to the letter. Each hospital/Trust may have different procedures for approval and you are advised to gain familiarity with them. If you are in the process of developing or updating protocols, we can recommend reading an article by Nightingale (2008), which takes the reader step by step through the creation of protocols for advanced and consultant practice.

Once created, protocols should be actively managed. For instance, they should be updated regularly; old protocols should be removed from the clinical area and archived, in accordance with hospital/Trust policies. On archiving, end dates should be indicated, as well as start dates. Staff should be made aware of which one is in use and be informed when new ones are introduced. If necessary, training should be made available for compliance with any new protocol competencies.

Knowing that patients can be different and that written protocols cannot cover all circumstances, it is important that healthcare workers know when they are allowed to deviate from the protocols. Some workers will not be allowed to do this; as such they must call for assistance from those who can, in line with Trust/hospital policy. For those who are allowed to deviate, it would be seen as good clinical practice to record, in writing, what different care has been provided. This would be in line with good legal practice, as there would be a written record of events for defending a claim should one arise. Accurate record keeping is of paramount importance and the following should be borne in mind when recording information:

- Information should be accurate, clear and comprehensive
- The narrative should be jargon free, or at the very least abbreviations and acronyms should be consistent with the discipline's vernacular
- The 'facts' should be recorded
- The narrative should not be altered – unless the change is indicated clearly and the insert is dated and signed
- The narrative should be signed and dated, electronically or personally
- The narrative should be written as soon as possible after the event.

CHAPTER 2

Do note that, as shown by Hammond v West Lancashire Health Authority (1998), claims can be lost because of poor record keeping!

Patient Group Directions – the special case protocol

Strictly speaking, Patient Group Directions (PGDs) are not protocols but, at first sight, they look as if they might be. PGDs are 'written instructions for the supply and administration of medicines' to 'categories' of patients. As with protocols, PGDs should be approved using formal local mechanisms, with the additional scrutiny of local medicines management committees. Details on PGDs and supplementary prescribing can be obtained in Hogg et al. (2007). They should be managed and archived similarly to protocols.

A final thought

Good clinical practice will result in care and management of patients being of an acceptable and reasonable standard. Engaging in such practice will minimize harm to patients and also minimize the chance of a legal negligence claim arising or being successful. Good clinical practice is consistent with good legal practice and, when seen in this fashion, the threat of litigation should not place an additional burden on healthcare workers when they deliver their reasonable standard of care.

References

Alderson, C.J., Hogg, P., 2003. Advanced radiographic practice – the legal aspects. Radiography 9 (4), 305–314.

Berlin, L., 1999. Malpractice issues in radiology, the missed cancer: perceptions and realities. Am. J. Radiol. 173, 1161–1167.

Bolam. Friern Hospital Management Committee V 1957. WLR 1, 582.

Bolitho. City and Hackney Health Authority V 1997. WLR 3, 1151.

Butt, P., 1998. Radiological negligence. Newsletter of Royal College of Radiologists 52, 14.

Hammond. West Lancashire Health Authority V 1998. Lloyds Rep. Med. 146.

Health Professions Council, 2007. Standards of proficiency (Radiographers). <http://www.hpc-uk.org/assets/documents/10000DBDStandards_of_Proficiency_Radiographers.pdf> Accessed 18-1-08.

Hogg, P., Hogg, D., Francis, G. et al., 2007. Prescription, supply and administration of medicines in therapy and diagnosis. Synergy 26–31.

Nightingale, J., 2008. Developing protocols for advanced and consultant practice. Radiography 14 (Supplement 1), e55–e60.

Statements for Professional Conduct from the Society and College of Radiographers, 2002. (reprinted 2004) ISBN 1871101166

Tawn, D.J., Squire, C.J., Mohammed, M.A., et al., 2005. National audit of the sensitivity of double contrast barium enema for colorectal carcinoma, using control charts. Clin. Radiol. 60, 558–564.

Introduction to patient preparation and pharmacology for gastrointestinal tract examinations

Alison Booth

Contents ||||||||||||||||||||||||||||||||||||||||||||||||||||||||||||||||||||||||||||||||

Introduction

The development of contrast media and patient preparations is interlinked with the development of image quality. As early as 1901, the use of air as a contrast medium was being discussed and *single contrast* meals became accepted practice in 1905. By 1917, the development of a reasonably reliable technique for imaging the colon meant that radiological descriptions of pathologies, such as carcinoma, tuberculosis, diverticulosis, megacolon and polyps, had been made. By the 1920s, it was stated that 'the examination of the stomach and intestinal canal has become one of the most important spheres of radiographic work' (Knox, 1923). Poor image quality limited the visualization of the gastrointestinal (GI) tract to more advanced pathologies such as strictures. Therefore, positive contrast studies predominated. However, with the improvements made in the 1960s in the detail available radiographically and fluoroscopically, the value of *double contrast* techniques was quickly advocated and became standard practice. It was quickly recognized that visualization of the mucosal lining of the GI tract was possible when using a double contrast technique and that the removal of artefacts within the system was essential to accurate diagnosis. As a result, a range of preparations and contrast media (positive and negative) has been developed and refined to support the requirement for increasingly high quality imaging, and an expanding variety of modalities and techniques are now used to visualize the GI tract.

This chapter discusses the principles of patient preparation and the pharmacology of preparations, contrast media and other pharmaceutical products currently used in the imaging of the GI tract.

Preparation

The earlier a GI abnormality is detected, the more the aim of treatment can be preventative rather than curative, and curative rather than palliative (National Institute for Clinical Excellence, 2004; Centre for Reviews and Dissemination, 2004). Maximizing diagnostic sensitivity and specificity in GI imaging is therefore a high priority. Diagnostic imaging is comprised of a series of events which are only ever as good as the weakest part of the process, making patient preparation as important a factor as any other. Diagnostic accuracy can be compromised by the presence of *artefacts*, such as food in the stomach or feces in the large bowel. These can mask or mimic pathology. It is therefore important that such artefacts are removed before an examination is carried out (Hendry et al., 2007; Pickhardt, 2007).

There are a number of important considerations when adopting a *preparation regime*. The process of clearance must leave the colon clean but not have any macro- or microscopic effects on the mucosa or compromise the patient's physiology (Holte et al., 2004). For example, the action of a bowel preparation on the mucosal lining of the bowel can affect the adherence of the barium solution used (Cittadini et al., 1999a, 1999b). The need to review the contrast used should be taken into account when a regime is adopted or amended. Efficacy of the preparation needs to be balanced with patient compliance and acceptability in respect of taste, volume and action (Chan et al., 1997; Brown and DiPalma, 2004; Hendry et al., 2007). While it may be desirable to have a single regime for all patients from an administrative point of view, patients vary in their physical ability and comorbidities which need to be considered along with the adverse effects and contraindications of the agents used (Beloosesky et al., 2003; Sweetman, 2007; British Medical Association and the Royal Pharmaceutical Society of Great Britain, 2008). Finally, the financial cost of laxatives available varies considerably and poor preparation has been shown to have increased consequential costs (Bartram, 1994; Rex et al., 2002).

Getting the preparation regime right is important from the patient, clinician and service provider perspectives, as can be seen in Box 3.1. An appropriate bowel preparation regime can reduce both patient anxiety and the burden on the healthcare system.

The more distal in the GI tract the examination, the greater the patient preparation required. Little or none is required for examinations of the salivary

---

BOX 3.1 Advantages of a successful bowel preparation regime

- Speeds diagnosis
- Improves specificity and sensitivity
- Helps limit investigation to a single examination
- Means shorter examination times, which can minimize patient discomfort, allow higher throughput of patients, and minimize radiation dose to patients and staff

glands, larynx, pharynx or esophagus (when imaged alone). For imaging the esophagus and stomach, generally a few hours' dietary restriction is all that is required.

For small bowel imaging, preparation varies by imaging modality. For a fluoroscopic examination of the small bowel, the patient may require a laxative the day before and to have nothing to eat or drink for approximately eight hours prior to examination. For other imaging procedures such as computed tomography (CT) enteroclysis and capsule endoscopy, preparation may be more intensive (Paulsen et al., 2006; Rajesh and Maglinte, 2006; Van Tuyl et al., 2007; Kalantzis et al., 2007).

There is no single ideal preparation regime for imaging of the small bowel and the colon, but the principal elements used are a combination of dietary restriction and a laxative bowel cleansing solution.

Diet

A standard dietary preparation is for a *low residue diet* two days before the examination, where advice is given on what may be eaten (e.g. white bread, poached, grilled or steamed fish, black tea or coffee, clear liquids). Fiber, the residue of plant cells, is resistant to hydrolysis by intestinal and pancreatic enzymes; therefore minimizing dietary fiber should reduce bulk in the colon and thereby reduce residual feces. High fiber foods such as brown bread, fruit, vegetables and potatoes should therefore be avoided.

No solid food is permitted the day before the examination but clear fluids are recommended, the volume depending on the type of laxative used. These should not be diet or low calorie drinks (unless the patient is diabetic) as sugary drinks help maintain energy levels.

Laxatives

Bowel cleansing solutions are classed as laxatives but are not used in the treatment of constipation. They are specifically designed to ensure the bowel is free of solid contents prior to colonic surgery, colonoscopy and radiological examination. There are a variety of products commercially available and they all carry similar warnings and contraindications (Table 3.1).

Known side effects from bowel cleansing agents include nausea, vomiting, abdominal pain (usually transient and reduced by taking more slowly), abdominal distension, and anal discomfort. Less frequently a rash and electrolyte disturbances are recognized side effects.

Laxatives are classified according to their mode of action, although the precise nature of the action is not always fully understood and there is some overlap between groups. The two types of laxatives used for bowel cleansing are stimulant and osmotic solutions.

Stimulant solutions increase intestinal motility by directly stimulating the nerve endings in the colonic mucosa. They can cause abdominal cramp and should not be used in patients with intestinal obstruction. Stimulant laxatives used in practice include bisacodyl (e.g. Dulcolax), sodium picosulphate (e.g. Picolax, Fleet, OsmoPrep, Picoprep) and members of the anthraquinone group, which includes senna (e.g. X-Prep). The use of strong stimulants such as cascara and castor oil is obsolete.

Table 3.1 Risk factors and contraindications for bowel preparation

Risk factors	Contraindication or caution advised	Potential risk
Pregnancy	Caution	Risks are unknown as there are no data evaluating the effects in pregnancy
Patients with heart disease and congestive cardiac failure	Caution	Hyperphosphatemia, hypocalcemia, hypernatremic dehydration and acidosis
Ulcerative colitis	Caution	Exacerbation of existing condition
Reflux esophagitis	Caution	Regurgitation or aspiration for oral examinations
Impaired gag reflex	Caution	Aspiration
Unconscious or semiconscious patients	Caution	Regurgitation or aspiration for oral examinations
Patients with renal impairment	Caution	Hyperphosphatemia, hypocalcemia, hypernatremic dehydration and acidosis
Pre-existing serious renal impairment	Contraindication	Renal failure
Gastrointestinal obstruction, gastric retention, ileus	Contraindication	Exacerbation of existing condition; perforation
Gastrointestinal ulceration, perforated bowel, toxic colitis, toxic megacolon	Contraindication	Exacerbation of existing condition; perforation

Data from Russmann et al., 2007; Zuccaro et al., 2007; Sweetman, 2007; British Medical Association and the Royal Pharmaceutical Society of Great Britain, 2008; US FDA, 2008

Osmotic solutions work by increasing intestinal osmotic pressure, which encourages the retention of water in the large bowel. They include the saline laxatives, magnesium citrate, magnesium hydroxide and sodium sulfate and macrogols, such as polyethylene glycol (PEG) solutions. The saline laxatives draw fluid from the body into the bowel to provide a wash out effect, while the inert polymers of ethylene glycol work to retain in the bowel the fluid with which the solutions were administered. Example brand names for these solutions include, Citramag, Klean-Prep, GoLytely, MoviPrep; there are many more. Choice of laxative will depend on the examination to be performed, for example, colonoscopy can be successfully performed even if the mucosa is 'wet', whereas double contrast barium enema (DCBE) and CT colonography (CTC) would normally require a 'dry' colon (Bartram, 1994).

The principles of preparation for CT and magnetic resonance (MR) colonography remain essentially the same as for DCBE and colonoscopy. However, this is an area where optimal preparation, contrast and imaging are still rapidly evolving. Currently, in addition to diet and laxative preparation, *fecal tagging* is used in many centers. This allows differentiation of fecal remnants in the colon and involves the patient taking a positive contrast orally in advance of the examination (Taylor et al., 2008). Development work is focusing on minimizing discomfort for patients, which may eventually reduce the need for extensive bowel preparation for these examinations (Lefere et al., 2004; Zalis et al., 2006).

Preparation for CT proctography generally involves a dilute barium suspension taken orally one hour prior to examination to outline the small bowel, and glycerine suppositories to evacuate the rectum 20 minutes beforehand (Harvey et al., 1999).

Psychological and physical considerations of patient preparation

The main colonic imaging examinations, including barium enema, colonoscopy and computed tomography colonography, require bowel preparation. Efficacy of the preparation needs to be balanced with patient compliance and acceptability in respect of taste, volume and action. It is not feasible to 'tailor' a bowel preparation regime for individual patients; therefore, a standard regime to suit most bowel habits is generally used. However, any regime adopted will only ever be as good as the patients' ability to understand and willingness to carry out the instructions for taking it. Issues for patients taking colon preparations include the complexity of preparing it, the taste and volume to be taken and the physical effects it has on them (potentially, this includes nausea, vomiting, bloating, cramps, headache, urgency and loss of sleep) (Gluecker et al., 2003).

Patients may already be anxious because they have symptoms that have made them visit a doctor and the expectation of pain and embarrassment of an examination of the GI tract may add to this. Detailed but concise *written instructions* should be provided in lay language for patients, together with details of what happens during the examination. Ideally, these should also be explained by the referring clinician to ensure the full cooperation of the patient (Department of Health, 2001). Once home with the preparation and instructions, patients often find questions they wish to ask, so contact details for someone who can answer queries and provide reassurance are essential.

Timing of preparation can affect patient experience. In a study comparing a preparation regime given in the morning to one group and the same given in the afternoon to another group, the preparation had similar efficacy when assessed overall. However, when the right side of the colon alone was assessed, preparation was significantly better in the morning group; the afternoon preparation was associated with loss of more working hours and sleep (Gupta et al., 2007).

Patient referral for a GI examination should include consideration not only of the clinical appropriateness of the test, taking into account the symptoms and potential risks from the test, but also from the physical and psychological perspective. Patients need to be capable of following the instructions, so special thought must be given to patients with a learning disability, English as a second language, ethnic or religious reasons why they may not be able and/or willing to undergo the examination after taking the prep (e.g. Muslim women wearing x-ray gown – male health professional undertaking the examination).

Physical barriers to complying with either the preparation or examination include immobility and incontinence, which can cause poor tolerance of bowel cleansing. Likewise strict dietary and purgative preparations in conditions such as diabetes could have serious consequences if not appropriately addressed. For elderly patients and those with diabetes, special effort should be made to ensure an early morning appointment and/or additional dietary advice to avoid adverse events such as dehydration and/or hypoglycemia (Lichtenstein et al., 2007). For example, patients with diabetes are advised that the clear fluids they drink should be sugar free and that they should check their blood sugar levels more frequently than usual. Elderly patients without home support or at risk of adverse effects from the preparation and those with learning difficulties may have to be admitted to a hospital ward for supervision. It should be noted, however, that in-patient preparation is often poorer than that of out-patients (Hendry et al., 2007).

Where a perfectly clean colon is the goal, it is not always achieved in all patients, so the presence of fecal matter has to be recognized at the time of the examination and, if necessary, the technique modified and extra views taken. Where *fecal residue* renders an examination suboptimal, the reporter needs to state this and the level of confidence they have in their findings, so the referring clinician can follow up patients appropriately. Occasionally, the preparation may be so poor that the examination has to be abandoned and the patient referred for re-preparation. This should not be taken lightly and detailed discussion with the patient to establish possible causes for failure of the preparation are essential, especially where there is fecal impaction. It has been known for patients to be re-prepared a couple of times, before a stricturing lesion is found. This increases the risk of perforation, a delayed diagnosis or an acute presentation for obstruction, reducing the chances of a favorable outcome (Centre for Reviews and Dissemination, 2004). In all such cases the anxiety, discomfort, inconvenience and risk of repeated preparation for the patient should not be underestimated; their general physical and mental wellbeing should also always be taken into consideration.

Minimal preparation CT (MPCT) colon was introduced in the early 1990s in the UK (Koo et al., 2006; Ganeshan et al., 2007). Understandably, patients prefer examinations that require less bowel preparation, and minimal preparation techniques in both CT and MR colonography have been developed (Florie et al., 2007; Tolan et al., 2007; Taylor et al., 2008). While these examinations may be suitable for the elderly and frail where evidence of large and structuring lesions is sought, they are far less reliable for detection of smaller lesions and polyps.

MRI colonography is a rapidly developing area of colon imaging and this is reflected in the variety of preparation regimes being used. The principles are similar to those used for CT colonography; however, the emphasis is on the use of fecal tagging with or without a cleansing agent. Minimizing the preparation required is a focus of current developments (Pickhardt, 2007; Kuehle et al., 2007; Taylor et al., 2008).

Contrast media

All medical imaging techniques work by detecting the differences in the physical properties of tissues within the body. Contrast media are used to accentuate those differences and enhance the detail on the resultant image. The ideal contrast medium is one that can be safely administered, does not alter the patient's physiology and only accentuates the tissues or organ specifically required.

Different contrast media are used with different imaging modalities. In x-ray examinations such as fluoroscopy and CT, *positive contrast media* are used. These contain elements with high atomic numbers, such as iodine and barium, and therefore absorb x-rays. *Negative contrast media*, such as air, may also be used to allow penetration by the x-rays. Occasionally, a combination provides the optimum imaging; for example, double contrast barium enemas involve the use of a positive (barium sulfate) and a negative (air or carbon dioxide (CO_2)) contrast agent to coat and distend the mucosal lining of the bowel which could not otherwise be seen. For CTC, in addition to the use of a contrast agent for fecal tagging and air or CO_2 to demonstrate the colon, *intravenous iodinated contrast medium* may also be used to highlight extracolonic structures (Tolan et al., 2007).

It is important to select the appropriate contrast media for the technique and area to be visualized, taking into account the contraindications associated with the contrast agent and any physical limitations on the part of the patient (e.g. age, morbidity) and compatibility with other agents used (e.g. laxatives for bowel preparation) (Bartram, 1994).

Positive contrast media

Water-soluble contrast media are iodinated organic compounds, particularly tri-iodinated benzene compounds, where iodine content is directly proportional to their *radiodensity*. While iodine content is related to effectiveness, safety is related to the *osmolality* of the solution, i.e. the number of particles present in a given weight of solution. The lower the osmolality, the less likely a reaction.

Water-soluble contrast media are classed as ionic or non-ionic, monomeric or dimeric and it is these properties that influence their use. *Ionic monomeric media* generally have a high osmolality, while *non-ionic dimeric media* have a low osmolality. For safety reasons, ionic contrast media are no longer in use; the incidence of severe reactions with non-ionic agents is 0.04% and very serious reactions is 0.004% (Katayama et al., 1990; Christiansen, 2005).

Administration and distribution within the body depend on the pharmacokinetic and physical properties of the individual contrast medium and are influenced by the viscosity, which is linked to the osmolality. Examples of contrast media in use for the imaging of the GI tract include iodixanol (Visipaque), a non-ionic dimeric, and iopromide (Ultravist), a non-ionic monomeric.

Intravenous iodinated contrast media should be used for the relevant licensed purpose and in line with the manufacturers' recommendations. The complications and *adverse effects* from the use of contrast media, particularly when administered intravenously, range from nausea and vomiting to anaphylactic shock. Patients considered at increased risk of an adverse event are listed in Box 3.2. Identifying these patients prior to examination allows preventative action such as *prophylaxis* or use of an alternative examination not requiring iodinated contrast media (Royal College of Radiologists, 2005; Tramèr et al., 2006). Use in patients who are pregnant, hyperthyroid or receiving interleukin-2 treatment should be avoided; however, there are no special precautions.

Diatrizoate meglumine (Gastrografin) is a water-soluble contrast medium that can be taken orally or given rectally for GI examinations. Its hyperosmotic properties mean it will draw fluid into the bowel lumen, which may be useful in patients who are constipated, but dangerous for patients presenting with a small bowel obstruction. It can also cause severe chemical pneumonitis if aspirated.

Barium sulfate preparations for the GI tract have to be of the right viscosity to wash residual mucus and food/fecal residue from the surface wall, but still be able to absorb residual fluid and adhere to the mucosal surface for the time the examination takes, without flocculating (clumping). It has to be radiopaque enough to demonstrate the mucosal detail; too dense and it could obscure lesions (Rubesin et al., 2000). There is a large range of preparations available either in powder or suspension form, with varying densities and with a variety of additives, such as suspending agents to ensure uniform coverage, dispersing agents to prevent bubble formation and flavors and sweeteners for products administered orally.

The use of barium sulfate is contraindicated in patients with gastrointestinal obstruction or perforation and should be avoided in those at risk of perforation (e.g. acute ulcerative colitis, post radiotherapy). The presence of barium sulfate in the abdominal cavity (e.g. perforation of the bowel) can lead to peritonitis, adhesions, granulomas and a high mortality rate (Sweetman, 2007). Although barium sulfate itself is inert, a range of hypersensitivity reactions to the additives contained in the preparation have been reported (Janower, 1986). Aspiration can lead to pneumonitis or granuloma formation (Sweetman, 2007).

Possible adverse effects following the administration of barium sulfate can include constipation and impaction, on occasion leading to fecoliths and appendicitis.

BOX 3.2 Patients at increased risk of an adverse event following the administration of intravenous contrast agents

- History of contrast media reaction
- Multiple allergies
- Documented severe allergy requiring therapy
- Asthma
- Those taking metformin
- Impaired renal function

Barium sulfate is the preferred medium for the GI tract as it is safe, dense, giving good quality imaging, and is less expensive than iodine-based media. The use of water-soluble agents is indicated where barium sulfate is not feasible or is potentially dangerous.

Negative contrast media

For barium meals, sodium bicarbonate powder is given together with some lemon juice which, in combination, generates CO_2, which distends the stomach to give a clearer view of the mucosal lining.

For barium enema examinations, air, if used, is manually pumped in to inflate the colon. Carbon dioxide from a pressurized cylinder is administered via a flow meter to prevent over inflation, or alternatively can be pumped into an empty enema bag which can then be squeezed manually to insufflate the bowel. *Insufflation* can cause abdominal pain and discomfort not only during the examination but afterwards, because residual gas in the small and large bowel produces colic. The advantage for patients of CO_2 over air is that it is absorbed more quickly so any discomfort is minimized. This can present a challenge to the operator as it can reduce the window of opportunity for optimal distension and imaging. Alternatively, *active drainage* of air following completion of the examination has been shown to reduce post-procedural pain and swelling (Farrow et al., 1995). The use of an *automated insufflator* to administer CO_2 for CT colonography is the preferred option (Pickhardt, 2007; Tolan et al., 2007).

The risk with the use of negative contrast agents is of perforation, particularly in the colon. Therefore, careful patient selection and use of good technique when using a hand pump for air, or an automated administration set for CO_2, combined with visual monitoring are recommended for patient safety.

Pain relief: antispasmodics, sedation and local anesthetics

Antispasmodics can be used to reduce both gut motility and patient discomfort during examinations that require distension, such as endoscopy, barium meal, barium enema and CTC. Hyoscine-N-butylbromide, *Buscopan*, is the most commonly used antispasmodic in the UK (NB it is not licensed for use in the USA). The contractions of the smooth muscle of the bowel wall are caused by a neurotransmitter called acetylcholine. These contractions are not under conscious control and are not usually felt but, if the muscles go into spasm, this can cause pain. Hyoscine stops the spasms in the smooth muscle by blocking the muscarinic or cholinergic receptors on the muscle cells that the acetylcholine would normally act on. This reduces the contractions, allows the muscle to relax and reduces the painful spasms and cramps. Hyoscine-N-butylbromide may cause temporary blurring of vision and cause the patient to have a dry mouth. Use is contraindicated in patients with *closed angle glaucoma* and should be avoided in patients with porphyria (Sweetman 2007; British Medical Association and the Royal Pharmaceutical Society of Great Britain 2008). Patients should be warned of the small possibility of exacerbating undiagnosed acute angle closure glaucoma. This is a very rare occurrence, but if they experience a pain in the eye, haloes around lights and blurred vision within 24 hours they must seek immediate medical attention. Buscopan can also increase the heart rate and caution should be used in patients with poorly controlled angina, heart failure or patients who are predisposed to tachycardia.

Glucagon is a polypeptide hormone identical to human glucagon that increases blood glucose and relaxes the smooth muscle of the gastrointestinal tract. Given intravenously, it is effective on the large bowel and, administered parenterally, it relaxes the smooth muscle of the stomach, duodenum, small bowel and colon (Eli Lilly, 2005). Glucagon is contraindicated in patients with known hypersensitivity to it and in patients with known insulinoma, pheochromocytoma or glucagonoma. Adverse reactions include nausea, vomiting, diarrhoea, hypokalemia (British Medical Association and the Royal Pharmaceutical Society of Great Britain, 2008). Where licensed for use, Buscopan is the preferred muscle relaxant as it is generally considered more effective and is considerably cheaper (Skucas, 1994; Rubesin et al., 2000).

The addition of peppermint oil to barium sulfate suspension has been shown to relieve spasm during barium enema and may be considered a simple, safe and cheap approach to reducing the number of patients who need to be given an intravenous antispasmodic agent (Sparks et al., 1995).

Sedation is commonly used during invasive GI procedures, such as endoscopy and stent placement. It relieves anxiety and causes temporary relaxation without putting the patient to sleep and has the advantage that most patients remember very little about the procedure afterwards. The type and dose of sedative given depends on the procedure and how anxious the patient is. The most common sedatives used are *benzodiazepines*, such as diazemuls or midasolam. Benzodiazepines work by acting on specific receptors in the brain causing the release of gamma aminobutyric acid (GABA). GABA is a neurotransmitter that acts as a natural 'nerve-calming' agent. It helps keep the nerve activity in the brain in balance, so as diazepam increases the activity of GABA in the brain, it increases its calming effect and results in sleepiness, a decrease in anxiety and relaxation of muscles.

With conscious sedation, it is sometimes possible for the patient to reach a deeper level of sedation than intended. For this reason, guidelines state that all patients should be monitored during conscious sedation, including their blood pressure, pulse and oxygen saturation (Royal College of Radiologists, 2003). The professional monitoring the patient's condition throughout the procedure should have training in monitoring breathing and heart function. Immediate corrective action is necessary if sedation becomes too deep. Anexate injection contains the active ingredient flumazenil, which reverses the effects of benzodiazepines by competing with them for the GABA receptors. Flumazenil binds to the receptors, preventing benzodiazepines from acting on them. This blocks their effects and causes sedation to be reversed.

Sedative drugs do not block the pain signals to the brain, so *local anesthesia* may be given as well, for example, during a percutaneous transhepatic cholangiogram (PTC). Local anesthetics, such as *lidocaine*, are used to numb the skin and generally are administered by injection superficially under the dermis, then deeper into tissue depending on requirements of the procedure.

In addition to any preparation required for the specific GI procedure, patients requiring sedation should be asked not to eat for six hours before the procedure. After the procedure patients are usually allowed to go home once most of the effects of the sedation have worn off. However, they are advised not to drive, drink alcohol, operate machinery or sign legal documents for at least 24 hours after the treatment.

The use of sedation and local anesthetics is common practice and is generally safe, however, after sedation, patients may get a headache, feel nauseous or be sick, and have feelings similar to those of a hangover. Most people have some amnesia about the procedure but, on rare occasions, can have unpleasant memories of the procedure. There is a very small risk of an unexpected reaction to the anesthetic (British Medical Association and the Royal Pharmaceutical Society of Great Britain, 2008; US FDA, 2008).

Prescribing, supplying and administration of drugs

Bowel preparations, contrast media and antispasmodics are classified as non-controlled *prescription only medicines* (POMs). Originally, only medically qualified professionals could prescribe POMs but, in recognition of the expertise and value of advanced roles of nurses and allied health professionals, prescribing rights have been extended (Medicines Act 1969; Department of Health, 1999, 2000). In particular, provision has been made for persons who are operators under the Ionising Radiation (Medical Exposure) Regulations 2000 (IRMER) to administer POMs given in connection with medical exposures under those regulations (SCoR, 2001; Department of Health, 2006).

In addition to writing a prescription (a legal document authorizing supply of a drug for a specific reason to a specific person), *prescribing* involves the supplying of a drug (by the pharmacy to the health professional or by a health professional to the patient) and the preparation and administration of a drug (whether self-administered by the patient or given by a health professional). These are separate actions and each should be undertaken within legislative and safety regulations. In order to confirm that local practice is safe and legal for everyone's benefit, it is necessary to consider each action for every examination. Having mapped this information, it is important to ensure that the appropriate personnel, who are trained and competent, are undertaking those actions and that any delegated responsibilities are appropriately documented.

Non-medical prescribing is complex and governed by legislation particular to each country. A range of non-medical prescribing models has been introduced internationally and interpretation may vary depending on local conditions (Emmerton et al., 2005). In the UK, *Patient Group Directions* (PGD) are written instructions for the supply or administration of a licensed medicine/s in an identified clinical situation, where the patient may not be individually identified before presenting for treatment (NeLM, 2008). PGDs are drawn up locally, to identify the situation and drugs covered, those permitted to operate under it, and the training, updates and monitoring of practice required (Department of Health, 2005; MHRA, 2008). Another model, used widely in the USA, is *prescribing by protocol*, where authority is formally delegated by a medical prescriber. The protocol gives explicit details of the activities that may be performed by the person receiving the delegated authority. Other models used in the UK are that of *supplementary prescribing*, which relates to a patient specific clinical management plan, and *independent prescribing*; there is currently no role for either of these in diagnostic radiography.

Non-medical prescribers need to be trained in the appropriate use, properties, adverse effects and contraindications of the pharmaceuticals they are prescribing; have an understanding of the legal framework they are working within; understand their accountability and responsibilities; understand the level of consent required, how to obtain that consent and the information the patient must be given. Once trained, non-medical prescribers are also required to work within the PGD or protocol and keep a record of their competence (MHRA, 2008; NeLM, 2008; NPC, 2009).

Any Patient Group Directions or protocols should be mutually agreed between the delegating prescriber and the non-medical prescriber. It should be within the skills of the health professional, who must act only within their own area of expertise and competence. The documentation must be signed by the delegating medical prescriber and the health professional involved and approved by the pharmacy and organization in which it is to be used, to ensure appropriate organizational insurance indemnity.

References

Bartram, C.I. 1994. Bowel preparation – principles and practice. Clin. Radiol. 49, 365–367.

Beloosesky, Y., Grinblat, J., Weiss, A., et al., 2003. Electrolyte disorders following oral sodium phosphate administration for bowel cleansing in elderly patients. Arch. Intern. Med. 163, 803–807.

British Medical Association and the Royal Pharmaceutical Society of Great Britain, 2008. British National Formulary (BNF) 55. <http://www.bnf.org/bnf/extra/current/450053.htm>

Brown, A.R., DiPalma, J.A., 2004. Bowel preparation for gastrointestinal procedures. Curr. Gastroenterol. Rep. 6, 395–401.

Centre for Reviews and Dissemination, 2004. The management of colorectal cancers. Eff. Health Care 8, 3.

Chan, C.C., Loke, T.K.L., Chan, J.C.S., et al., 1997. Comparison of two oral evacuants (Citromag and Golytely) for bowel preparation before barium enema. Br. J. Radiol. 70, 1000–1003.

Christiansen, C., 2005. X-ray contrast media – an overview. Toxicology 209 (2), 185–187.

Cittadini, G., Sardanelli, F., De Cicco, E., et al., 1999a. Do magnesium ions influence barium mucosal coating of the large bowel? Eur. Radiol. 9, 1135–1138.

Cittadini, G., Sardanelli, F., De Cicco, E., et al., 1999b. Bowel preparation for the double-contrast barium enema: how to maintain coating with cleansing? Clin. Radiol. 54, 216–220.

Department of Health, 1999. Review of prescribing, supply and administration of medicines. HMSO, London.

Department of Health, 2000. Health services circular 2000/026. Patient group directions (England Only). <http://www.dh.gov.uk/en/PublicationsAndStatistics/LettersAndCirculars/HealthServiceCirculars/DH_4004179> Accessed 06 Sept 2008.

Department of Health, 2001. Good practice in consent implementation guide: consent to examination or treatment. Crown copyright. <http://www.dh.gov.

uk/en/Publicationsandstatistics/Publications/PublicationsPolicyAndGuidance/DH_4005762> Accessed 06 Sept 2008.

Department of Health, 2005. Supplementary prescribing by nurses, pharmacists, chiropodists/podiatrists, physiotherapists and radiographers within the NHS in England. A guide for implementation. Department of Health Gateway reference: 4941. <http://www.dh.gov.uk/en/Publicationsandstatistics/Publications/PublicationsPolicyAndGuidance/DH_4110032> Accessed 06 Sept 2008.

Department of Health, 2006. Statutory instrument no. 2807 the medicines for human use (administration and sale or supply) (miscellaneous amendments) order 2006. HMSO, London.

Eli Lilly & Co, 2005. Information for the physician: glucagon for injection (rDNA origin). <http://pi.lilly.com/us/rglucagon-pi.pdf> Accessed 07/09/08

Emmerton, L., Marriott, J., Bessell, T., et al., 2005. Pharmacists and prescribing rights: review of international developments. J. Pharm. Pharm. Sci. 8 (2), 217–225.

Farrow, R., Jones, A.M.M., Wallace, D.A., et al., 1995. Air versus carbon dioxide insufflation in double contrast barium enemas: the role of active gaseous drainage. Br. J. Radiol. 68, 838–840.

Florie, J., Birnie, E., Van Gelder, R.E., et al., 2007. MR colonography with limited bowel preparation: patient acceptance compared with that of full-preparation colonoscopy. Radiology 245 (1), 150–159.

Ganeshan, A., Upponi, S., Uberoi, R., et al., 2007. Minimal-preparation CT colon in detection of colonic cancer, the Oxford experience. Age & Ageing 36 (1), 48–52.

Gluecker, T.M., Johnson, C.D., Harmsen, W.S., et al., 2003. Colorectal cancer screening with CT colonography, colonoscopy, and double-contrast barium enema examination: prospective assessment of patient perceptions and preferences. Radiology 227 (2), 378–384.

Gupta, T., Mandot, A., Desai, D., et al., 2007. Comparison of two schedules (previous evening versus same morning) of bowel preparation for colonoscopy. Endoscopy 39 (8), 706–709.

Harvey, C.J., Halligan, S., Bartram, C.I., et al., 1999. Evacuation proctography: a prospective study of diagnostic and therapeutic effects. Radiology 211, 223–227.

Hendry, P.O., Jenkins, J.T., Diament, R.H., 2007. The impact of poor bowel preparation on colonoscopy: a prospective single centre study of 10 571 colonoscopies. Colorectal Dis. 9 (8), 745–748.

Holte, K., Nielsen, K.G., Madsen, J.L., et al., 2004. Physiologic effects of bowel preparation. Dis. Colon Rectum 47, 1397–1402.

Janower, M.L., 1986. Hypersensitivity reactions after barium studies of the upper and lower gastrointestinal tract. Radiology 161, 139–140.

Kalantzis, C., Triantafyllou, K., Papadopoulos, A.A., et al., 2007. Effect of three bowel preparations on video-capsule endoscopy gastric and small-bowel transit time and completeness of the examination. Scand. J. Gastroenterol. 42 (9), 1120–1126.

Katayama, H., Yamaguchi, K., Kozuka, T., et al., 1990. Adverse reactions to ionic and non-ionic contrast media. Radiology 175, 621–628.

Knox, R., 1923. Radiography and radio-therapeutics, Part 1: Radiography, fourth ed. A&C Black, London.

Koo, B.C., Ng, C.S., King-Im, J.U., et al., 2006. Minimal preparation CT for the diagnosis of suspected colorectal cancer in the frail and elderly patient. Clin. Radiol. 61 (2), 127–139.

Kuehle, C.A., Langhorst, J., Ladd, S.C., et al., 2007. Magnetic resonance colonography without bowel cleansing: a prospective cross sectional study in a screening population. Gut 56 (8), 1079–1085.

Lefere, P., Gryspeerdt, S., Baekelandt, M., et al., 2004. Laxative-free CT colonography. Am. J. Roentgenol. 183, 945–948.

Lichtenstein, G.R., Cohen, L.B., Uribarri, J., 2007. Bowel preparation for colonoscopy – the importance of adequate hydration. Aliment. Pharmacol. Ther. 26 (5), 633–641.

Medicines Act, 1969. HMSO, London.

Medicines and Healthcare products Regulatory Agency (MHRA). <http://www.mhra.gov.uk/index.htm> Accessed 04 Sept 2008.

National electronic Library for Medicine (NeLM), Patient Group Directions (PGD). <http://www.portal.nelm.nhs.uk/PGD/default.aspx> Accessed 04 Sept 2008.

National Institute for Clinical Excellence, 2004. Guidance on cancer services: improving outcomes in colorectal cancers: the research evidence for the manual update, National Institute for Clinical Excellence. <www.nice.org.uk> Accessed 04 Sept 2008.

National Prescribing Centre (NPC), Non-medical prescribing. <http://www.npc.co.uk/prescribers/nmp.htm> Accessed 16 May 2009.

Paulsen, S.R., Huprich, J.E., Fletcher, J.G., et al., 2006. CT Enterography as a diagnostic test tool in evaluation small bowel disorders: review of clinical experience with over 700 cases. Radiographics 26, 641–662.

Pickhardt, P.J., 2007. Screening CT colonography: how I do it. Am. J. Roentgenol. 189, 290–298.

Rajesh, A., Maglinte, D.D.T., 2006. Multislice CT enteroclysis: technique and clinical applications. Clin. Radiol. 61, 31–39.

Rex, D.K., Imperiale, T.F., Latinovich, D.R., et al., 2002. Impact of bowel preparation on efficiency and cost of colonoscopy. Am. J. Gastroenterol. 97, 1696–1700.

Royal College of Radiologists Board of the Faculty of Clinical Radiology, 2005. Standards for iodinated intravascular contrast agent administration to adult patients, Royal College of Radiologists, London.

Royal College of Radiologists Board of the Faculty of Clinical Radiology, 2003. Safe sedation, analgesia and anaesthesia within the radiology department, Royal College of Radiologists, London.

Rubesin, S.E., Levine, M.S., Laufer, I., et al., 2000. Double-contrast barium enema examination technique. Radiology 215 (3), 642–650.

Russmann, S., Lamerato, L., Marfatia, A., et al., 2007. Risk of impaired renal function after colonoscopy: a cohort study in patients receiving either oral sodium phosphate or polyethylene glycol. Am. J. Gastroenterol. 102, 2655–2663.

Skucas, J., 1994. The use of antispasmodic drugs during barium enemas. Am. J. Roentgenol. 162, 1323–1325.

Society and College of Radiographers, 2001. Radiographer prescribing: a vision paper. Society and College of Radiographers, London.

Sparks, M.J.W., O'Sullivan, P., Herrington, A.A., et al., 1995. Does peppermint oil relieve spasm during barium enema? Br. J. Radiol. 68, 841–843.

Sweetman, S.C. (Ed.), 2007. Martindale: the complete drug reference, thirtyfifth ed. Pharmaceutical Press, London, pp. 1327–1341, 1526–1564, 1690–1727.

Taylor, S.A., Slater, A., Burling, D.N., et al., 2008. CT colonography: organisation, diagnostic performance and patient acceptability of reduced-laxative regimens using barium based faecal tagging. Eur. Radiol. 18 (1), 32–42.

Tramèr, M.R., von Elm, E., Loubeyre, P., et al., 2006. Pharmacological prevention of serious anaphylactic reactions due to iodinated contrast media: systematic review. Br. Med. J. doi:10.1136/bmj.38905.634132.AE.

Tolan, D.J.M., Armstrong, E.M., Burling, D., et al., 2007. Optimization of CT colonography technique: a practical guide. Clin. Radiol. 62 (9), 819–827.

US Food and Drug Administration (FDA), Center for Drug Evaluations and Research (CDER), 2008. <http://www.fda.gov/cder/index.html> Accessed 06 Sept 2008.

Van Tuyl, S.A.C., Den Ouden, H., Stolk, M.F.J., et al., 2007. Optimal preparation for video capsule endoscopy: a prospective, randomized, single-blind study. Endoscopy 39 (12), 1037–1040.

Zalis, M.E., Perumpillichira, J.J., Magee, C., et al., 2006. Tagging-based, electronically cleansed CT colonography: evaluation of patient comfort and image readability. Radiology 239, 149–159.

Zuccaro, G., Connor, J.T., Schreiber, M., 2007. Colonoscopy preparation: are our patients at risk? Am. J. Gastroenterol. 102, 2664–2666.

Further reading

Barrs-Thomas, J., 2005. X-rays and radiopaque drugs. Am. J. Health Syst. Pharm. 62 (19), 2026–2030.

Barrs-Thomas, J., 2006. Overview of radiopaque drugs: 1895–1931. Am. J. Health Syst. Pharm. 63 (22), 2248–2255.

Brookes, D., Smith, A. (Eds.), 2006. Non-medical prescribing in healthcare practice: a toolkit for students and practitioners. Palgrave Macmillan, London.

Chapman, A.H., Adell, J.F., Atkin, W. (Eds.), 2004. Radiology and imaging of the colon. Springer-Verlag, Berlin.

Department of Health and NHS National Practitioner Programme, 2006. A guide to mechanisms for the prescribing, supply and administration of medicines. Medicines Matters. HMSO, London.

Laufer, I., Levine, M.S., 1999. Double contrast gastrointestinal radiology, third ed. Saunders, London.

Reeders, J.W.A.J., Rosenbusch, G. (Eds.), 1994. Clinical radiology and endoscopy of the colon. Thieme, Stuttgart.

Rex, D.K., Johnson, D.A., Lieberman, D.A., et al., 2000. Colorectal cancer prevention 2000: screening recommendations of the American College of Gastroenterology. Am. J. Gastroenterol. 95, 868–877.

Applied anatomy and physiology of the gastrointestinal tract (GIT)

Julie M. Nightingale

Contents ||||||||||||||||||||||||||||||||||||||||||||||||||||||||||||||||||||||||||||||

Introduction

A range of imaging techniques can be employed to visualize the anatomy, physiology and pathology of the GI tract. Fluoroscopic studies have been the traditional method of imaging mucosal detail and structural abnormalities complementing endoscopic and cross-sectional techniques. The software developments in cross-sectional imaging are increasing its capability to provide an alternative imaging option.

For any health professional involved in either referring patients or performing and/or interpreting GI tract imaging studies, a firm underpinning of normal anatomy and physiology and commonly encountered anatomical variants is essential. This includes not only the gross anatomical features clearly visualized on the images, but also the relevant relations, histology, circulation, innervation and lymphatic drainage. An understanding of the embryological development of the GI tract is also helpful in explaining some normal variants and congenital abnormalities encountered in clinical practice, as is an appreciation of the effects of aging upon the individual components of the GI tract. This chapter will explore some of the fundamental underpinning knowledge of GI anatomy and physiology required for successful imaging studies.

Overview

The *gastrointestinal (GI) tract*, also known as the *alimentary canal*, commences at the buccal cavity of the mouth and terminates at the anus. It can be divided into an *upper GI tract* (consisting of mouth, pharynx, esophagus and stomach) and *a lower GI tract* (small and large intestines). The three primary functions of the GI tract are the ingestion of food and water, the digestion of food and absorption of nutrients and the expulsion of waste matter. These primary functions are carried out in conjunction with the *accessory digestive organs* such as the salivary glands, pancreas, liver and gall bladder. Further detailed exploration of the accessory abdominal organs is outside the remit of this book, but suitable references are suggested at the end of the chapter.

Embryology of the GI tract

As the newly implanted embryo reaches the fourth week of gestation it begins to fold ventrally (anteriorly) in two directions. The head and tail end of the embryo curl towards each other and the sides of the embryo begin to fold ventrally towards each other. A constriction results between the embryo and the greater part of the yolk sac, trapping a small part of the yolk sac within the embryo (Figure 4.1A). The constriction corresponds to the future *umbilicus*. The trapped part of the yolk sac becomes the *primitive digestive tube* (Lewis, 2000).

Further anterior growth of the cranial end of the embryo results in folding of the *buccopharyngeal membrane* and this causes a diverticulum of the digestive yolk sac to form – this becomes the *foregut*. Another diverticulum also extends from the caudal end, becoming the *hindgut*. The remaining primitive digestive tube is known as the *midgut*. For the first four weeks of gestation, a wide communication exists between the digestive tube and the main yolk sac, but this gradually narrows to form the *vitelline duct*. This usually regresses but, where it remains after birth, it is known as a *Meckel's diverticulum*, found in approx 2% of individuals (Lewis, 2000). The diverticulum is a 5 cm long blind-ended pouch projecting from the ileum in the affected adult, approximately 1 metre from the ileocecal valve (Lewis, 2000).

The primitive gut is well vascularized, receiving blood from the aorta via the *celiac trunk* (foregut), the *superior mesenteric artery* (midgut) and the *inferior mesenteric artery* (hindgut) (Figure 4.1B).

In the fifth gestational week, the primitive gut grows rapidly and reorganizes into the permanent GI tract structures (Table 4.1). This progression is traditionally divided into three stages:

- Herniation of the midgut outside the eventual abdominal wall and into the proximal part of the umbilical cord. This is a normal migration of the midgut which occurs because there is insufficient room in the abdomen due to the relatively massive liver and kidneys at this stage in development (Moore and Persaud, 2007)
- Further growth, repositioning and rotation of organs, with a return of the midgut to the abdomen by the 10th week (additional room is created in the abdominal cavity by a decrease in the relative size of the liver and kidneys)
- Organs return to their final positions within the abdomen by the 12th week of gestation.

Table 4.2 outlines the three stages and considers some congenital anomalies that can be seen as a result of developmental problems during these three stages. In particular, midgut rotational abnormalities are relatively common and can be seen in Figure 4.2.

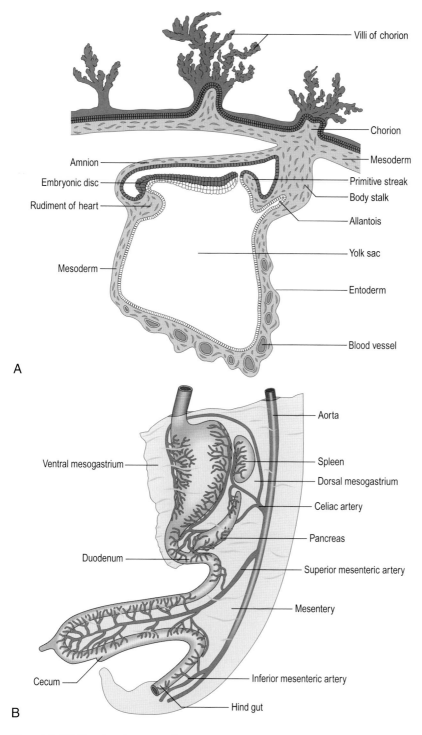

A

B

Figure 4.1 (A) The development of the primitive digestive tube. The embryonic disk curves ventrally trapping some of the yolk sac within it. This forms the primitive digestive tube. (B) The embryological gut and its blood supply. (From an original drawing in Gray's Anatomy).

Table 4.1 Embryological development of the permanent GI structures

Primitive digestive tube	Arterial supply	Venous return	Lymphatic drainage	Innervation	Eventual adult organs
Foregut	Celiac trunk: gastric, splenic, pancreatico-duodenal arteries	Portal venous system	Prevertebral celiac nodes (sited at the origin of the celiac artery)	Epigastric	Pharynx, esophagus, stomach, 1st and 2nd parts of duodenum, liver, gall bladder, upper border of pancreas, spleen
Midgut	Superior mesenteric artery (SMA)	Portal venous system	Prevertebral SMA nodes (sited at the origin of the celiac artery)	Superior mesenteric plexus	3rd and 4th parts of duodenum, jejunum, ileum, cecum, appendix, ascending colon, hepatic flexure, proximal 2/3rds of transverse colon
Hindgut	Inferior mesenteric artery (IMA)	Portal venous system	Chyle cistern (cisterna chyli)	Inferior mesenteric plexus	Distal 1/3rd of transverse colon, splenic flexure, descending colon, sigmoid colon, rectum, anal canal (proximal part)

Table 4.2 The process of development of the gut and subsequent related anomalies

Development stage	Gestational week	Outline of development	Congenital anomalies resulting from adverse development
Stage 1	5th–8th week	The midgut loop, mesentery and the SMA 'herniate' into umbilical cord The midgut loop rotates 180 degrees counter-clockwise	**Atresia** – usually esophageal (1/4000 births), duodenal or anal **Mesenteric cysts** **Diverticula** – congenital, incl. ileal (Meckel's) and jejunal **Duplication** – e.g. of colon (rare)
Stage 2	10th–12th week	Midgut returns to abdominal cavity and rotates a further 90 degrees Small intestine lies to the right of the cavity Cecum is still outside the abdomen, but gradually enters the abdomen and rests in the RUQ	**Congenital omphalocele** – intestines fail to return to abdomen (hernia) **Non-rotation** – colon left side, cecum midline, small bowel left **Incomplete rotation** – cecum LUQ, fixed colon (may lead to volvulus) **Reversed rotation** – transverse colon posterior to duodenum **Malrotation** – leading to increased risk of volvulus and obstruction
Stage 3	By 12th week	Cecum descends into the RIF Ascending and descending colon becomes anchored by peritoneum to the posterior abdominal wall Ligament of Treitz develops (duodeno-jejunal flexure) Small bowel mesentery retracts to its permanent position	**Cecal anomalies** – undescended/mobile/hyperdescended cecum **Colon/ileocecal mesentery** – laxity and hypermobility increasing risk of volvulus **Internal hernias** – where colonic fixation is incomplete

SMA, superior mesenteric artery; RUQ, right upper quadrant; LUQ, left upper quadrant; RIF, right iliac fossa

Embryology of the GI tract

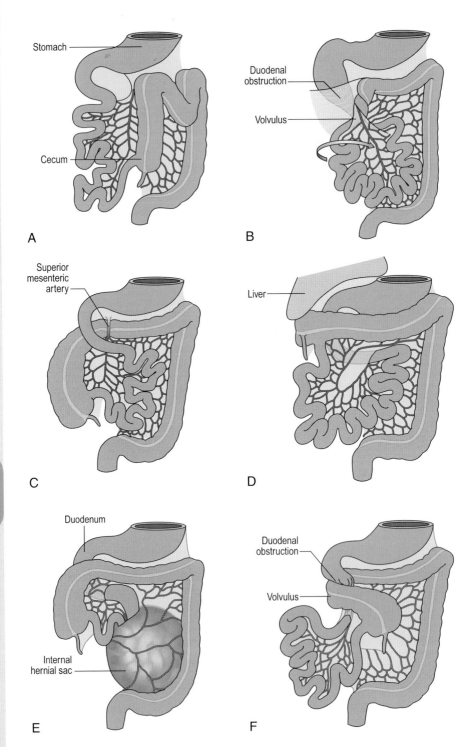

Figure 4.2 Abnormalities of midgut rotation. (A) Nonrotation; (B) Mixed rotation and volvulus (twisting) of the intestines; (C) Reversed rotation; (D) Subhepatic cecum; (E) Paraduodenal hernia; (F) Midgut volvulus. (Reproduced from Moore KL and Persaud TVN, Before we are Born: Essentials of Embryology and Birth Defects, 7th edn. Saunders, Philadelphia, 2007.)

Histology of the GI tract

The GI tract displays a uniform histology throughout its length, with subtle differences between regions corresponding to functional specialization. The GI tract is divided into four concentric layers surrounding the lumen as shown in Figure 4.3 (mucosa, submucosa, muscularis externa and serosa or adventitia).

The innermost layer is known as the *mucosa*, which surrounds the lumen of the GI tract. It has both a protective function (from injury and infection), as well as a digestive function (chemical breakdown, absorption and secretion). The mucosa can be further subdivided into three layers. The *epithelium* is the innermost layer, in contact with the ingested material. It is supported structurally and nutritionally by the *lamina propria*, a layer of loose irregular connective tissue, well supplied by blood capillaries and lymphatic tissue. The outermost subdivision of the mucosa is a thin layer of smooth muscle known as the *muscularis mucosae*. This smooth muscle throws the mucosa into small folds, increasing the absorptive surface area and encouraging the turbulence of the fluid contents (chyme). The mucosal layer is highly specialized within each organ of the GI tract, reflecting the different functions and chemical environments (Table 4.3).

The *submucosa* is a dense layer of connective tissue containing numerous blood vessels, lymphatics and nerves, which branch into the mucosa and the muscularis externa. This layer contains a network of nerves forming part of the enteric nervous system, known as the *submucosal* (or *Meissner's*) *plexus*. This plexus is primarily responsible for initiating chemical secretion.

The *muscularis propria (externa)* generally consists of two smooth muscle layers; however, in the esophagus, striated (skeletal) muscle replaces the smooth muscle in the proximal third. Throughout the rest of the GI

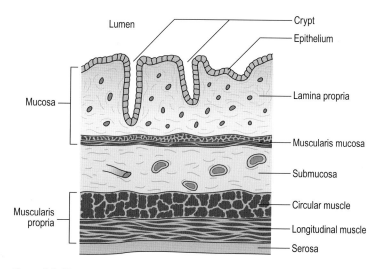

Figure 4.3 Histology of the GI tract.

Table 4.3 Mucosal differentiation throughout the GI tract

GI tract organ	Cellular composition of mucosa	Mucosal features
Mouth	**Stratified squamous epithelium** for protection	The epithelium is partially **keratinized** on gums and hard palate. A muscularis mucosae is not present
Pharynx	**Columnar ciliated epithelium** (nasal part) **Stratified squamous epithelium** (oral and laryngeal parts)	Mucosa is continuous with lining of auditory tubes, nasal cavities, mouth and larynx Beneath mucosa are mucous glands which secrete mucus – numerous around the orifices of the auditory tubes
Esophagus	Thick layer of **stratified squamous epithelium**. Transition to columnar epithelium at gastro-esophageal junction	Thrown into longitudinal folds which disappear on distension Beneath mucosa are mucous glands which secrete mucus through long ducts
Stomach	Single layer of **columnar epithelium** with occasional goblet (mucus secreting) cells and gastric glands (acid and enzyme secreting)	Thick, smooth and 'velvety' layer. Small shallow depressions cover the surface and are the ducts of the gastric glands. During contraction, the mucosa is thrown into mainly longitudinal folds called **rugae**, which disappear on distension. When distended, the geometric surface pattern of the stomach becomes visible, with shallow grooves creating subdivisions known as **areae gastricae**
Small intestine	Columnar epithelium	Thick and highly vascular in proximal intestine, but thinner and less vascular in distal small intestine Thrown into permanent **circular folds (valvulae conniventes)**. Very large in duodenum, reducing gradually in size to the ileum, where they disappear. The folds slow the passage of food and provide an increased absorptive area Millions of small vascular processes projecting into the lumen **(intestinal villi)** hugely increase the absorptive area. Contain lacteals to drain products of fat digestion. Largest and most numerous in duodenum, reducing gradually in size and number towards the distal ileum Abundant **intestinal glands (crypts of Lieberkuhn)** scattered throughout the intestinal mucosa **Solitary lymphatic nodules** scattered throughout, but most numerous in the distal ileum **Aggregated lymphatic patches (Peyer's patches)** again largest and most numerous in the ileum

Table 4.3 Mucosal differentiation throughout the GI tract—cont'd

GI tract organ	Cellular composition of mucosa	Mucosal features
Large intestine	**Columnar epithelium** (absorbs water), interspersed with **goblet cells** (mucus secreting) and **enterochromaffin cells** (hormone secreting) **Stratified squamous epithelium** in distal anal canal	Pale, smooth lining with no villi. Contains shallow intestinal glands **Solitary lymphatic nodules** abundant in cecum and appendix. Colonic mucosa can be thrown into mucus-filled grooves in a geometric pattern known as **areae colonicae**

tract, the inner circular muscle layer has smooth muscle fibers lying in a concentric fashion around the circumference of the GI tract, while the outer longitudinal muscle layer has fibers orientated parallel to the direction of the GI tract. (Note that in the stomach there is also an additional innermost oblique layer of muscle fibers, mainly limited to the cardiac end of the stomach). In between the two layers lies a second enteric nerve plexus, known as the *myenteric* (or *Auerbach's*) *plexus*. This plexus is responsible for coordinating motility (movement) of the GI tract, including peristalsis, whereby coordinated contractions of the two muscle layers assist in propelling the food bolus along the lumen.

In the colon, the longitudinal muscle layer is incomplete, being gathered into three 1 cm thick bands called the *teniae coli*, with only a thin layer of muscle in between. These bands (the teniae omentalis, libera and mesocolica) converge on the base of the appendix, run the full length of the colon, fanning out into a continuous layer surrounding the rectum (Figure 4.4). Contraction of the teniae coli gathers up the colon in a concertina effect, the resulting sacculations being known as *haustral pouches* or *haustrations*. These are clearly defined and fixed in the proximal colon, but require active contraction in the distal colon, where the teniae are thinner (see Chapter 16).

The outermost layer of the GI tract wall is known as the *adventitia* and, in the esophagus, it is a tough layer of loose connective tissue. Within the abdominal cavity, the adventitia is covered by mesothelium, along with a thin connective tissue layer, forming a serous membrane, or *serosa*. This delicate membrane secretes a small quantity of serous fluid, which helps to lubricate the organs as they move during peristalsis. The serous membrane is derived from the innermost (visceral) layer of *peritoneum*, which lines the abdominal cavities and suspends the organs or anchors them in place. The serosa completely surrounds most of the abdominal GI tract (such as the jejunum and ileum), enabling it to move relatively freely, but it covers some parts of the duodenum and colon only partially, thus anchoring them in place along the posterior abdominal wall. Some parts of the serosa are lined with small fat-filled connective tissue pouches known as *epiploic appendages*, particularly common along the transverse colon.

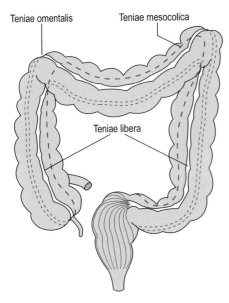

Teniae omentalis   Teniae mesocolica

Teniae libera

Figure 4.4 Location of the teniae coli. The three bands of longitudinal muscle converge on the appendix and fan out to envelop the rectum. The teniae libera travels anterior to the ascending and descending colon, but inferiorly on the transverse colon. Teniae mesocolica runs posteromedially in the ascending and descending colon and posterosuperiorly in the transverse. Teniae omentalis lies anterosuperiorly in the transverse colon, but travels posterolaterally in the ascending and descending colon.

Oral cavity

The oral cavity (mouth) is designed to support chewing, swallowing and speech. Two rows of teeth are embedded within the maxilla above and the mandible below and are surrounded by the gums (*gingivae*). The functions of the mouth are also facilitated by the hard and soft palate above, the floor of the mouth below, the cheeks laterally, the tongue, and the upper and lower lips externally (Figure 4.5). Two separate sets of teeth are grown in humans: the *primary dentition* (deciduous teeth) develops during early childhood and consists of 20 teeth. The *secondary dentition* (permanent teeth) gradually replaces the deciduous set with 32 adult teeth. These teeth are adapted for different functions, including cutting (incisors), tearing (canines), crushing (premolars) and grinding (molars).

The tongue is a specialized skeletal muscle connected to the hyoid bone. It has an important role concerned with sensation of taste, formation of speech, chewing (shaping the food bolus) and swallowing.

The large posterior opening into the oropharynx is bounded by the *pillars of Fauces* laterally, the soft palate superiorly and the upper surface of the tongue inferiorly. The pillars of Fauces are two vertical pairs of columns of mucous membrane at the back of the mouth, housing the *palatine tonsils*.

Several other openings within the oral cavity are associated with the salivary ducts. Three pairs of *salivary glands* secrete saliva into the oral cavity in response to food stimuli (Figure 4.6). *Saliva* is composed of primarily water (approximately 98%), in combination with ions, salivary amylase (which

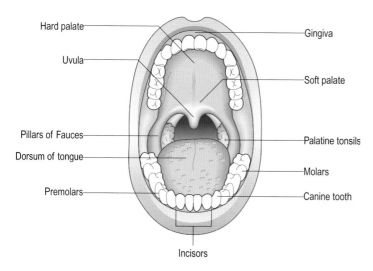

Figure 4.5 **Anterior view of the oral cavity.**

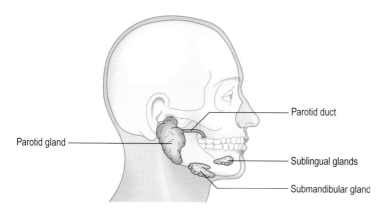

Figure 4.6 **Location of the salivary glands.**

begins the breakdown of starch to sugars), lysozymes (antibacterial), as well as trace quantities of urea (a waste product). The saliva lubricates the food and helps to form it into a bolus suitable for swallowing.

The large paired *parotid glands* are situated within the subcutaneous tissue of the face, anterior and inferior to the ear. They excrete saliva into the mouth via the *parotid duct* (Stensen's duct), emptying into the cheek at the parotid papilla situated opposite the second upper molar tooth. The *sublingual glands* are situated under the tongue, secreting their saliva and a high quantity of mucus via multiple openings through the buccal mucosa. The *submandibular glands*, situated in the floor of the mouth close to the ramus of the mandible, secrete the largest quantity of saliva via the 5 cm long submandibular duct (Wharton's duct) through a small papilla alongside the frenulum (vertical strip of tissue in the midline of the underside of the tongue). One of the larger sublingual ducts joins with the submandibular duct to empty at the frenulum.

The pharynx

The pharynx is a complex anatomical structure serving as a gateway to both the digestive and respiratory passageways. During respiration, the pharynx provides a patent airway from the nose and mouth through to the larynx. During swallowing (*deglutition*) it provides a passageway from the mouth to the esophagus, while ensuring that the bolus cannot enter the airway. The pharynx also has important functions in relation to speech, choking, vomiting and yawning (Rubesin, 1999).

The pharynx is a 12.5 cm long funnel-shaped tube of skeletal muscle, extending from the base of the skull (CV1) to the lower border of the cricoid cartilage (CV6). It lies anteriorly to the cervical vertebral bodies and their associated muscles and connective tissues. The buccopharyngeal fascia (surrounding the mouth and pharynx musculature) is only loosely attached to the prevertebral layer of muscle, forming the retropharyngeal space. This potentially distendable space runs from the base of skull through to the posterior mediastinum in the thorax and is therefore an important route of spread for infection and metastases.

The pharynx lies posteriorly to the nasal cavities, the oral cavity and the larynx. Laterally lie the muscles of the neck, the lateral portions of the hyoid bone and thyroid cartilage and the carotid sheath (Rubesin, 2000).

The pharynx is composed of three coats: an outer muscular coat, a central fibrous coat and an inner mucous coat. The fibrous coat is thicker in the superior portions of the pharynx and is almost absent in the inferior portions. It creates attachment for some of the important muscles of the pharynx, known as the constrictor muscles. The mucous coat is continuous with the linings of the pharyngo-tympanic tubes, the nasal cavities, the mouth and the larynx. In the nasal portions, it is covered by ciliated columnar epithelium, elsewhere it consists of stratified squamous epithelium.

The upper part of the pharynx is supplied by branches of the facial and maxillary arteries, while the lower pharynx is supplied by the ascending pharyngeal artery and branches of the superior thyroid artery. Lymphatic drainage is via the retropharyngeal and paratracheal nodes, or direct to the deep cervical nodes.

In humans, the pharynx can be divided into three parts: the nasopharynx, the oropharynx and the laryngopharynx (hypopharynx) (Figure 4.7). The *nasopharynx*, a permanently patent respiratory tract structure lying behind the nasal cavity, is normally excluded from the digestive tract by the soft palate. During swallowing, the bilateral *pharyngo-tympanic (Eustachian) tubes*, which connect the middle ears to the nasopharynx, open up to allow equilibrium of air pressures on either side of the tympanic membrane. During respiration, this passageway is closed. Within the posterior walls of the nasopharynx lie the *pharyngeal tonsils*, or adenoids, which are most prominent during childhood. These can create a nodular appearance on radiological examination and, if enlarged, can interfere with speech and respiration.

The *oropharynx* extends from the soft palate to the level of the hyoid bone, although this is a seemingly arbitrary description, as the hyoid bone and soft palate position changes during speech, respiration and swallowing (Rubesin, 1999). The oropharynx communicates anteriorly with the oral cavity, with the anterior wall made up of the base of the tongue and the

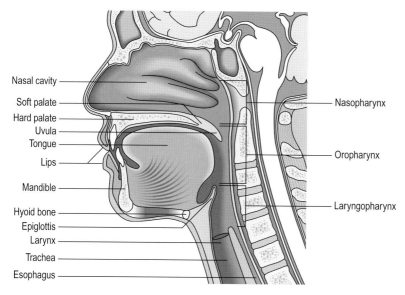

Figure 4.7 Median sagittal section through oral cavity and pharynx.

Labels (top to bottom, left): Nasal cavity, Soft palate, Hard palate, Uvula, Tongue, Lips, Mandible, Hyoid bone, Epiglottis, Larynx, Trachea, Esophagus

Labels (right): Nasopharynx, Oropharynx, Laryngopharynx

valleculae. The *valleculae* are paired cup-shaped spaces sitting behind the tongue, separating the tongue from the *epiglottis*, a leaf-shaped cartilage which is essential in closing off the respiratory passages during swallowing. The valleculae are not permanent structures, disappearing on swallowing as the epiglottis inverts. The *aryepiglottic folds* form the upper lateral margins of the epiglottis. The lateral wall of the oropharynx is made up of the palatine tonsils, *tonsillar fossa* and faucial pillars.

The *laryngopharynx* opens anteriorly into the triangular entrance of the larynx. It is indented anteriorly by the laryngeal structures, resulting in two grooves running anterolaterally in the laryngopharynx – these are known as the *piriform sinuses*. The lower end of the laryngopharynx is collapsed in the anteroposterior direction except when a food bolus passes. Radiologically, the laryngopharynx is indented by the cricoid cartilage and the *cricopharyngeus muscle*. When tonically contracted, this muscle assists in forming the *upper esophageal sphincter*.

The shape of the pharynx is determined by the underlying muscles as well as the indentation of cartilages as described above. The pharynx is divided into two muscle layers: an inner longitudinal layer and an outer circular layer. The outermost layer forms a ring of constricting muscles, which are incomplete anteriorly. These *constrictor muscles* are divided into superior, middle and inferior bands, which serve to push the food bolus sequentially through the pharynx (Figure 4.8). The internal layer of longitudinal muscle is closely associated with major folds of mucosa, resulting in the appearance of longitudinal striations on the lateral and posterior walls on contrast studies. Transverse patterns along the anterior wall result from redundant mucosa overlying the arytenoid and cricoid cartilages (Rubesin, 1999). *Killian's dehiscence* is a triangular area in the wall of the pharynx, lying in the midline between the inferior constrictor muscle and the cricopharyngeus muscle. It is of clinical significance as it represents a potentially weak spot where a pulsion diverticulum (Zenker's diverticulum) is more likely to occur.

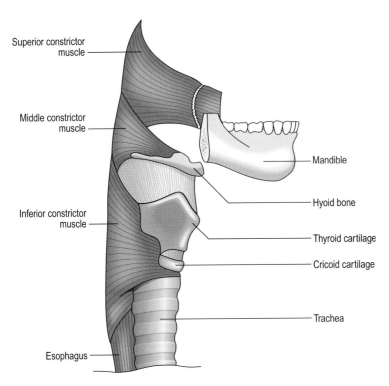

Superior constrictor muscle

Middle constrictor muscle

Inferior constrictor muscle

Esophagus

Mandible

Hyoid bone

Thyroid cartilage

Cricoid cartilage

Trachea

Figure 4.8 Constrictor muscles – anterolateral view of the pharynx.

Pharyngeal function depends on the interplay of the intrinsic muscles of the pharynx and larynx, along with the extrinsic muscles of the pharynx, arising from the base of skull, neck, tongue, mandible and hyoid bone. The mechanism of swallowing, known as *deglutition*, depends on a complex sequence of muscular contraction coordinated by six cranial nerves and three cervical nerves (Jones, 2000), enabling passage of the food bolus into the esophagus, while protecting the airway. In preparation for swallowing, the pharynx is drawn upwards and sideways, so increasing its transverse diameter. Anterior and superior movement of the tongue and larynx open the pharynx anteroposteriorly. When the food bolus is passed into the pharynx, the elevator muscles relax, the pharynx descends and the constrictor muscles begin to contract sequentially, so conveying the bolus into the esophagus. The process of deglutition is commonly divided into an *oral* (voluntary) stage, followed by involuntary *pharyngeal* and esophageal phases. These phases will be discussed in detail in Chapter 7.

The esophagus

The esophagus is a muscular tube (approximately 23 cm long), commencing at the base of the laryngopharynx (CV6) and descending through the superior and posterior mediastinum of the thoracic cavity immediately anterior to the vertebral column. It passes through the diaphragm to enter the abdominal cavity, connecting with the stomach at the *cardiac orifice* (TV11).

The esophagus can therefore be divided into arbitrary divisions known as the cervical, thoracic and abdominal portions (see Table 4.4 of relations), although in radiological reports the esophagus is often delineated into upper, middle and lower thirds. As the esophagus traverses through these regions of the body, the associated anatomical relations, blood supply, venous return, innervation and lymphatic drainage will change accordingly (Tables 4.4 and 4.5). While the course of the esophagus is predominantly vertical, it also follows the curve of the vertebral column anteroposteriorly, and changes course laterally at several vertebral levels (Figure 4.9). A number of anatomical and physiological indentations occur along its course (Table 4.6).

The esophagus has four coats: an external fibrous coat (adventitia), a muscular coat, a submucosal coat and an internal mucous coat. The muscular coat comprises an outer longitudinal coat and inner circular muscles, continuous with the inferior pharyngeal constrictor muscles and the circular muscles of the stomach. The muscle fibers are striated in the upper esophagus and smooth in the lower two thirds. The submucosal coat contains numerous glands secreting mucus, protecting and lubricating the epithelium and aiding the passage of the food bolus. The mucosa is lined

Table 4.4 Anatomical relationships of the esophagus

Region	Anterior	Posterior	Right	Left
Cervical	Thyroid gland Trachea Left recurrent laryngeal nerve	Vertebral column Longus colli muscle	Right common carotid artery Right recurrent laryngeal nerve Thyroid gland	Left inferior thyroid artery Left common carotid artery Thyroid gland Thoracic duct
Thoracic	Trachea (to T5) Left main bronchus Pericardium (left atrium) Diaphragm	Vertebral column Longus colli muscle Right intercostal arteries Thoracic duct (crosses to left at T5) Hemiazygos vein Aorta (inferiorly)	Right pleura Azygos vein Vagus nerve Thoracic duct (inferiorly)	Aortic arch Left subclavian artery Thoracic duct Left pleura Left recurrent laryngeal nerve Descending thoracic aorta (inferiorly)
Abdominal	Left lobe of liver Lesser omentum Anterior vagal trunk	Vertebral column Posterior vagal trunk Left crus of diaphragm	Lesser omentum Right crus of diaphragm Inferior vena cava	Greater omentum Left crus of diaphragm

Table 4.5 Circulation, lymphatics and innervation of the esophagus

Region	Cervical	Thoracic	Abdominal	Notes
Arterial supply	Inferior thyroid artery	Upper intercostal arteries (superiorly) Descending paired aortic branches: bronchial and esophageal	Esophageal branches of left gastric artery (from celiac artery) Left inferior phrenic artery (from abdominal aorta)	Longitudinal plexus of vessels formed
Venous return	Inferior thyroid vein (to brachiocephalic and superior vena cava)	Azygos branches	Azygos and hemiazygos (through esophageal opening), left gastric vein – portal vein to liver	Note the porto-systemic anastomosis in the distal esophagus – potential implications for spread of cancer and esophageal varices with portal hypertension
Lymphatic drainage	Deep cervical nodes	Superior and posterior mediastinal nodes	Left gastric and preaortic nodes	Forms a longitudinal plexus within submucosa. Travels long distances – implications for spread of cancer
Innervation	From vagus and sympathetic trunks, forming an esophageal plexus Recurrent laryngeal nerves	Vagus and greater splancnic nerve fibers form the esophageal plexus	Vagus and greater splancnic nerve fibers form the esophageal plexus	Some somatic nerves in the upper esophagus (skeletal muscle) Most fibers are parasympathetic (e.g. vagus) A few sympathetic fibers initiate vasoconstriction

by stratified squamous epithelium and is orientated in longitudinal folds which disappear on distension (Lewis, 2000).

The passage of a food bolus from the pharynx into the esophagus is regulated by the *upper esophageal sphincter*. This sphincter is formed primarily by contraction of the cricopharyngeal muscle (the horizontal portion of the

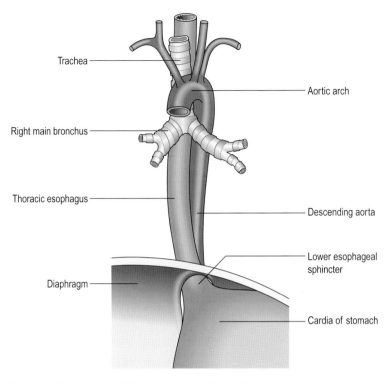

Figure 4.9 **Anterior view of the esophagus and its relations.**

Labels: Trachea, Aortic arch, Right main bronchus, Thoracic esophagus, Descending aorta, Lower esophageal sphincter, Diaphragm, Cardia of stomach

Table 4.6 Normal indentations of the esophagus

Level of constriction	Anatomical impression
CV6	Inferior constrictor muscle impression
TV4	Crossing of the aortic arch
TV5–6	Crossing of the left main bronchus
TV10	Passage through the diaphragm at the esophageal hiatus

inferior constrictor muscle). The *lower esophageal sphincter* is not a true muscular sphincter mechanism, but is defined as a high-pressure zone measuring 2–4 cm in length in the esophago-gastric region (Ott, 2000).

At rest, the esophageal body is in a collapsed state, with the upper and lower esophageal sphincters closed to prevent retrograde flow of ingested food contents. When swallowing is initiated, the esophagus propels the food bolus from the pharynx into the stomach, aided by peristalsis, as well as gravity with upright posture. *Peristalsis* is the rhythmic contraction of smooth muscles, creating a pressure wave, thus propelling the food bolus along the GI tract. Peristalsis is normally initiated by circular muscles, which contract behind the food bolus to prevent retrograde flow. This is followed by longitudinal muscle contraction, driving the bolus forwards. The *primary peristaltic wave* is initiated when the food bolus enters the pharynx. The upper esophageal sphincter relaxes almost immediately, with relaxation of the lower esophageal sphincter occurring several seconds later. This wave moves through the esophagus in approximately 6–8 seconds (Ott, 2000). Once the food bolus reaches the stomach, the lower esophageal sphincter returns to its resting tone to help prevent refluxing of stomach contents. If a food bolus gets stuck, or moves slower than the primary wave, the distension stimulates local stretch receptors in the esophagus, which initiate a *secondary peristaltic wave*. This secondary wave works behind the bolus to drive it forwards and continues until the bolus enters the stomach. In contrast to these peristaltic waves, occasionally *tertiary* or *non-peristaltic waves* can be seen. These waves occur spontaneously or during swallowing, and while they may be non-specific, they may also be associated with structural or motility disorders of the esophagus (Ott, 2000).

The stomach

The stomach lies within the epigastric, umbilical and left hypochondriac regions of the abdomen (Figure 4.10) and is the most dilated part of the GI tract. Its shape and position varies from person to person and within the phase of digestion, but is classically said to represent a 'J' shape. The stomach presents two openings, two curvatures and two surfaces for description purposes (Figure 4.11). The esophagus communicates with the stomach via the *cardiac orifice*, situated to the left of the midline at approximately TV10. The left border of the esophagus is continuous with the greater curvature of the stomach, while the right border is continuous with the lesser curvature. This right esophageal border meets the stomach at a sharp angle, known as

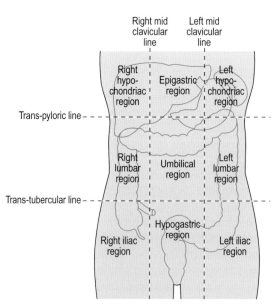

Figure 4.10 The nine regions of the abdomen. The abdomen can also be divided into four equal quadrants: left and right upper and lower quadrants.

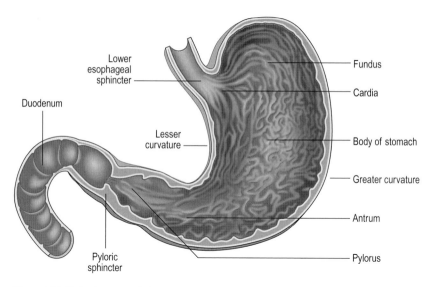

Figure 4.11 Major features of the stomach (anterior view).

the *cardiac incisura*. The inferior opening of the stomach is the *pyloric orifice*, communicating with the duodenum, lying to the right of the midline at the level of the upper border of LV1.

The *lesser curvature* extends from the cardiac to the pyloric orifices, creating the right or posterior border of the stomach. Close to the pyloric end there is a sharply angulated notch, known as the *incisura*. The *lesser curvature* is attached to two layers of the *hepatogastric ligament*, which suspends the stomach from the lower border of the liver. The greater curvature is up to five times as long as the lesser curve and is covered at its commencement with peritoneum. The left part of the curvature is attached to the *gastrolienal ligament* (connecting it to the spleen), while the anterior portion of the curve gives rise to the two layers of the *greater omentum*. This peritoneal reflection lies underneath the anterior abdominal wall. A storage area for fat, it is often termed the 'fatty apron'.

The two surfaces of the stomach vary in position with different degrees of stomach distension, thus are termed the anterosuperior and posteroinferior surfaces. The left side of the *anterosuperior surface* is in contact with the diaphragm (separating it from the left lung), the pericardium and the 7th–9th ribs. The right side is related to the left lobe of the liver and the anterior abdominal wall. The whole surface is covered with peritoneum. The posteroinferior surface is related to several structures forming the *stomach bed*, in which the stomach rests. These structures include the diaphragm, the spleen, the left adrenal gland, the left colic flexure and the upper part of the transverse mesocolon. During a double contrast barium examination, the fully distended stomach can become compressed by these extrinsic organs. This is particularly noticeable in a thin patient.

The stomach can be subdivided into a left portion or *body*, a superior portion or *fundus* and a right portion or *antrum*, as shown in Figure 4.11. The circulation, innervation and lymphatic drainage of these subdivisions is demonstrated in Table 4.7. When erect the fundus is often distended with gas.

Table 4.7 Circulation, innervation and lymphatic drainage of the stomach

Region	Anterosuperior surface	Posteroinferior surface	Greater curvature	Lesser curvature	Notes
Arterial supply	Short gastric artery (fundus) Gastric arterial anastomoses	Gastric arterial anastomoses	From splenic artery: right gastro-omental artery (inferiorly), anastomoses with left gastro-omental artery (superiorly) Also supply the omentum	From celiac trunk: left gastric artery (superiorly) Anastomoses with right gastric artery (branch of hepatic artery) (inferiorly)	Stomach receives blood supply from all 3 branches of the celiac trunk (hepatic, splenic and left gastric arteries). Main arteries supply the curvatures, then form anastomoses which supply the surfaces
Venous return	Drain towards curvatures	Drain towards curvatures	Right gastro-omental veins to the superior mesenteric vein Left gastro-omental vein to splenic vein	Left and right gastric and esophageal arteries to portal vein Note the porto-systemic anastomosis	Larger veins follow course of the arteries of the same name All veins drain eventually to the portal vein to the liver
Lymphatic drainage	Drain to the greater and lesser curvatures	Drain to the greater and lesser curvatures	Pancreaticosplenic nodes to celiac nodes Right gastro-omental nodes to pyloric nodes – celiac nodes	Gastric group: left gastric nodes to left celiac nodes Right gastric and pyloric nodes to hepatic and celiac nodes	Lymph channels follow the arterial courses All nodes eventually drain to celiac nodes, preaortic nodes and to the cisterna chyli
Innervation	Left vagus – hepatic branches supply anterior stomach and pylorus. Increase motility, open pylorus, initiate gastric secretions	Right vagus – celiac branches supply posterior wall			Sympathetic supply – greater splanchnic nerves (thoracic) – decrease motility, vasoconstriction, close pylorus

The wall of the stomach consists of four coats as outlined previously. The serous coat is derived from peritoneum, completely enveloping the stomach except at the curvatures where the omenta attach – this creates a small space through which nutrient vessels and nerves pass (Lewis, 2000). The muscular coat consists of an outer longitudinal layer, with fibers continuous with those of the esophagus and distally with the duodenum and pyloric sphincter. The circular fibers are continuous with the esophageal muscles and are most abundant within the pylorus, forming the sphincter. The oblique fibers lie internal to the circular layer, mainly limited to the cardiac region. The submucosa is loose connective tissue, connecting muscular with mucosal layers. The mucosal layer is thick and is thrown into numerous longitudinally-orientated bands called *rugae*. These bands are most visible towards the pylorus and greater curvature and disappear upon distension. There is a sharp change from stratified epithelium in the distal esophagus to *columnar epithelium* with mucos-secreting *goblet cells* in the stomach.

A network of shallow grooves divides the mucosa up into gastric areas approximately 1–5mm in diameter (*areae gastricae*). This surface pattern can be seen in barium studies as a faint honeycomb appearance in approximately 70% of patients (Levine and Laufer, 1999). Small shallow depressions on the mucosal surface are the openings of the gastric pits, into which several gastric glands spill their contents. Mucus-secreting cells secrete *alkaline mucus* which sticks to the columnar epithelium, creating a 1 mm thick protective barrier. Secretion of hydrochloric acid by parietal cells creates a hostile environment within the stomach lumen of around pH 1–4, and this, coupled with the secretion of gastric enzymes which begin the digestion of proteins, put significant stresses upon the stomach mucosa. A number of factors combine to help to reduce the chances of autodigestion of the stomach lining (Table 4.8), which would result in ulceration and potential perforation.

The function of the stomach is to receive the food bolus from the esophagus and begin the breakdown of large food molecules into smaller components that will eventually be absorbed in the small intestine. Strong mechanical activity called *mixing waves* help to churn the stomach contents,

Table 4.8 Factors which assist in preventing stomach autodigestion

Factor	Action
Mucus-secreting cells line the epithelium with alkaline mucous	Provide a physical and chemical barrier to attack by HCL
Pepsin produced in an inactive form (pepsinogen)	To prevent digestion of the protein based cell walls in gastric glands
Pepsinogen and hydrochloric acid produced and secreted separately	Pepsinogen only converted to active form pepsin in presence of HCL – will only occur once released from gastric glands into the lumen
Gastric mucosa has a high mitotic index (cell turnover)	Rapid replacement of damaged cells
Rich blood supply to gastric lining	Repair damage and high cell turnover

HCL, hydrochloric acid

reducing food particles in size and helping to mix them with the chemical secretions from *gastric juice*. Up to 3 litres of gastric juice can be secreted per day. While the low pH environment stops the action of salivary amylase, it also promotes the conversion of the inactive *pepsinogen* to the enzyme pepsin. *Pepsin* begins the process of protein digestion, converting proteins to polypeptides. Other secretions include *intrinsic factor* from the parietal cells, which work to promote the absorption of vitamin B12 (vital to prevent pernicious anemia) from the small intestine. In infants, an enzyme known as *rennin* is also secreted, which emulsifies milk so that other enzymes can break it down further.

Within the epithelium lie scattered *endocrine cells*, secreting hormones either to promote or inhibit gastric activity. Gastric secretions are increased in the presence of the hormone *gastrin*, which also increases gastric motility. Other hormones have a lesser effect, tending to decrease gastric emptying (e.g. cholecystokinin) or decrease gastric acid secretion and motility (e.g. secretin, gastric inhibitory peptide and enteroglucagon) when the intestines are full. The stomach is also capable of absorbing some ions, water and lipid-soluble compounds such as aspirin, alcohol and caffeine.

The small intestine

The small intestine is a convoluted tube, reported to have a mean length of 6.38 metres (Herlinger, 2001), which gradually diminishes in size from its commencement at the pyloric sphincter of the stomach to its termination at the ileocecal valve. The small intestine resides within the central and lower parts of the abdomen, bordered superiorly and laterally by the large intestine, while the greater omentum lies anteriorly. The small intestine is suspended from the vertebral column by a fold of peritoneum called the *mesentery of the small intestine*.

The small intestine can be divided into three parts known as the duodenum, jejunum and ileum. The *duodenum* is the shortest, widest and most fixed part of the small intestine, forming a 25 cm C-shaped curve around the head of the pancreas (Figure 4.12). From the diagram it can be seen that the

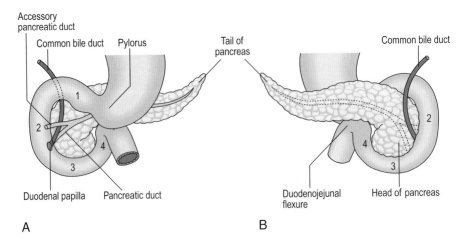

A

B

Figure 4.12 Parts of the duodenum and their relationship with the pancreas. (A) Anterior view; (B) posterior view.

duodenum can be subdivided into 1st part (superior), 2nd part (descending), 3rd part (transverse) and the 4th part (ascending), uniting with the jejunum at the abrupt *duodenojejunal flexure*. The 1st part of the duodenum is relatively mobile, being surrounded by peritoneum; however, the inferior portions of the duodenum are fixed in position. The ascending portion and the duodenojejunal flexure are suspended from the left crus of the diaphragm by the *ligament of Treitz*. The relations of each part of the duodenum are seen in Table 4.9.

Table 4.9 Relations of the duodenum

	Anterior	Posterior	Left	Right	Superior	Inferior
1st part	Quadrate lobe of liver, gall bladder	Common bile duct, portal vein, hepatic artery, gastroduodenal artery, lesser sac, head of pancreas			Quadrate lobe of liver, gall bladder	Head of pancreas
2nd part	Right lobe of liver (superiorly), transverse colon (medially), small intestine (inferiorly)	Hilum of right kidney, right ureter, renal vessels, inferior vena cava, psoas muscle	Head of pancreas, common bile duct	Right colic flexure		
3rd part	Superior mesenteric artery, vein and nerve	Right crus of diaphragm, inferior vena cava, right psoas muscle, right gonadal artery + vein, right ureter, vertebra			Head of pancreas	
4th part	Root of mesentery, coils of the jejunum	Left border aorta, left psoas muscle, left gonadal artery + vein, left renal artery + vein, inferior mesenteric vein, sympathetic branches		Aorta		Mesentery

The majority of the duodenum is only partially covered by peritoneum, thus resulting in it lying within the *retroperitoneal cavity*. The 2nd part houses within its medial wall the opening of the common bile duct and pancreatic duct at the *duodenal ampulla* (ampulla of Vater), situated approximately 7–10 cm below the pylorus (Lewis, 2000). The *accessory pancreatic duct* sometimes pierces the mucosa 2 cm above and in front of the ampulla.

The gastric contents (*chyme*) enter the duodenum in small quantities via the pyloric valve. Pancreatic juices and bile can, under the influence of various hormones, enter the duodenum via the ampulla and mix with the chyme. *Bile* is produced within the liver and stored in the gall bladder and, when secreted into the duodenum, it emulsifies fats. *Pancreatic enzymes*, which require an alkaline environment in which to function, continue the process of protein digestion. They also begin the breakdown of fats into fatty acids and break down starches to simpler sugars.

The duodenal mucosa comprises simple columnar epithelium, with openings of *duodenal glands* (Brunner's glands) from the submucosa, which secrete mucus and duodenal juices. The duodenal glands are most numerous in the 1st part of the duodenum.

The *circular folds* (valvulae conniventes) are large valvular flaps projecting into the lumen of the small intestine. They are absent within the 1st part of the duodenum, but gradually increase in size and number throughout the rest of the duodenum. The folds retard the passage of the partly digested food and create a greater surface area for absorption.

The duodenum derives its blood supply from the right gastric artery and superior and inferior pancreaticoduodenal arteries, with venous drainage returning to the superior mesenteric vein and splenic vein.

The *jejunum* commences at the duodenojejunal flexure and leads into the *ileum*, terminating at the *ileocecal valve*. The jejunum and ileum are suspended by the mesentery to the posterior abdominal wall, ensuring considerable mobility to enable peristalsis to occur. This mesenteric small intestine is the least accessible part of the GI tract for radiological and endoscopic investigation. The lumen diameter gradually decreases from the jejunum to the distal ileum, as does bowel wall thickness. The *terminal ileum* is the most distal part of the ileum, lying within the pelvis, then crossing into the right iliac fossa where it opens into the medial side of the large intestine at the ileocecal valve.

The jejunum and ileum have a number of similar features, making it difficult to state categorically where the transition from one to another occurs. However, some subtle mucosal changes are seen as one moves from the proximal to distal ends of the small intestine and many of these may be identified radiologically and endoscopically. Table 4.10 outlines these distinguishing features, including the presence or absence of circular folds and single and aggregated lymphatic nodules (known as *Peyer's patches*) and the presence and type of intestinal villi.

The *intestinal villi* are highly vascular processes projecting from the mucous membrane of the intestinal wall. They are largest and most numerous in the duodenum and jejunum, becoming gradually smaller and more sparse within the ileum. The villi create a huge surface area for absorption of the products of digestion, with blood capillaries and lacteals (fat transport) in close approximation with the intestinal fluids (chyle) within the

Table 4.10 Distinguishing features of the jejunum and ileum

Feature	Jejunum	Ileum
Abdominal position	Left upper/middle abdominal portions	Right middle and lower abdominal portions
Length	Proximal 2/5th (2.5 meters)	Distal 3/5th (3.8 meters)
Caliber	Wider, normally up to 3.5 cm	Gradually narrows, normally up to 2.5 cm
Bowel wall thickness	Wider – 2 mm	Thinner – 1 mm
Vascularization	More vascular, with deeper color as a result	Slightly less vascular, lighter in color
Presence of circular folds	Large and thick	Small and absent in distal ileum
Presence of intestinal villi	Very long villi and most numerous	Short villi and sparse (especially in terminal ileum)
Presence of lymphatic patches (solitary aggregated nodules)	No Peyer's patches in upper part, few in lower part. Some single nodules	Peyer's patches larger and more numerous. Abundant single nodules
Presence of intestinal glands	Numerous	Numerous

Adapted from Herlinger (2001). Note that variations exist in measurements related to the type of procedure (e.g. barium study or cross-sectional imaging).

intestine. *Intestinal glands*, commonly known as the crypts of Lieberkuhn, are found throughout all of the small intestine in large numbers. They secrete a range of enzymes which continue the process of breaking down complex structures into simpler molecules which are suitable for absorption via the intestinal villi.

The small intestine has a rich blood supply, with the jejunum and ileum deriving their blood supply from intestinal branches of the superior mesenteric artery. These branches anastomose to form a rich plexus which runs within the submucosa. Venous drainage is via the superior mesenteric vein, through to the portal vein and liver. Lymphatics of the jejunum and ileum drain from the mucous membrane (lacteals) and from the muscular coat to mesenteric nodes.

The large intestine

The large intestine is approximately 1.5 meters long from cecum to anus. It lies peripheral to the loops of the jejunum and ileum, being generally more fixed and of greater caliber than the small intestine. With the exception of the appendix and anal canal, the different parts of the large intestine feature the same histology. In most patients, the mucosal surface appears smooth and featureless (Laufer, 2000). The mucosal layer possesses *columnar epithelium* in conjunction with intestinal glands or crypts, which often group together around shallow grooves. This may, in some patients, result in a geometric surface pattern similar to that found in the stomach and known as the *areae colonicae* or *innominate grooves*. These grooves frequently fill with mucus from goblet cells (Reeders and Rosenbusch, 1994). The columnar epithelium absorbs water and water-soluble substances, such as electrolytes, very readily, with over 90% of water being absorbed in the colon. The large intestine displays sacculations known as *haustra*, resulting from contraction of the muscularis mucosa and the concertina effect created by the teniae coli. The *teniae coli* are three thickened bands of longitudinal muscle, arising from the base of the appendix and travelling the length of the colon (see Figure 4.4). They fan out at the rectosigmoid junction to cover the rectum in a complete band. The haustra are believed to cause turbulence of passing chyme and slow the passage of the digested matter.

From the right iliac fossa, the cecum extends as the ascending colon (Figure 4.13) before it turns abruptly to the left, beneath the liver, at the hepatic flexure. Crossing the abdomen, the transverse colon reaches the left hypochondriac region where, at the splenic flexure, it continues downwards as the descending colon, then forming small bends known as the sigmoid colon. The sigmoid colon passes along the posterior wall of the pelvis where, at the level of the sacral prominentary the rectosigmoid junction merges into the rectum. The rectum is a dilated part of the intestine, connecting with the anal canal and anus. The main relations of each part of the large intestine are identified in Table 4.11.

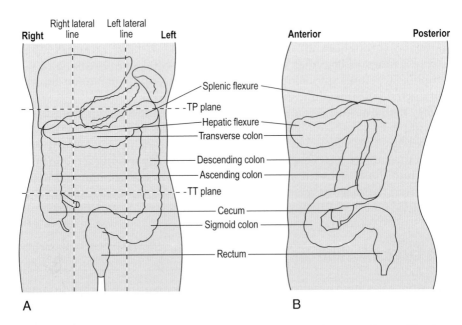

Figure 4.13 Gross anatomy of the large intestine. (A) Anterior view, demonstrating position in relation to abdominal organs and abdominal regions. (B) Lateral view, demonstrating the anterior position of the transverse and sigmoid colon, with the rectum, ascending and descending colon lying posteriorly. (Adapted from Reeders and Rosenbusch, 1994.)

Table 4.11 Relations of the large intestine

	Anterior	Posterior	Lateral	Medial	Superior	Inferior
Cecum	Anterior abdominal wall (occasionally greater omentum and small intestine coils)	Iliacus, psoas major muscle		Terminal ileum, appendix		Inguinal ligament
Ascending colon	Coils of ileum	Posterior abdominal wall, iliacus, quadratus lumborum, right kidney, right paracolic gutter, nerves and lymphatics	Right paracolic gutter	Terminal ileum		Cecum
Hepatic flexure				Gall bladder	Right lobe of liver	
Transverse colon	Greater omentum, peritoneum, descending colon (distally)	2nd part of duodenum, head of pancreas, coils of small intestine			Liver, gall bladder, greater curvature of stomach, spleen	Small intestine
Splenic flexure					Spleen, tail of pancreas	
Descending colon	Coils of small intestine, peritoneum	Left paracolic gutter, left kidney, transverse abdominus, quadratus lumborum	Left paracolic gutter	Left kidney		
Sigmoid colon	Small intestine, bladder (male), uterus (female)	Iliacus and psoas muscles, external iliac vessels, left piriformis, left sacral plexus				
Rectum	Proximally: bladder (male), uterus (female), sigmoid colon Distally: fundus of bladder, seminal vesicles and ducts, prostate (male), posterior wall of vagina (female)	Proximally: superior hemorrhoidal vessels, left piriformis, left sacral plexus Distally: sacrum, coccyx, levator ani			Sigmoid colon	Anal canal

CHAPTER 4 ▊▊▊▊ The large intestine

Situated within the right iliac fossa, the *cecum* is a dilated pouch extending superiorly to the upper border of the ileocecal valve, where it continues as the ascending colon (Figure 4.14). The cecum is approximately 6.25 cm in length and 7.5 cm in width, although its size can vary (Lewis, 2000). It may also vary considerably in both shape and position, due to a complete covering of peritoneum in many cases (Lewis, 2000). The *apex* of the cecum in 90% of individuals is pushed to the left toward the ileocecal junction and gives rise to the *vermiform appendix* (Lewis, 2000). The appendix is a long narrow blind-ended tube, varying between 2 and 20 cm in length and 0.5–1 cm in width (Reeders and Rosenbusch, 1994), occupying variable intraperitoneal and retroperitoneal positions (see Figure 4.14). Histologically, the mucosa and submucosa of the appendix demonstrate numerous lymph follicles, particularly in children. Over time the appendiceal lumen obliterates with fibrous tissue in many adults (Reeders and Rosenbusch, 1994; Balthazar, 2000).

The *terminal ileum* opens into the posteromedial border of the large intestine, where the cecum and colon meet. The opening is guarded by the *ileocecal valve*, comprising two horizontal lips of mucosa and circular muscle fibers projecting into the lumen of the large intestine (see Figure 4.14). This valve is thought to act as a sphincter, preventing contents of the ileum from passing too quickly into the cecum. It is also thought to assist in the prevention of reflux of cecal contents back into the small intestine (Zuidema and Yeo, 2002).

The *ascending colon* is continuous with the cecum, though is of smaller caliber. It is normally fixed to the posterior abdominal wall by a covering of peritoneum on its anterior and lateral surfaces. Lateral to the ascending colon lies the *right paracolic gutter*. The shallow *hepatic flexure* leads into the *transverse colon*. Normally completely invested in peritoneum, it is suspended from the lower border of the pancreas by the *transverse mesocolon*. The transverse

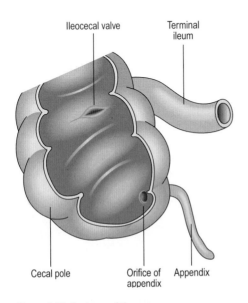

Figure 4.14 Features of the cecum.

colon forms an arch passing anteriorly and inferiorly, resulting in the mid transverse colon normally being a more anterior structure than the ascending and descending colon and the flexures (Figure 4.13).

The *splenic flexure* forms an acute angle, such that the distal transverse colon often lies in close contact with (and anterior to) the proximal descending colon. The splenic flexure normally lies higher than the hepatic flexure (which is limited by the bulk of the liver) and is attached to the diaphragm by the *phrenicocolic ligament*.

The *descending colon* is of a smaller caliber than the proximal colon and is normally covered on its anterior and lateral surfaces with peritoneum. This anchors it in place deep in the posterior abdomen. Lateral to the descending colon lies the *left paracolic gutter*.

The *sigmoid colon* commences within the left iliac fossa, curving inferiorly and medially to lie within the pelvis. The sigmoid colon is entirely surrounded by peritoneum, forming the *sigmoid mesocolon*. The middle loops of the sigmoid colon are highly mobile, whereas the junctions with the descending colon and with the rectum are fixed in position. Distally, the sigmoid curves anterior to the sacrum to join with the rectum at the rectosigmoid junction, approximately at the level of the 3rd sacral vertebra.

The rectum lies within the sacrococcygeal curve and presents two anteroposterior curves along its length. The upper curve has its convexity posteriorly, while the lower curve (into the anal canal) has its convexity anteriorly. Smaller lateral curves are also noted (Figure 4.15). Rectal length is approximately 12 cm, but the width expands from a similar caliber to the sigmoid colon at its commencement, to a dilated *rectal ampulla* distally. The main features of the rectum can be seen in Figure 4.15. The rectum lacks any haustration, but normally displays three permanent *semilunar transverse folds*. Two folds are situated to the left of the rectal wall and the middle fold is situated to the right. The middle fold is the largest and may be referred to as the *valve of Houston*. These folds are 12 mm in width (Lewis, 2000) and are thought to help to slow the transit (Reeders and Rosenbusch, 1994) and support the weight of fecal matter while in the rectum (Lewis, 2000). The peritoneum covers the anterior and lateral sides of the upper third of the rectum and only the anterior wall of the middle third. At this level, the peritoneum forms the *recto-uterine recess* (females) or *rectovesical recess* (males), also known as the *pouch of Douglas*. The lower third is not covered with peritoneum (sub-peritoneal), which reflects over the seminal vesicles in the male and the posterior vaginal wall in the female (Figure 4.16).

The *anal canal* measures approximately 2.5–4 cm in length (Lewis, 2000) and is directed postero-inferiorly from the *anorectal junction* to the anus. In the upper half of the lumen are found between 6 and 10 vertical vascular folds known as the *anal columns (of Morgagni)*, separated by grooves known as *anal sinuses*. These fuse distally in a transverse saw-toothed margin called the *dentate line* (see Figure 4.15). Above the dentate line, the mucosa is covered with columnar epithelium, but below the line this changes into *keratinized epithelium*, similar to skin tissue. Anal closure is the result of a double sphincter mechanism. The *internal sphincter* is formed from a thickening of circular intestinal muscle fibers, while surrounding this the *external sphincter* is formed from striated (skeletal) muscle, which is under voluntary control.

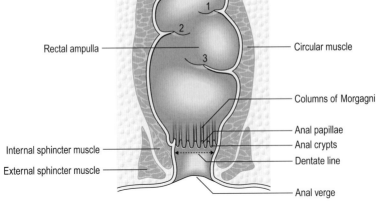

1 – Left upper valve of Houston
2 – Right middle valve of Houston
3 – Left lower valve of Houston

Rectal ampulla

Circular muscle

Columns of Morgagni

Anal papillae
Anal crypts
Dentate line

Internal sphincter muscle

External sphincter muscle

Anal verge

A Anterior view

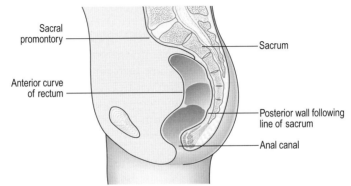

Sacral promontory

Sacrum

Anterior curve of rectum

Posterior wall following line of sacrum

Anal canal

B Lateral view

Figure 4.15 Features of the rectum and anal canal. (A) Anterior view demonstrating the rectum and anal canal. Note that the number and position of rectal valves may vary. (B) Lateral view demonstrating relationship with the sacrum and coccyx posteriorly. In males, the bladder lies anteriorly and, in females, the vaginal canal and uterus lie anteriorly.

The *levator ani* is the major muscle of the perineum, supporting the rectum in a muscular sling. In particular, one part of the levator ani, the *puborectal sling*, is important in maintaining rectal continence.

The large intestine is supplied by three arterial systems: the *superior mesenteric artery* (SMA) and the *inferior mesenteric artery* (IMA), both major branches of the abdominal aorta, and the *internal iliac arteries*. The branches of these major arteries supply different parts of the intestine, although the exact nature of the supply is variable. However, the branches of the SMA will supply the right colon from the cecum to the mid transverse colon in the majority of cases (Reeders and Rosenbusch, 1994) and the IMA branches supply the left colon from the distal transverse colon through to the mid rectum. Branches of the external iliac and internal iliac arteries supply the mid rectum

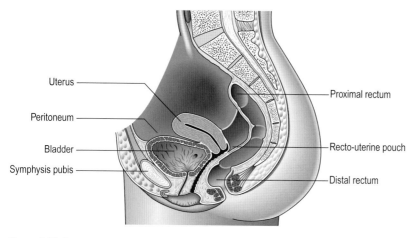

Figure 4.16 Peritoneal covering of the rectum (female). The peritoneum reflects over the superior surface of the bladder, the anterior and superior surface of the uterus in females and covers the upper third of the rectum on its anterior and lateral sides. A peritoneal pouch forms known as the recto-uterine pouch in the female and, in the male, the recto-vesical pouch (pouch of Douglas).

through to the anal canal. However, the IMA and internal iliac branches form an extensive intramural and extramural network around the anorectum.

The circulation noted above can form many anastomotic connections, which may serve as a collateral circulation in the event of a blockage (arterial occlusion). The *intermesenteric arcade (of Riolan)* is formed by a branch of the left colic artery (IMA) anastomosing with the middle colic artery (SMA) near to the splenic flexure. This vascular arc would only be noticed arteriographically if an occlusion is present on one side (Reeders and Rosenbusch, 1994). The *marginal colonic artery (of Drummond)* is a paracolic anastomosis along the mesenteric (centrally facing) border of the colon. It connects the five arteries of the SMA and may extend from the cecum to the sigmoid colon. The marginal artery gives rise to the *vasa recta*, which pierce the colon perpendicularly to supply the wall with blood. The *Griffith's point* is the site of a critical anastomosis between the marginal artery and other vessels at the site of the splenic flexure (Figure 4.17). This anastomosis is said to be absent in 43% of individuals (Reeders and Rosenbusch, 1994), resulting in a site that may have low resistance to ischemic events.

Veins usually follow a similar course to arteries of the same name. The cecum and proximal (right) half of the colon drains into the *superior mesenteric vein* (SMV). The left half of the colon drains into the *inferior mesenteric vein* (IMV) (commencing as the superior rectal veins), which enters the splenic vein, then joins with the SMV to form the portal vein. The portal vein drains blood into the liver sinuses.

The distal rectum and anal canal are both encircled by internal and external (subcutaneous tissue) *venous networks*. These usually drain to the inferior and middle rectal veins, draining via the hypogastric veins to the inferior vena cava. The blood flow from the distal rectum and anus does not, therefore, enter the liver. This should be a consideration when investigating tumor spread from this region.

The large intestine

CHAPTER 4

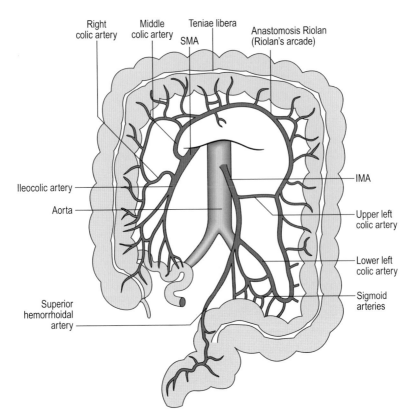

Figure 4.17 Major arteries supplying the large intestine. The colon is shown with the transverse portion raised so that the arteries may be seen more clearly. Note the Riolan anastomosis between branches of the superior mesenteric artery (SMA) and the inferior mesenteric artery (IMA). This is a potential area of reduced blood supply.

References

Balthazar, E.J., 2000. Diseases of the appendix. In: Gore, R.M., Levine, M.S. (Eds.), Textbook of gastrointestinal radiology, vol. 1, second ed. WB Saunders, Philadelphia.

Herlinger, H., 2001. Anatomy of the small intestine. In: Maglinte, D., Herlinger, H., Bernbaum, B. (Eds.), Clinical imaging of the small intestine, second ed. Springer-Verlag, New York.

Jones, B., 2000. Functional abnormalities of the pharynx. In: Gore, R.M., Levine, M.S. (Eds.), Textbook of gastrointestinal radiology, vol. 1, second ed. WB Saunders, Philadelphia.

Laufer, I., 2000. Barium studies of the colon. In: Gore, R.M., Levine, M.S. (Eds.), Textbook of gastrointestinal radiology, vol. 1, second ed. WB Saunders, Philadelphia.

Levine, M.S., Laufer, I., 1999. Stomach. In: Levine, M.S., Rubesin, S.E., Laufer, I. (Eds.), Double contrast gastrointestinal radiology, third ed. WB Saunders, Philadelphia.

Lewis, W.H. (Ed.), 2000. Gray's anatomy of the human body (Gray, H., Ed.). Lea & Febiger, Philadelphia, 1918; revised and re-edited by Warren H Lewis for Bartleby.com, 2000. <www.bartleby.com/107/> Accessed 10.12.07.

Moore, K.L., Persaud, T.V.N., 2007. Before we are born: essentials of embryology and birth defects, seventh ed. WB Saunders, Philadelphia.

Ott, D.J., 2000. Motility disorders of the oesophagus. In: Gore, R.M., Levine, M.S. (Eds.), Textbook of gastrointestinal radiology, vol. 1, second ed. WB Saunders, Philadelphia.

Reeders, W.A.J., Rosenbusch, G., 1994. Clinical radiology and endoscopy of the colon, Thieme Medical Publishers, New York.

Rubesin, S.E., 1999. Pharynx. In: Levine, M.S., Rubesin, S.E., Laufer, I. (Eds.), Double contrast gastrointestinal radiology, third ed. WB Saunders, Philadelphia.

Rubesin, S.E., 2000. Pharynx: normal anatomy and examination techniques. In: Gore, R.M., Levine, M.S. (Eds.), Textbook of gastrointestinal radiology, vol. 1, second ed. WB Saunders, Philadelphia.

Stradling, S. (Editor-in-Chief), 2005. Gray's Anatomy. The anatomical basis of clinical practice, 39th ed. Churchill Livingstone, Edinburgh.

The large intestine

CHAPTER 4

Symptoms of upper gastrointestinal disease

Christopher Wong

Contents

Introduction

Symptoms of the upper gastrointestinal tract are very common. The prevalence of upper gastrointestinal symptoms in Western populations is estimated to be 20–40%. The majority of people will have no clinically significant or benign causes. A small proportion (2%) will be caused by upper gastrointestinal cancers. It is estimated that approximately 3–4% of a general practitioner's workload will consist of patients with upper gastrointestinal complaints but, on average, a single general practitioner will only see one patient with esophageal cancer in 5 years, one gastric cancer in 3 years and one pancreatic cancer in 4 years. It is therefore important to maximize the yield of investigations by identifying those patients who are more likely to have pathology. In 2002, guidelines were issued by The British Society of Gastroenterology with this aim. In this chapter, we will discuss commonly encountered symptomatology and investigations.

Upper gastrointestinal investigations

The mainstay of upper gastrointestinal investigations comprises: *endoscopic*, including gastroscopy, endoscopic retrograde cholangiopancreatography (ERCP); *radiologic*, including contrast swallow studies, ultrasonography, computed tomography, magnetic resonance imaging, positron emission tomography; and a *combination* of both endoscopic and radiologic in the form of endoscopic ultrasonography.

Dyspepsia

Dyspepsia is a general term used to refer to upper abdominal (including retrosternal) pain. This is a general non-specific term and is sometimes interchanged with indigestion. Dyspepsia is very common and is estimated to affect some 25% of the population. Using dyspepsia in its broadest sense, its cause may be functional, ulcer, gastroesophageal reflux disease, gallstones and cancer. *Functional* refers to failure to function normally related to either the muscles of the organ or the nerves that control the organ. The symptoms of dyspepsia are varied and, in 2006, an *updated symptom criteria* was proposed further to define this. The Rome III committee was published and the definition of dyspepsia was again refined (Tack et al., 2006). They have defined functional dyspepsia as symptoms originating in the gastroduodenal region in the absence of any organic, systemic or metabolic disease that is likely to explain these symptoms. This is further refined into two new symptom classes: *epigastric pain syndrome*, referring to epigastric pain/burning and *postprandial distress syndrome*, which is meal-induced symptoms.

The Rome III criteria are, in reality, of little use to clinicians in everyday practice. The management of such a patient has been rationalized by the National Institute of Clinical Excellence (NICE). Briefly, the *initial management* should focus upon excluding causes of dyspepsia from medications, excluding alarm symptoms and *Helicobacter pylori* (*H. pylori*) infection. A short course of *proton pump inhibitor* may be prescribed and the effect monitored. Persistence of symptoms or appearance of alarm symptoms will require urgent endoscopic investigation (British Society of Gastroenterology, 2004).

NICE recommends that:

routine endoscopic investigation of patients of any age, presenting with dyspepsia and without alarm signs, is not necessary. However, in patients aged 55 years and older with unexplained and persistent recent-onset dyspepsia alone, an urgent referral for endoscopy should be made.

Gastro-esophageal reflux disease (GERD)

This condition is caused by stomach contents refluxing into the esophagus. The most common refluxate is gastric acid and sometimes bile may also be the refluxing agent. Reflux occurs infrequently in many people and usually does not cause major harm or concerns as the refluxate returns to the stomach rapidly. *Esophagitis* and symptoms of retrosternal pain occur when there is persistent acid or bile reflux in the esophagus (Weatherall et al., 1996).

The symptoms of GERD include 'heartburn' or retrosternal pain. This is commonly described as a *burning pain* behind the sternum. The pain may radiate to the jaw and arms mimicking a cardiac event. The pain is worse when lying down and acid and bile may reach the mouth when bending down or carrying out exercises. In some cases, the sensation of food sticking may be described. This is often confused with dysphagia.

GERD may be accompanied by esophagitis, Barrett's esophagus and, in some occasions, the esophageal mucosa may be normal (non-erosive reflux disease).

Treatment of GERD includes lifestyle modifications (stop smoking, reduce alcohol intake, refrain from spicy foods, caffeine and weight reduction in those who are overweight). If conservative therapy fails then *anti-reflux surgery* is indicated (see common gastrointestinal surgery).

The recommendation for treatment for GERD is similar to dyspepsia. A 4–8 weeks course of full dose proton pump inhibitors (PPIs), followed by maintainence therapy if indicated. If RED flag signs are present then the patient should undergo a gastroscopy.

Alarm (RED flag) symptoms

The British Society of Gastroenterology (2005) published guidelines for referral for suspected upper gastrointestinal cancers. In that, they listed:

- Chronic gastrointestinal bleeding
- Iron deficiency anemia
- Progressive unintentional weight loss
- Progressive difficulty swallowing, dysphagia
- Persistent vomiting
- Epigastric mass
- Suspicious barium meal.

Ninety-nine percent of upper gastrointestinal cancers occur over the age 45 years with 90% of gastric cancers occurring above 55 years. The chance of a dyspeptic patient age under 55 years of having a cancer is one in a million.

Chronic gastrointestinal bleeding may result from the upper and lower gastrointestinal tract (see Chapter 10). Chronic gastrointestinal tract bleeding may result in normocytic or microcytic *anemia*. Patients who have upper gastrointestinal bleeding may complain of black offensive smelling stool (*melena*). *Iron deficient anemia* is commonly found. It has been estimated that gastrointestinal cancers are found in approximately 10% of patients presenting with iron deficient anemia and approximately 4% are from the upper gastrointestinal tract (James et al., 2005; Killip et al., 2007). Unintentional weight loss is defined as decrease of 5% or more in body weight within a 6–12 month period. It may be caused by organic, psychosocial and unknown etiologies. Of these, approximately 25% are caused by malignancies (Lankisch et al., 2001; Metalidis et al., 2008). Weight loss in gastrointestinal malignancy may be caused by reduced nutrient intake caused by physical obstruction of food intake (dysphagia and vomiting), anorexia, early satiety and other tumor hormonal factors.

Dysphagia is difficulty in swallowing and may be further refined to impedance in swallowing solids and liquid (see Chapter 7). Though it may be difficult, dysphagia should be distinguished from globus sensation, which is a feeling of having a lump in the throat, which is unrelated to swallowing and occurs without impaired transport.

Dysphagia may occur in esophageal tumors (malignant and benign), pharyngeal pouch, peptic stricture, pharyngeal web, connective tissue diseases (scleroderma), achalasia, diffuse esophageal spasm, extrinsic compression from enlarged left atrium, aortic aneurysm, aberrant subclavian artery, retrosternal thyroid, cervical bony exostosis and thoracic tumor.

Vomiting may occur in complete or severe dysphagia and in gastric outlet obstructions. *Gastric outlet obstruction* may be caused by functional (e.g.

diabetic gastroparesis) or mechanical (gastric cancers and peptic ulceration) conditions. Early satiety and fullness are common in gastric and head of pancreas cancers. About 50–60% of gastric outlet obstruction is caused by malignancy with 50% of these from pancreatic cancers (Kaw et al., 2003). Patients may complain of a mass in the epigastrium from a distended stomach or from the cancer itself.

Peptic ulcers

Peptic ulcers include gastric and duodenal ulcers. This is characterized by a disruption of the mucosa of the gastrointestinal tract and is a result of the imbalance between mucosal defense (water-insoluble mucous barrier, local production of bicarbonate) and offensive factors (increased gastric acid secretion, *H. pylori* infection, non-steroidal anti-inflammatory drugs (NSAIDs) and mucosal ischemia).

Helicobacter pylori is a gram-negative urease-producing spirochete that was linked to gastric ulcers and gastritis in 1983. The urease neutralizes the acidic environment and causes mucosal inflammation, ulceration as well as increasing gastric acid production. As a result the duodenum is exposed to higher levels of acid.

Symptoms of peptic ulcer disease are variable but may include nausea, anorexia, weight loss, hunger pain, melena, upper abdominal pain that may be improved (duodenal) or worsened (gastric) with food ingestion and antacids. The pain of peptic ulcer disease correlates poorly with the severity of active ulceration or gastritis. *Complications* of peptic ulcers include bleeding/ hemorrhage, perforation and obstruction. Investigations of choice for peptic ulcer disease include *gastroscopy* that will allow for diagnosis as well as obtaining tissue for histological differentiation of benign ulcers from malignant gastric cancers. Other investigations that are acceptable, especially in elderly and frail individuals, include double contrast study, although it may not detect small ulcers. As well as guidance given for treatment of dyspepsia (see dyspepsia), NICE recommends:

'offering *H. pylori* eradication therapy to *H. pylori*-positive patients who have peptic ulcer disease. For patients using NSAIDs with diagnosed peptic ulcer, stop the use of NSAIDs where possible. Offer full-dose PPI or H_2 receptor antagonist (H_2RA) therapy for 2 months to these patients and, if *H. pylori* is present, subsequently offer eradication therapy'

Diarrhea

Diarrhea is defined as frequent passage of watery stools. Diarrhea may be acute or chronic (lasting more than 2 weeks) (Table 5.1). Nausea, vomiting, anorexia, weight loss, passing blood per rectum, dehydration, abdominal pain and fever may also accompany diarrhea.

Investigations are usually required in severe and chronic diarrhea. The type of investigation is guided by the medical history and suspected cause of the diarrhea.

Infectious diarrhea: the most common cause of diarrhea is infective which may be bacterial (salmonella, staphylococci, *Escherichia coli*, *Clostridium difficile*), viral (Norovirus, rotavirus, Norwalk virus, cytomegalovirus) and

Table 5.1 Common causes of diarrhea

Causes	Investigations
Infectious diarrhea Bacterial Viral Parasites Antibiotics	Stool culture within 3 days of onset
Food intolerance Celiac disease Lactose intolerance	Anti-tissue transglutaminase, anti-endomysium, anti-gliadin antibodies, lactose intolerance test Gastroscopy
Inflammatory bowel disease Crohn's disease Ulcerative colitis	Contrast studies – small bowel, large bowel, CT scan Gastroscopy, colonoscopy, enteroscopy Capsule endoscopy
Pancreatic insufficiency Chronic pancreatitis Cystic fibrosis Pancreatic surgery Pancreatic cancer	Fecal fat, fecal elastase, pancreolauryl test. Ultrasound scan, CT scan, ERCP, MRCP
Metabolic Thyrotoxicosis Diabetes	Thyroid function test, random, fasting glucose, glucose tolerance test
Irritable bowel disease	Investigations are not always necessary for diagnosis of irritable bowel disease. However, gastroscopy, colonoscopy and ultrasound abdominal scans are often employed
Dumping syndrome	Contrast study, blood glucose

less common in developed countries, parasites (*Giardia lamblia, Entamoeba histolytica* and *Cryptosporidium*). The majority of diarrhea is self-containing and resolves after a few days.

The value of *stool culture* is limited. A large study of 59,500 specimens only yielded a positive result in 6.4% of cases. A timely stool culture is crucial to confirming or excluding infective causes (<3 days infective, <4 days parasitic from onset) (Valenstein et al., 1996).

Food intolerance: blood and breath tests may be used for food intolerance in addition to gastroscopy and radiological studies.

Celiac disease is a common condition, affecting about 1 in 100–300 adults in the UK, that is caused by intolerance to gluten. Anti-endomysial, anti-gliadin and anti-tissue transglutaminase antibodies as well as IgG and IgA levels are used for detecting celiac disease before gastroscopy to obtain *tissue biopsy* for confirmation which remains as the gold standard for confirming celiac disease. *Radiological studies* (abdominal CT, small bowel enema) for celiac disease are used for detecting complications of the disease (intussusception (usually intermittent), ulcerative jejunitis, osteomalacia, cavitating lymph node syndrome and an increased risk of malignancies such as lymphoma, adenocarcinoma and squamous cell carcinoma) rather than as a diagnostic tool (Buckley et al., 2007).

Lactose intolerance is the inability of the body to digest lactose, which is a sugar commonly found in milk and diary products. A degree of lactose intolerance is found in approximately 75% of the population. Hydrogen breath test, lactose/milk intolerance test, small bowel biopsy and stool acidity tests are used to detect lactose intolerance. Radiology does not have much role in managing this condition.

Inflammatory bowel disease: Crohn's and ulcerative colitis are discussed in Chapter 16. Investigations include gastroscopy, colonoscopy, enteroscopy, small bowel enema and abdominal CT scan.

Pancreatic insufficiency: pancreatic insufficiency is caused by insufficient exocrine pancreatic function, in other words, the inability of the pancreas to produce adequate digestive enzymes. The causes of pancreatic insufficiency include cystic fibrosis, chronic pancreatitis, pancreatic surgery and pancreatic cancer.

Investigations of pancreatic insufficiency include radiological imaging of the pancreas (ultrasound, CT, MRI scans, endoscopic retrograde cholangiopancreatography). The function of the pancreas may be assessed by fecal fat, fecal elastase, pancreolauryl test.

Metabolic: thyrotoxicosis (hyperthyroidism) may cause diarrhea. The patient will often display symptoms of anxiety, raised heart rate, history of weight loss. Investigations include a simple blood test for thyroid function.

Diabetes can cause autonomic neuropathy of the gastrointestinal tract resulting in diabetic diarrhea. Other symptoms of diabetic diarrhea include steatorrhea (pale fatty stool) and malabsorption. Diagnosis of diabetic diarrhea is by exclusion and investigations include gastroscopy, colonoscopy, small bowel enema and hydrogen breath test.

Dumping syndrome: this syndrome is a collection of gastrointestinal and systemic symptoms. It can be caused by any surgery (vagotomy, pyloroplasty, gastrojejunostomy and laparoscopic Nissan fundoplication) to the stomach that affects the delivery of food into the small intestines.

Investigations for dumping syndrome include gastroscopy and barium swallow and follow through.

Jaundice

Jaundice is characterized by the skin and sclera turning yellow. This is caused by increased level of bilirubin in the blood. Patients may complain of darkened urine in obstructive jaundice. The causes of jaundice can be pre-hepatic (hemolysis), hepatic (hepatitis, liver cirrhosis) and post-hepatic (obstructive jaundice from gallstones, cholangiocarcinoma, pancreatic cancer).

Investigation for jaundice is dependent on the cause and will include blood tests to check for liver function, anemia from hemolysis, malaria, sickle cell anemia, spherocytosis, hepatitis screen, autoimmune antibodies, ceruloplasmin, transferritin. Radiological investigations include transabdominal and endoscopic ultrasound, CT, MRI scan, fibro scan and liver biopsy.

Nausea and vomiting

Nausea and vomiting are symptoms that can accompany many conditions (Table 5.2). It is important to take a detailed medical history that will help direct the investigations. In general, vomitus that does not contain bile is

Table 5.2 Common causes of nausea and vomiting

Causes	Investigations
Acute gastritis • Infections: bacterial, viral and parasitic infections of the gastrointestinal tract • Peptic ulcer disease	Stool cultures if appropriate Empiric treatment with proton pump inhibitors if no alarm symptoms present Gastroscopy
Central causes • Pregnancy • Motion sickness • Migraine, pain • Brain tumors, concussions, infections e.g. meningitis, encephalitis • Noxious stimuli, emotional stress • Eating disorder	CT scan of brain if appropriate

Diseases
• Diabetes: gastroparesis, hyperglycemia and hypoglycemia
• Gallstones disease
• Pancreatitis
• Gastro-esophageal reflux disease
• Esophageal diverticula:
  • pharyngeal pouch (Zenker's diverticulum)
  • mid-esophageal (traction) diverticulum
  • epiphrenic (pulsion) diverticulum
• Renal disease
• Some forms of cancer
• Myocardial infarction, angina
• Septicemia
	Gastroscopy
	Contrast studies
	Abdominal ultrasound
	Serum lipase or amylase
	Serum urea and electrolytes
	Electrocardiogram
	Tumor markers
	Blood cultures

Gastrointestinal causes
• Gastrointestinal malignancies that may or may not be causing obstruction
  • esophagogastric cancer
  • small bowel cancer
  • large bowel cancer
• Gastrointestinal obstruction
  • hernia
  • adhesions
  • volvulus
• Megaduodenum (Wilkie's syndrome, superior mesenteric artery compression)
	Gastroscopy/colonoscopy
	Contrast studies
	CT scan
	Endoscopic ultrasound
	Duplex scan

Medications • Any drug treatments can cause nausea and vomiting	

likely to be *but not always* of less serious nature (central causes). Vomitus that contains bile is taken to be more significant and may suggest an obstruction somewhere beyond the second part of the duodenum (bowel obstruction, pancreatic cancer).

Investigations may include blood tests, stool culture, abdominal x-rays, ultrasound, contrast gastrointestinal studies, CT/MRI scans and endoscopy.

References

British Society of Gastroenterology, 2004. Dyspepsia: managing dyspepsia in adults in primary care. http://www.nice.org.uk/Guidance/CG17

British Society of Gastroenterology, 2005. Referral for suspected cancer. A clinical practice guideline. June.

Buckley, Brien, J., Ward, E., et al., 2007. The imaging of coeliac disease and its complications. Eur. J. Radiol. 65 (3), 483–490.

James, M.W., Chen, C.M., Goddard, W.P., et al., 2005. Risk factors for gastrointestinal malignancy in patients with iron-deficiency anaemia. Eur. J. Gastroenterol. Hepatol. 17 (11), 1197–1203.

Kaw, M., Singh, S., Gagneja, H., et al., 2003. Role of self-expandable metal stents in the palliation of malignant duodenal obstruction. Surg. Endosc. 17 (4), 646–650.

Killip, S., Bennett, J., Mara, D., et al., 2007. Iron deficiency anemia. Am. Fam. Physician 1, 671–682.

Lankisch, P., Gerzmann, M., Gerzmann, J.F., et al., 2001. Unintentional weight loss: diagnosis and prognosis. The first prospective follow-up study from a secondary referral centre. J. Intern. Med. 249 (1), 41–46.

Metalidis, D., Knockaert, H., Bobbaers, S., et al., 2008. Involuntary weight loss. Does a negative baseline evaluation provide adequate reassurance? Eur. J. Intern. Med. 19 (5), 345–349.

Tack, J., Talley, N.J., Camilleri, M., et al., 2006. Functional gastroduodenal disorders. Gastroenterology 130, 1466–1479.

Valenstein, P., Pfaller, M., Yungbluth, M., 1996. The use and abuse of routine stool microbiology: a College of American Pathologists Q-probes study of 601 institutions. Arch. Path. Lab. Med. 120, 206–211.

Weatherall, D.J., Ledingham, J.G.G., Warrell, D.A. (Eds.), 1996. Diseases of the oesophagus. Oxford Textbook of Medicine, Oxford.

Investigation of salivary gland disease

Vivian E. Rushton

Contents

Introduction

Salivary gland tissue has been shown to display a wide diversity of pathology encompassing inflammatory, obstructive, infectious, neoplastic and systemic disease. Inflammatory and obstructive disease within salivary gland tissue accounts for the majority of patients seeking treatment for their symptoms whereas the incidence of salivary gland tumors is extremely low.

This pathology division is reflected in the radiological techniques employed when imaging patients with salivary gland disease. For those patients presenting with *inflammatory disease*, plain film radiography, either alone or in combination with contrast studies and/or ultrasonography, often comprises 'first-line' imaging. These techniques provide the high resolution images with which to detail the presence of salivary calculi and allow the clinician to document accurately any significant changes within the ductal architecture of the gland. For those patients in whom a *mass lesion* is suspected then computed tomography (CT) and magnetic resonance imaging (MRI) are the imaging modalities of choice.

The presenting symptoms of the patient are often very useful in determining the type of abnormality present. *Typical symptoms* of inflammatory disease are swelling of the salivary gland allied with mealtimes and the sight and smell of food followed by a gradual reduction of the swelling having eaten. The latter is highly suggestive of either obstruction by a calculus or an inflammatory induced ductal stricture which indirectly compromises salivary flow. In some cases, the patient may additionally complain of pain, a bad taste and pus may or may not be evident at the duct orifice. These symptoms and signs are indicative of current inflammatory disease. Finally, a number of patients may present with a dry mouth, the causes of which are wide ranging.

The aim of this chapter is to provide details of the most common radiographic techniques with which to image salivary gland pathology, whilst also providing the reader with an overview of each of the other competing investigations and the rationale for their use.

Sialography

The technique employs the use of contrast media to delineate the fine anatomy of the *salivary gland ductal system*. Patient symptoms will range from pain, which may be acute or chronic in its presentation, to a generalized recurrent or discrete swelling which is often present at mealtimes. Some patients are referred with a dry mouth which relates to a myriad of clinical conditions including autoimmune diseases, drug therapy and previous radiotherapy.

Indications

- Possible obstruction within the salivary duct system. Sialography should *only* be carried out after a plain radiographic examination to exclude or confirm the presence of either calcified or non-calcified sialoliths (i.e. calculi) or the presence of foreign bodies
- An evaluation of the extent of irreversible ductal damage
- To enable the differentiation between a variety of disease entities, i.e. chronic sialadenitis, Sjögren's disease, sialosis etc
- An evaluation of fistulae, ductal trauma and ductal strictures

Contraindications

- A calculus close to the duct orifice
- Sialography should not be performed if the salivary gland is infected
- Sialography is best avoided in cases of known iodine hypersensitivity

The presence of an *acute inflammatory episode* would be confirmed clinically by the presence of pain and swelling of the salivary gland. Similarly, a *chronically inflected salivary gland* with pus emanating from the salivary duct orifice would also contraindicate sialography until the infection had been controlled by appropriate antibiotic therapy.

Complementary and competing investigations

Ultrasonography

Newer ultrasound equipment exhibits high spatial resolution. This factor, combined with the relative superficial anatomical position of the salivary gland tissue relative to the ultrasound probe, allows the operator to obtain high definition images. Similarly, the superficial topography of the salivary gland tissue also permits fine-needle aspiration biopsy and core biopsy techniques to be performed with relative ease for both the patient and the operator (Bialek et al., 2006).

The technique has become commonplace in clinical practice when assessing generalized swellings or the presence of a mass within the salivary glands.

Advantages of the technique

- Non-invasive
- Does not involve the use of ionizing radiation
- Can differentiate between intra- and extra-glandular lesions
- Use of color Doppler enables identification of vessels
- More sensitive than CT in identifying small lesions
- Can identify calculi >2 mm
- Enables fine-needle aspiration biopsy of lesions to be undertaken (Bradley, 1993)

Disadvantages of the technique

- Difficulties encountered in identifying lesions confined primarily to the deep lobe of the parotid gland
- Margins of deep lobe lesions may be difficult to identify in their entirety. Needs additional investigation using CT and/or MRI to evaluate fully the extent of the lesion

Computed tomography (CT)

The technique can be used to diagnose swellings both associated with the salivary glands themselves and those structures extrinsic to the glands.

Advantages of the technique

- Allows three-dimensional imaging
- Allows the identification of calcified sialoliths
- Enables the clinician to determine the extent of the disease
- Allows differentiation between cellulitis and abscess formation
- Allows differentiation between pathology in particular compartments in the suprahyoid neck, i.e. between the parotid and masticator space
- Determines the nature of the margins and the content of the lesion
- Determines whether the lesion is intra- or extra-capsular
- Has high sensitivity for the detection of salivary gland tumors
- CT sialography allows better delineation of the major duct architecture
- IV contrast highlights pathology

Disadvantages of the technique

- Fine anatomy of intra-glandular ducts is not well imaged
- Provides no information on salivary gland function
- Stenson's duct seen only if markedly dilated
- Facial nerve normally not seen
- High dose to the patient
- Difficulties in differentiating benign salivary gland lesions from low-grade malignancies as both exhibit smooth margins
- Streak artefacts from adjacent metal dental restorations. However, these can be reduced by using an increased angled coronal scan geometry

Magnetic resonance (MR)

Advantages of the technique

- No use of ionizing radiation
- Major vessels identified by flow voids
- Facial nerve and ductal architecture can be identified on certain sequences
- T1 and T2 images allow differentiation between normal and abnormal salivary gland tissue
- Allows differentiation between malignant and benign lesions as margins more sharply resolved by MR
- Use of a variety of imaging sequences allows the clinician to optimize the diagnosis without the routine use of contrast agents
- MR sialography allows an assessment of the ductal architecture without the use of contrast
- Dynamic contrast enhancement studies have been shown to differentiate between different pathological lesions whilst also allowing glandular functional activity to be derived (Roberts et al., 2008)

Disadvantages of the technique

- Often difficult to distinguish a solid mass from a cyst unless there are contrast-enhanced images
- Calcifications better seen on CT
- Focal bone erosion cannot be assessed

Radioisotope imaging (sialoscintigraphy)

Advantages of the technique

- Allows an evaluation of both parenchymal function and the rate of excretion of saliva from each of the salivary glands simultaneously
- Allows the clinician to assess salivary gland tumors that can highly concentrate ^{99m}Tc pertechnetate, i.e. Warthin's tumor and oncocytoma
- Allows analysis of the results using time-activity curves and quantitative parameters such as percentage secretion to be derived
- Employed in those rare cases where aplasia of one or more major salivary glands is suspected

Disadvantages of the technique

- High dose to the patient
- Provides no information on ductal architecture or gland anatomy
- No information available on the pathology within the salivary gland tissue
- When used, it is arguable whether there is any impact on patient management

Conclusion

There are many imaging modalities available to the clinician and the decision to choose a particular examination will be decided following a thorough clinical history and examination of the patient.

Preoperative assessment of the patient and room preparation

The type of room used will be dependent on where the examination is performed. Sialography may well be performed in the *dental chair* in some institutions while, in others, a *dedicated angiography room* (Figure 6.1) may be used to conduct the examination.

Patient identification is confirmed by the operator and a brief clinical and medical history is taken to confirm the clinical signs and symptoms and also to allow justification of the radiographic examination.

If the patient's *clinical history* is suggestive of current infection within the salivary gland under consideration, then a thorough *clinical examination* should be conducted to verify the diagnosis. Both current infection and a prior history of an allergy to iodine would contraindicate sialography. If the presence of a calcified sialolith (a salivary stone) is suspected from the patient's history, then either ultrasonography or plain films should be undertaken to ascertain this prior to sialography.

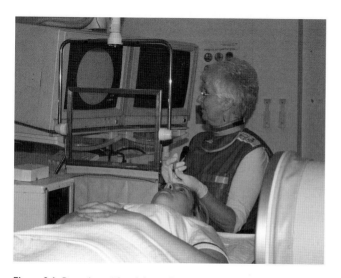

Figure 6.1 Room layout for sialography.

Plain intraoral films for identifying calcified sialoliths

For the submandibular salivary gland:

1 To assess the distal aspects of the submandibular duct: an *anterior lower true occlusal* (with soft tissue exposure) (Rushton, 2005)

2 To assess the proximal aspects of the submandibular duct: (a) the *lower posterior oblique occlusal* (with soft tissue exposure) (Rushton, 2005) or (b) a *true lateral view*: the patient's index finger is used to depress the floor of the mouth so that the displaced calculus is visualized below the inferior cortex of the mandible.

An alternative method to the lower posterior oblique occlusal has been devised by Semple and Gibb (1982) for those patients who have a shortneck or limited neck movement. For those patients who cannot tolerate intraoral placement of dental films, a *sectional panoramic radiograph* related to the side under consideration or an extra-orally positioned occlusal film can be used (Harkin, 1983).

For the parotid salivary gland:

1 An *intraoral (size 2: 31×41 mm)* dental film placed in the buccal sulcus overlying the parotid orifice and supported by the finger of the patient.

2 An *anteroposterior radiograph* of the face with the patient inflating the cheek in order to detect calcified sialoliths within Stenson's duct or the gland itself.

While additional lateral views may be employed, the presence of a calculus can be obscured by the density of bone and tooth tissue inherent within the image.

The basic equipment to perform sialography

The basic equipment to perform sialography is as follows:

- Sialographic cannulas: Rabinov-type catheters are produced by several companies with graded sizes ranging from 0.012 to 0.032 inch (0.03–0.08 cm). The largest size (0.032) cannula (Figure 6.2) has a rounded tapered closed end with bilateral side ports and is usually used for parotid sialography. The remaining cannulas are straight with an open end and are used for both submandibular sialography and for the narrow parotid orifice.
- In those cases in which a fistula has formed, either from trauma or the result of long-term infection, a higher caliber catheter (4 French) can be employed to perform a successful sialogram without reflux of contrast.

The remaining equipment (Figures 6.3 and 6.4) comprises:

- A 5 ml syringe
- Gauze pads
- A flexible high intensity light
- ×4 magnifying loupe
- Water-soluble contrast agent (typically Omnipaque 300 or equivalent)
- Micropore© tape
- Citric acid solution (or lemon juice) to act as a sialogogue.

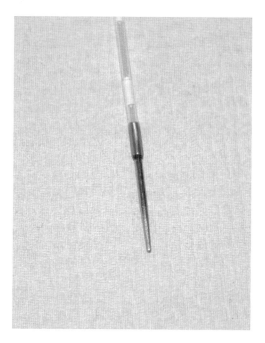

Figure 6.2 0.032 Rabinov catheter.

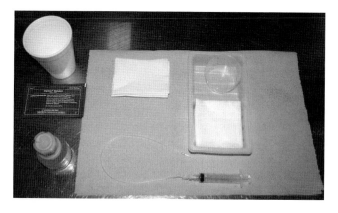

Figure 6.3 Basic equipment for sialography.

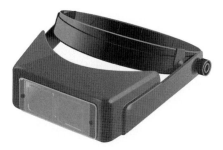

Figure 6.4 Magnifying loupe.

The standard procedure

- The patient is positioned supine on the table
- The orifice of the salivary gland under consideration is identified using a high intensity light. A combination of drying of the mucosa adjacent to the duct orifice, massaging the gland, the use of a sialogogue and/or the use of magnification often helps to identify the duct orifice
- If needed, the orifice can be enlarged using lacrimal dilators, although the Rabinov catheter itself is a more effective tool for this purpose
- The appropriate sized Rabinov catheter is attached to a 5 ml syringe, previously filled with water-soluble contrast media ensuring that there are no air bubbles within the solution. The latter can give a false-positive diagnosis for mucous plugs if inadvertently injected into the gland
- Following placement of the catheter, the orifice of the duct usually forms a tight seal around its circumference
- The patient is asked gently to support the plastic tube between their anterior teeth and also by pursing their lips around it.
- The tubing is stabilized using a Micropore© non-allergenic adhesive strip taped onto the patient's forehead. The latter also ensures that the operator's hands are not within the primary beam
- The x-ray tube is appropriately positioned relative to the salivary gland under investigation

For the parotid gland: 0.5–1.0 ml of contrast medium is injected slowly. Subsequent films would include an *oblique lateral radiograph* to ensure adequate filling with contrast and a *PA view* centered on the gland under investigation. Finally, an *evacuation film* should be performed after removing the catheter. If any contrast is still retained within the gland then a sialogogue should be administered.

For the submandibular gland: 0.2–0.5 ml of contrast medium is injected slowly. Films would include an *oblique lateral,* a *true lateral* and a *mandibular true occlusal.* Finally, an *evacuation film* should be performed after removing the catheter, followed by a sialogogue if contrast is still retained within the gland.

Variation of the standard technique

Hydrostatic sialography

The technique was developed to overcome the under or overfilling of salivary glands when injecting contrast using hand pressure and without the obvious benefit of monitoring the flow of contrast into the gland radiographically. The technique relies upon the positive pressure from a reservoir of contrast positioned 70–90 cm above the orifice of the salivary gland to overcome the natural pressure of the gland itself. Refinements of the technique have included the use of a constant infusion pump supplying contrast at a rate of between 0.01 and 1.0 ml/min with a transducer to record pressure.

Subtraction radiography

Post processing subtraction of bony structures provides the clinician with high definition sialographic images with which to evaluate the salivary gland ductal system. The equipment used is commonplace in digital imaging suites consisting of a C-arm, a 17 cm (smallest film/largest magnification) field image intensifier and a 512×512 matrix. The exposure sequence used is identical for both the parotid and the submandibular glands. It consists of one frame per second on a subtracted run followed by single acquired images. The contrast is hand injected allowing the operator to control visibly the volume of contrast entering the gland preventing overfilling.

For the parotid gland, the standard views are: a *true lateral* and an *anteroposterior* view followed by an emptying view post catheter removal. If emptying is delayed, then a sialogogue is given and a further lateral view is obtained. For the submandibular gland, the *true lateral* is the view of choice both for contrast filling of the gland, the emptying film and after the sialogogue has been administered (Ilgit et al., 1992; Buckenham et al., 1994).

Advantages of the technique:

- Subtraction of bony and air containing overlapping structures enables evaluation of the gland with superior quality images
- Contrast resolution is higher
- Post processing facilities enhance the image
- Demonstration of gland architecture requires less contrast and a reduced likelihood of extravasation
- Reduced exposure and shorter exposure times

Basket retrieval of mobile calculi

Basket retrieval techniques can be effectively employed for smaller mobile calculi or for calculus fragments in the middle and proximal thirds of the submandibular duct and in any region of the parotid main duct using fluoroscopic control.

Balloon dilatation of strictures

This technique employs the use of a 1.8F angioplasty balloon catheter to bypass the stricture using digital subtraction radiography (Figure 6.5).

Aftercare

There are no special requirements for after-care post sialography.

Image interpretation

Before commencing sialography, the pattern of the normal anatomy of the *parotid gland* (Figure 6.6) and the *submandibular gland* (Figure 6.7) should be thoroughly understood.

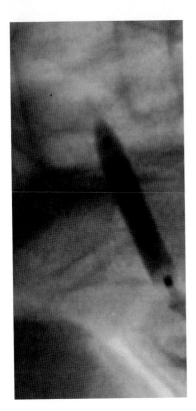

Figure 6.5 Balloon dilatation of a stricture.

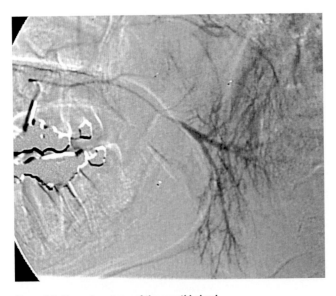

Figure 6.6 Normal anatomy of the parotid gland.

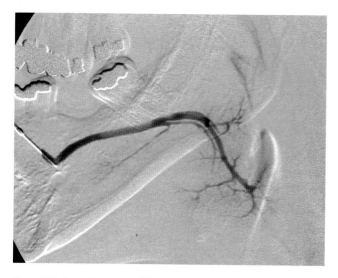

Figure 6.7 Normal anatomy of the submandibular gland.

The clinical presentation of patients requiring sialography can be summarized as follows:

- Obstructive sialadenitis
- Autoimmune sialadenitis
- Trauma and post-trauma evaluation
- Presence of tumor.

Obstructive sialadenitis

Obstructive sialadenitis is the result of recurrent infection within the salivary gland which usually results in a combination of both ductal strictures and dilation. The sialographic examination displays the extent of ductal damage within the gland due to these repeated inflammatory episodes. For those patients with grossly distorted ducts (Figure 6.8), gland removal is often the treatment of choice. Conversely, those patients with a localized focal stricture might well benefit from balloon dilatation. In addition, the status of the salivary gland ductal system in which a stone has recently been passed can also be assessed.

The sialographic findings of obstructive sialadenitis are:

- Minimal to grossly deformed ductal system
- Areas of focal strictures and dilation of the main duct, the so-called 'string of sausages' appearance (Figure 6.9)
- Involvement of the secondary duct system.

Autoimmune sialadenitis

The majority of patients presenting with this condition will be suffering from Sjögren's syndrome (Roberts et al., 2008). The patients present with salivary gland enlargement and classification of the sialographic findings relate primarily to the size of the dilated secondary ducts. Punctate

Image interpretation

CHAPTER 6

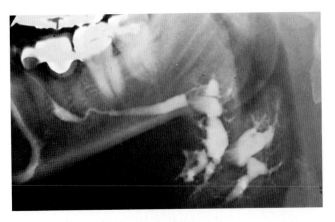

Figure 6.8 Obstructive chronic sialandenitis.

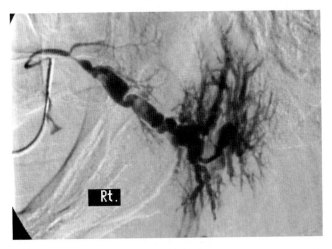

Figure 6.9 Focal strictures and dilation of the main duct appearing as the so-called *'string of sausages'*.

sialectasis is used to describe cases with dilation less than 1 mm in diameter, globular sialectasis for those between 1 and 2 mm and for those cases with non-uniform duct diameter greater than 2 mm, the term cavitatory sialectasis is used (Figure 6.10).

Trauma and post-trauma evaluation

Sialography can be extremely useful in identifying the site and extent of duct and/or glandular trauma. Common findings are the presence of a fistula (Figure 6.11) or complete occlusion of the duct.

Presence of tumor

Sialography can often highlight the presence of a salivary gland mass, although MR and CT would be the imaging modality of choice if a mass lesion was suspected. The sialographic signs of a mass lesion are:

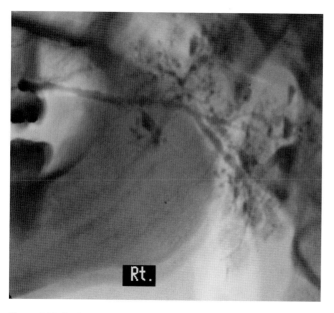

Figure 6.10 Cavitatory sialectasis evident in this patient with Sjögren's syndrome.

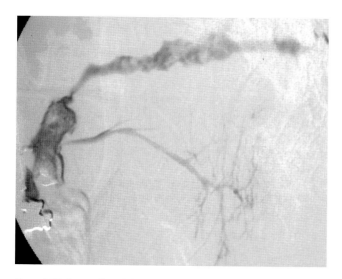

Figure 6.11 Laceration of the main duct of the parotid gland. The use of a larger cannula allowed an assessment of the detriment to the main duct and the gland itself. Contrast can be seen extravasating into soft tissue

- *'Ball in hand'* appearance due to ductal splaying around an expanding mass lesion (Figure 6.12)
- Ductal cut off caused by a mass compressing and occluding the duct
- Ductal irregularities due to the presence of an infiltrating lesion and contrast pooling within the gland.

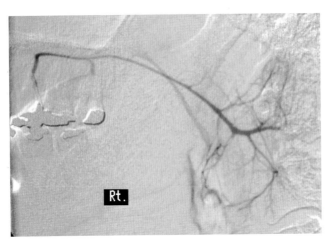

Figure 6.12 The ducts associated with the inferior aspects of the parotid gland display a '*ball in hand*' appearance due to ductal splaying around an expanding mass.

References

Bialek, E.J., Jakubowski, W., Zajkowski, P., et al., 2006. US of the major salivary glands: anatomy and spatial relationships, pathological conditions and pitfalls. Radiographics 26, 745–763.

Bradley, M.J., 1993. Ultrasonography in the investigation of salivary gland disease. Dentomaxillofac. Radiol. 22, 115–119.

Buckenham, T.M., George, C.D., McVicar, D., Moody, A.R., Coles, G.S., 1994. Digital sialography: imaging and intervention. Br. J. Radiol. 67, 524–529.

Harkin, P., 1983. Demonstration of submandibular calculi. Radiography 49, 84.

Ilgit, E.T., Cizmeli, O., Isit, S., et al., 1992. Digital subtraction sialography: technique, advantages and results in 107 cases. Eur. J. Radiol. 15, 244–247.

Roberts, C., Parker, G.J.M., et al., 2008. Glandular function in Sjögren's syndrome: assessment with dynamic contrast enhanced MR imaging and tracer kinetic modelling-initial experience. Radiology 246, 845–853.

Rushton, V.E., 2005. Section 10: dental radiography. In: Whitely, A.S. (Eds.), Clark's positioning in radiography, twelth ed. Hodder Arnold Publication.

Semple, J., Gibb, D., 1982. The posterior-anterior lower occlusal view – a routine projection for the submandibular gland. Radiography 48, 122–124.

Further reading

Blair, G.S., 1973. Hydrostatic sialography: an analysis of the technique. Oral Surg. 36, 116–130.

Buckenham, T.M., Page, J.E., Jeddy, T., 1992. Technical report: interventional sialography – balloon dilatation of a Stenson's duct stricture using digital subtraction sialography. Clin. Radiol. 45, 34.

Luyk, N.H., Doyle, T., Fergusson, M.M., 1991. Recent trends in imaging the salivary glands. Dentomaxillofac. Radiol. 20, 3–10.

McGurk, M., Escudier, M.P., Brown, J.E., 2005. Modern management of salivary calculi. Br. J. Oral. Surg. 92, 107–112.

Murray, M.E., Buckenham, T.M., Joseph, A.E.A., 1996. The role of ultrasound in screening patients referred for sialography: a possible protocol. Clin. Otolaryngol. 21, 21–23.

Videofluoroscopy

Roger D. Newman

Contents ||||||||||||||||||||||||||||||||||||||||||||||||||||||||||||||||||||||||

Introduction

Videofluoroscopy of swallow (VFS) is defined by the Royal College of Speech and Language Therapists (RCSLT) (2006) as a modification of the standard barium swallow examination used in the assessment and management of oropharyngeal swallowing disorders. This instrumental swallowing evaluation is often described as the 'gold standard' for the assessment of dysphagia (Daniels et al., 1997; Robbins et al., 1999). Dysphagia is defined as a disorder of swallowing food (solid and/or liquid) from the mouth to the stomach (Logemann, 1998). Swallowing disorders can occur at every age and have various etiologies. Swallowing dysfunction can be caused by head and neck pathologies (e.g. inflammations and tumors of the oral cavity, oropharynx and larynx), neurological diseases and injuries (e.g. strokes, multiple sclerosis, motor neurone disease (MND), Parkinson's disease, tumors and head injury) or other illnesses (e.g. psychological/functional, or as a side effect of medication). As stated by the RCSLT in their Policy Statement (2006), VFS can be used for assessment, treatment and management of swallowing where the suspected condition or disease process impacts upon swallow function and may result in a risk of death, pneumonia, dehydration, malnutrition and psychosocial issues related to discomfort and difficulty in eating and drinking.

Videofluoroscopy has the additional benefit of providing an objective baseline to which future examinations can be compared as a measure of improvement and enabling management strategies to be formulated. Martino et al. (2000) reinforced the importance of videofluoroscopy by stating that the validity of most other assessments and screening tools is often measured against videofluoroscopy and none comes close to VFS in terms of sensitivity and specificity. This chapter will provide the basis to enable a greater understanding of the videofluoroscopic procedure and the predisposing factors necessary to create a successful fluoroscopy team.

Purpose and benefits

Being both a time consuming and costly examination, it is vital that the actual VFS procedure runs as smoothly as possible. Communicating the plans of the procedure to all staff involved and prior explanation to the patient/carer will ensure minimal time delay. This should in turn prevent the patient and staff feeling rushed and anxious, both of which may result in a suboptimal examination. Patients must be fully informed about the VFS procedure prior to the examination. Consideration should be given to providing information in accessible spoken, written and/or visual formats, including the nature, purpose and likely effects of the examination (RSCLT 2006). Logemann (1998) categorically states that:

> nutrition is never jeopardised during the course of management of the patient's swallowing problem. Thus, from the day of the initial evaluation, the swallowing therapist must interact closely with the patients, patient's physicians, nursing staff, and dietician to outline the best program to maintain nutrition and increasingly improve the patient's swallowing function.

Also known as a modified barium swallow, a VFS is simply that – an adjustment to the traditional barium swallow. One modification is that low density contrast is utilized which highlights flow through the oropharynx much better than high density used in traditional barium swallows (where increased coating of the mucosal wall is desired). Further modifications are associated with the volumes and consistencies of the contrast agents provided, together with the speed at which they are given, attempting to replicate the consistencies of everyday food and fluid. This then demonstrates any dysfunction of oropharyngeal deglutition, enabling treatment and therapy aims to be devised. The primary aims of the VFS as described by the RCSLT (2006) are seen in Box 7.1.

As is stated by RCSLT (2006): 'Patients must undergo an appropriate clinical assessment of swallowing by a Speech and Language Therapist (SLT) prior to VFS being undertaken'. The widely accepted standard procedure is for all patients to undergo a *clinical swallowing evaluation* (CSE) prior to completion of VFS. This will serve to fulfil many purposes, inclusive of enabling the aims of VFS to be established; assessment of candidate suitability for VFS; full explanation of the procedure (inclusive of aims of outcome); and obtaining of consent.

In addition, RCSLT (2006) state that an SLT-led CSE prior to VFS will also 'assist in determining the nature and severity of the swallowing disorder and other factors contributing to the conduct of the VFS, such as cognition, presence of the carer, feeding arrangements, positioning and anxiety etc.' It will also aid communication within the VFS to alert the radiographer and other multidisciplinary team (MDT) members what the plans for the procedure are and how they are to be completed. Communication with the patient during the VFS is imperative so that they are aware of every step of the procedure. The pre-VFS CSE should have prepared them with instructions, but anxiety and confusion can compound any complications and, if not treated

BOX 7.1 Purpose of videofluoroscopy as defined by RCSLT (2006)

- Evaluation of oropharyngeal structures
- Evaluation of swallowing physiology, including lip and tongue function, velopharyngeal closure, base of tongue retraction, hyolaryngeal elevation, pharyngeal contraction, upper esophageal sphincter function and airway protection mechanisms
- Assessing swallow function in relation to a variety of consistencies of food and liquid
- Detecting the presence of, and response to aspiration, whether silent (no coughing reflex) or overt
- Assessing the impact of therapeutic interventions on swallowing physiology, safety and efficiency
- Timing of swallow events where appropriate equipment is available
- Ongoing assessment and monitoring of dysphagia over time
- Biofeedback. This involves the correlation of videofluoroscopy and intraluminal manometry, in addition to taught techniques of safer swallowing for volitional augmentation in order to modify impaired swallowing
- Patient, carer and health professional education
- Contributing to the diagnostic profile (e.g. in suspected Parkinson's disease) in the context of the multidisciplinary assessment

accordingly, can waste the examination completely by altering the results from those aimed to be achieved, e.g. *positional modification*. The patient should be instructed clearly and concisely, by demonstration if necessary. If they do not complete the desired instruction they may aspirate contrast to such an extent that the examination has to be abandoned. Potential dangers of aspiration such as *choking* and *pneumonia* are also factors which correct communication should avoid.

The radiographer or radiologist should work closely with the speech therapist, where present, to ascertain the requirements for fluoroscopic screening and spot films – VFS is 'one moment in time' and it is essential to capture each stage of the swallowing process. Good communication by the different team members will reduce both time and radiation exposure. Post-examination communication with the patient is vital to enable understanding of the importance of positional/texture modification. If necessary the video/DVD recording can be used for visual feedback to demonstrate this more clearly.

It must be noted that patients rarely present with an *isolated dysphagia*. As previously mentioned, dysphagia usually arises as a result of a wide range of pathologies, which often have other associated motor, sensory and emotional/psychological problems. These must all be taken into account when planning and arranging a VFS. A patient who is bedbound and unable to support themselves in an upright position may not be a suitable candidate for a VFS due to poor strength and/or restricted movement, but accommodating alterations to the procedure are possible. This includes specialist seating equipment, physical supports or simple altered position of the x-ray table. It must be noted that within a VFS the ideal initial position for examination is a *lateral* view but, for a bedbound patient who is only able to manage *supine* positioning, *anterior-posterior* (AP) viewing may be the only possibility. Within a fluoroscopy suite equipped with a C-arm, manipulation of the x-ray tube to the side of the patient will enable lateral viewing but, in the traditional screening room, this is not possible and viewing is limited to AP positioning. While this has benefits for assessment of *laterality of deficit*, full assessment of *laryngeal penetration* and *aspiration* is not as clear as in the lateral position.

While the VFS is, as previously mentioned, the 'gold standard' within swallowing assessment, these *motor, sensory* and *emotional/psychological* constraints often limit the procedure and, in some cases, inhibit the examination. Langmore et al. (1991) summarize those groups of patients where VFS cannot be utilized:

- Patients who are in intensive care and cannot be easily moved to the fluoroscopy suite
- Patients who are unable to be positioned adequately on the fluoroscopy platform or table because of a severe weakness, limited mobility, or contractures
- Patients who are very ill and unable to tolerate the risk of aspirating even very small quantities of food
- Patients who need an immediate examination.

It is within these cases that other forms of objective assessment of swallowing would prove beneficial.

Contrast agents

The types of positive contrast media used within VFS fall into two main categories – *barium based* and *iodine based*. The positive contrast agents increase the atomic number of the area to be demonstrated in relation to the surrounding tissue and x-rays are considerably attenuated by these types of contrast agents.

The benefits of barium sulfate are reported to be that it is *non-toxic, relatively cheap* and *inert*. Farrow and Stevenson (1997) state that barium is an excellent contrast agent for the GI tract provided that is where it stays. Barium aspirated into the lungs is usually harmless and can be expectorated either spontaneously or aided by a physiotherapist. However, barium is thought to cause inflammation and infection if aspirated into the lungs where expectoration is poor or suction is not available and should therefore be avoided if there is a significant risk of this occurring. However, there is extremely minimal evidence to support this, resulting in many institutions continuing to utilize barium as the contrast of choice. In cases where aspiration is suspected and the reason for it is the primary purpose of the investigation, administering small volumes initially would therefore be reasonable to limit the amount of contrast entering the airway.

Within a national health service VFS clinic, barium sulfate is the contrast agent of choice due to its reasonable cost and non-toxicity. It also mixes well with other food agents to alter its viscosity to enable holistic assessment of the oropharyngeal swallow with different consistencies. Meijing et al. (1992) argue that contrast viscosity is directly related to its density and can affect bolus transition at the oropharyngeal stage. However, during most VFS investigations, capability to manage altered consistencies is one of the key factors under investigation and, although lower density barium is preferred in case of aspiration, no modifications to the preparation (other than changes to viscosity) are seen to be necessary if high density barium is used.

The iodine-based contrast agents act as a 'carrier' molecule for the iodine, as when used alone as a contrast agent, iodine is toxic. Gastromiro® has therefore been introduced as a water-soluble iodine-based contrast agent designed specifically for GI use and, being water based, has the benefit of being recommended where there is suspected leakage into the lungs, pleural cavity or peritoneal cavity due to the fact that re-absorption is rapid and generally innocuous. Patients who have undergone specialist surgery, e.g. *laryngectomy* and have a *tracheo-esophageal speaking valve* would also benefit from Gastromiro® as fistula formation is prevalent and aspiration could result. Due to the fact that barium also contains particles dissolved in water, these may block such a valve making it ineffective.

In terms of bolus consistency, barium has the benefit of mixing easily with foodstuffs to provide modification where the difficulty with the oropharyngeal swallow is with one particular texture. For example, if a patient demonstrates immediate aspiration with water-consistency barium and a chin tuck is ineffective, the barium can be made slightly thicker (e.g. with yoghurt/custard) to a 'runny honey' consistency to reduce the speed of bolus transition both within the mouth and the pharynx, providing the patient with increased control in order to trigger a swallow at an appropriate time, thus reducing the potential for aspiration. As an alternative, two to three consistencies of barium can also be made up with water at the beginning of the examination, leaving some of each set aside to trial in the event of difficulties with a true water consistency.

Other consistencies can be created by mixing barium with real foods such as rice pudding to provide a puree consistency. Mixing barium with foodstuffs the patient is both familiar with and likes the taste of can prove very beneficial, especially in the case of patients with cognitive disorders and dementia. Various barium biscuit recipes are also available to enable the patient to be trialled with one texture alone – or alternatively a normal biscuit/slice of bread may have a barium puree spread onto it. The latter may not be as palatable and is less likely to demonstrate bolus preparation. Several companies now produce their own ready-mixed contrast agents for VFS, increasing standardization and reducing the time required for the preparation of fluids and foods in advance.

Management strategies

Observation of swallowing function during a VFS may identify an inappropriate swallow, for example where the patient aspirates small quantities of fluid, or has residual pooling of contrast agent following the swallow. In these cases, it may be appropriate for the speech therapist or radiographer to trial under fluoroscopy control a number of modifications to the patient's swallow. Table 7.1 outlines the potential modifications and therapy techniques available to the therapist during the VFS and the reasons for their use. If successful, these modifications can then be explained to patients and carers so that they can be employed when eating and drinking, thus enabling oral intake to commence safely. It is imperative that the patient/carer follows the modification advice given at all times to prevent later difficulties and potential aspiration occurring.

Table 7.1 The role of positional modifications to the VFS procedure

Positional modification	Disorder and presentation
Chin tuck Chin is tucked down so the patient is 'looking into their lap'	Reduced base of tongue movement – residue in the valleculae Delayed pharyngeal trigger – overspill of contrast into the pharynx prior to onset of the swallow Laryngeal penetration – contrast evident in the laryngeal inlet and/or resting on the vocal cords Aspiration – residue evident in the airway below the true vocal cords
Chin lift Chin is lifted up so the patient is looking up to a 45° angle	Poor lip seal – anterior spillage of contrast Reduced oral strength – poor formation and manipulation of the bolus, often resulting in anterior spillage or premature overspill Nasal regurgitation – contrast noted to enter the nasopharynx
Head turn Patient turns the head to the affected side if the damage is unilateral (e.g. unilateral pharyngeal weakness post-CVA)	Unilateral pharyngeal wall disorder – residue in the affected pyriform fossa Reduced opening of the cricopharyngeal sphincter – residue in the pyriform fossae (often bilateral)
Lean/head tilt Patient leans or tilts their head to the stronger side	Oral *and* pharyngeal weakness – residue noted in the mouth and pharynx on the same side
Lie down Patient reclines beyond 45° angle	Reduced laryngeal elevation – residue at the entrance to the larynx Bilateral pharyngeal weakness – equal amounts of residue evident in bilateral pyriform fossae after swallowing

CVA, cerebrovascular accident

Multidisciplinary working in VFS

As has previously been outlined, there is a need for close communication between all members of the VFS team. This can include radiologists, radiographers, speech and language therapists and radiology nurses and assistant practitioners. Standardization of the procedure is important (allowing modifications where necessary), particularly as patients may be examined more than once to check response to treatment following a baseline assessment. Even where the examination was conducted by different staff members, consistency of approach is essential. This consistency is achieved by working within an agreed protocol, which is a detailed framework in which a patient is managed (College of Radiographers, 1999). Owen et al. (2004)

state that, in the context of imaging and therapy, the primary purpose of the protocol is to provide clear indication of how certain categories of patients will be managed and by whom.

When considering VFS, Power et al. (2006) exemplify through research the lack of clarity and blurring of roles that can exist between SLTs, radiographers and radiologists. Distinct role definition via the formation of a protocol ensures that the professional roles are outlined and minimizes risk to the patient(s) and staff involved. An evidence-based protocol also displays good clinical practice and offers a degree of medico-legal protection for staff undertaking delegated roles (Nightingale, 2008). Within protocol development, all professionals involved in the VFS procedure should contribute to enable precise documentation of the details of the procedure and the respective individuals' responsibilities.

Skills for Health (2005) published excellent working competences and core skills to enable professionals involved in VFS to offer the highest quality to patients, by demonstrating what is required of the VFS team. The implications of this workforce competence are that the team involved in examination must be just that – *a team*. It is impossible to complete a VFS without a strong team involvement and knowledge of other's working. The SLT and the radiographer must collaborate with each other to enable the patient to receive the highest quality of examination, from organization of the clinic to completion of the procedure with final reporting. An area which demonstrates the need for understanding of each other's role within the Skills for Health competencies, is listed within the section entitled 'Clinical Knowledge and Technical Knowledge'. Historically, the SLT involved within VFS would have the clinical knowledge and the radiographer would have the technical knowledge. While it is accepted that within VFS the SLT will always have an increased clinical knowledge of the 'anatomy and physiology of related structures of the areas being examined', and the radiographer will have the increased 'working knowledge of production, interactions and properties of x-rays', there are definite areas of cross-over which are now accepted as being important to the safe and efficient running of such an MDT clinic. These include the SLT having 'a working knowledge of harmful effects of radiation to the human body' and the radiographer having a 'working knowledge of signs and symptoms of aspiration' (direct quotations from Skills for Health, 2005). When forming a local protocol and developing guidelines for clinical expertise required of the clinicians within the VFS, the working competence document offered by Skills for Health (2005) is a highly useful tool for reference. Despite its name of a working competence, it should also be considered as national standards, as without these credentials the VFS clinic would not benefit the patient.

Image interpretation

The normal anatomy and physiology of the swallowing mechanism is best demonstrated through simple illustration of the structures involved (Figure 7.1, see color insert).

Logemann (1998) distinguishes four phases of deglutition: the oral preparatory phase; the oral phase; the pharyngeal phase and the esophageal phase.

The oral preparatory phase consists of food entering the mouth, masticated if necessary, being mixed with saliva and formed into a bolus. It is at this stage that the individual distinguishes taste, temperature and volume of food. This stage is completely voluntary and movements involved include those of the lips, tongue, mandible and cheeks. The airway remains open and the soft palate lowered at this stage and the individual is able to breathe through the nose (Figure 7.2).

The oral phase (also voluntary) consists of lip closure and increased pressure of the buccal musculature (cheeks), plus anterior–posterior 'wave-like' motion of the tongue against the hard palate forcing the prepared bolus to be propelled to the base of the tongue. Nasal breathing remains possible throughout this stage as the soft palate has not yet been raised and the airway is still open (Figure 7.3).

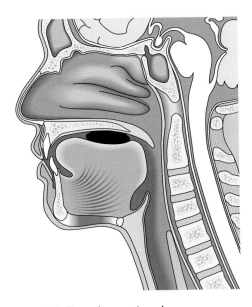

Figure 7.2 The oral preparatory phase.

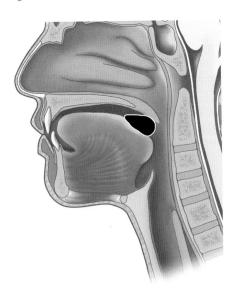

Figure 7.3 The oral phase.

The pharyngeal phase is the first stage of the 'voluntary to involuntary' swallowing mechanism. The soft palate is raised and articulates with the posterior pharyngeal wall to ensure none of the bolus enters the nasopharynx. The base of the tongue raises and forms a seal with the posterior pharyngeal wall, while the pharyngeal constrictor muscles contract at the same time to meet the base of tongue. This propels the bolus through positive pressure inferiorly as the swallow is triggered. As an involuntary reflexive response, the hyoid bone is drawn in a superior–anterior triangular motion which, in turn, elevates the larynx to form a seal with the lowered epiglottis. The vocal cords adduct to form an additional airway seal to prevent the passage of food. The cricopharyngeus, situated posterior in relation to the larynx at the proximal esophagus within the pharynx, also relaxes facilitating bolus entry into the esophagus (Figure 7.4).

It is during this stage that many disorders are commonly observed. These may be due to neurological dysfunction (motor and/or sensory) causing barium pooling or residue with subsequent overspill into the laryngeal inlet with secondary aspiration (Figure 7.5); structural abnormality, e.g. pharyngeal pouch (Figure 7.6); or the presence of a foreign body such as a tracheostomy tube which can 'anchor' the larynx in place and reduce elevation necessary to create complete airway protection (Figure 7.7).

The esophageal phase of the swallow is completely involuntary. Once the cricopharyngeus has constricted behind the bolus, the esophageal peristaltic wave commences which transports the bolus to the lower esophageal sphincter into the stomach (Figure 7.8).

The esophageal phase of swallowing can give rise to many disorders, but those presenting most like a true 'aspiration-based' disorder may arise from

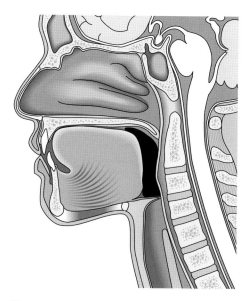

Figure 7.4 The pharyngeal phase.

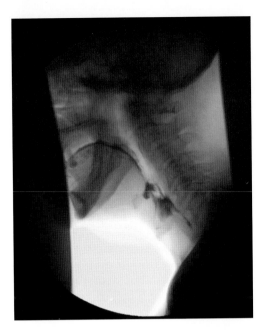

Figure 7.5 Lateral view showing significant pooling in valleculae and pyriform fossae with secondary overspill into the laryngeal inlet and penetration to the level of the true vocal cords. No aspiration evident.

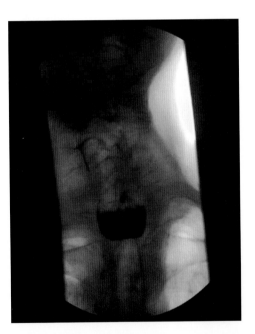

Figure 7.6 Slight coating of contrast in the bilateral valleculae and a small amount of residue in the right pyriform fossae, with a large pharyngo-esophageal pouch at the level of C7–T2.

a tracheo-esophageal fistula, where fluids, foodstuffs (and during videofluoroscopy an x-ray contrast) enter the airway through a small 'puncture' between the esophageal and tracheal walls (Figure 7.9). They may in childhood be caused by congenital abnormality but, in adulthood, they are usually

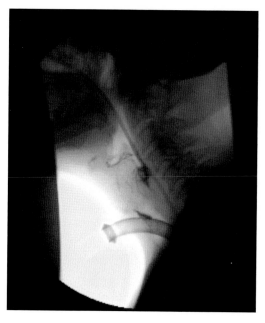

Figure 7.7 Incomplete pharyngeal clearance with slight residue in the pyriform fossae; overspill of contrast along the anterior wall of the laryngeal vestibule, plus aspiration of the bolus into the airway with contrast clearly visible sitting on superior surface of the tracheostomy tube.

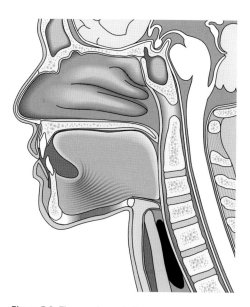

Figure 7.8 The esophageal phase.

as a result of radiation burns, spread of tumor or the sequela of surgical procedures, e.g. laryngectomy.

Logemann (1998) later states that the radiographic study may be done to examine the physiology of the swallowing mechanism or to evaluate the effectiveness of a particular treatment strategy or the effects of recovery, and

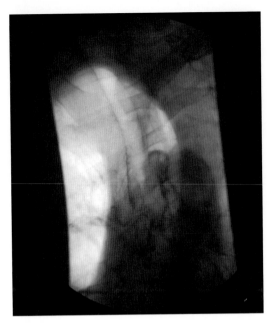

Figure 7.9 Large tracheo-esophageal fistula evident in the mid-esophagus with secondary pouring of contrast into the right main bronchus, coating the distal bronchial tree.

to identify the presence and cause of dysphagia. This therefore highlights the need for the aims of the VFS to be completed prior to the procedure so that the clinician has a plan in mind as to what to prepare, what to feed the patient and what to look for. If there are no specific aims, e.g. effect of lateral head turn, the patient may be placed at some degree of danger of unnecessary aspiration due to incorrect head positioning.

Familiarizing yourself with the normal anatomical features and common anatomical variants of the structures involved in swallowing, plus other structures of the head and neck as shown in Figure 7.1 (e.g. level and positioning of cervical and thoracic spine in relation to cricopharyngeus etc.) will undoubtedly help to increase understanding as to the interpretation of images obtained during a videofluoroscopy. In addition to this, observation of a normal oropharyngeal swallow during videofluoroscopy/barium swallow, as in the timing, strength and location of trigger of swallow, bolus management at each of the stages listed and anatomical shift during swallowing will help to appreciate and evaluate the images obtained when difficulties with the swallow arise. Accurate interpretation is essential by the team to allow the therapist, medical team and, inevitably, the patient manage the dysphagia in a safe and productive manner. This then gives rise to repeat examinations to evaluate the change/improvement and increase skills even further.

Acknowledgments

Many thanks to Matt Briggs, Medical Artist from Royal Preston Hospital, for help in the preparation of the figures.

References

College of Radiographers, 1999. Clinical governance. College of Radiographers, London.

Daniels, S.K., McAdam, C.P., Brailey, K., Foundas, A.L., 1997. Clinical assessment of swallowing and prediction of dysphagia severity. Am. J. Speech. Lang. Patho. 6 (4), 17–23.

Farrow, R., Stevenson, G.W., 1997. Gastrointestinal tract. In: Armstrong, P., Wastie, M.L. (Eds.), Diagnostic and interventional radiology in surgical practice. Chapman & Hall, London.

Langmore, S.E., Schatz, K., Olson, N., 1991. Endoscopic and videofluoroscopic evaluations of swallowing and aspiration. Ann. Otol. Rhinol. Laryngo. 100, 678–681.

Logemann, J.A., 1998. Evaluation and treatment of swallowing disorders, second ed. Austin, PRO-ED.

Martino, R., Pron, G., Diamant, N., 2000. Screening for oropharyngeal dysphagia in stroke: insufficient evidence for guidelines. Dysphagia 15 (1), 19–30.

Meijing, L., Brasseur, J.G., Kern, M.K., Dodds, W.J., 1992. Viscosity measurements of barium sulfate mixtures for use in motility studies of the pharynx and esophagus. Dysphagia 7, 17–30.

Nightingale, J., 2008. Developing protocols for advanced and consultant practice. Radiography doi:10.1016/j.radi.2008.04.001.

Owen, A., Hogg, P., Nightingale, J., 2004. A critical analysis of a locally agreed protocol for clinical practice. Radiography 10, 139–144.

Power, M., Laasch, H.U., Kasthuri, R.S., Nicholson, D.A., Hamdy, S., 2006. Videofluoroscopic assessment of dysphagia: a questionnaire survey of protocols, roles and responsibilities of radiology and speech and language therapy personnel. Radiography 12, 26–30.

Robbins, J.A., Coyle, J.L., Rosenbek, J.C., Roecker, E.B., Woods, J.L., 1999. Differentiation of normal and abnormal airway protection during swallowing using the penetration-aspiration scale. Dysphagia 14 (4), 228–232.

Royal College of Speech and Language Therapists, 2006. Videofluoroscopic evaluation of oropharyngeal swallowing disorders (vfs) in adults: the role of speech and language therapists. RCSLT Policy Statement.

Skills for Health, 2005. Direct and report on video fluoroscopic examinations of the oro-pharynx and oesophagus using contrast media. <http://www.skillsforhealth.org.uk/tools/view_framework.php?id=103> Accessed 19.11.07.

Further reading

Logemann, J.A., 1998. Evaluation and treatment of swallowing disorders, second ed. Austin, PRO-ED.

Logemann, J.A., 1993. Manual for the videofluorographic study of swallowing, second ed. Austin, PRO-ED.

Acknowledgments

CHAPTER 7

Fluoroscopic examinations of the pharynx, esophagus and stomach

Robert L. Law

Contents ||||||||||||||||||||||||||||||||||||||||||||||||||||||||||||||||||||||||||||||

Introduction

Roentgen's first publication on the discovery of x-rays and the x-ray absorption characteristics of metals and salts was in 1895. The potential for fluoroscopic examination of the upper gastrointestinal tract with contrast medium was raised immediately after Roentgen's seminal paper. In 1896, the German physician Wolf Becher utilized Roentgen's work to develop the concept of using contrast medium to provide an image of the stomach (Thomas, 1998).

Walter Bradford Cannon, a physiologist at Harvard University, studied digestion in animals using bismuth and x-rays. Using heavy metal salts mixed with food, Cannon studied gastrointestinal motility, tracing the fluoroscopic appearance of contrast through the alimentary tract. Changing from bismuth to barium in 1924, Cannon adapted the study for humans (Sebastian, 1999).

Despite the advances in medical technology, contrast fluoroscopy and the use of barium, in particular, continues to have a significant role in the imaging of the upper gastrointestinal tract. In this chapter, we will discuss the barium swallow, double contrast barium meal and the role of water-soluble contrast media.

The barium swallow

The barium swallow is a simple, safe and effective examination for patients with symptoms of dysphagia. It can provide a significant amount of information both on its own or complementary to endoscopy or esophageal motility studies (Esfandyari et al., 2002; Hansmann and Grenacher, 2006).

The clinical indications for a barium swallow are high (pharyngeal) or low (esophageal/esophago-gastric) dysphagia, the root cause being either neuromuscular or mechanical. Common causes for high and low dysphagia are given in Table 8.1.

The objective of the barium swallow is for the practitioner to:

- Demonstrate the presence or absence of aspiration or tracheo-esophageal fistula
- Image from the initiation of deglutition to the clearance of barium from the hypopharynx
- Image the distended esophagus, gastro-esophageal junction and gastric fundus in double contrast
- Observe and gauge the normality or otherwise of esophageal motility
- Confirm gastric emptying.

The optimum objectives can be aided by using a CO_2 impregnated contrast agent such as 100% w/v Baritop 100 (Sanochemia UK).

Pharyngeal and esophageal swallow technique

Where possible, the barium swallow should be performed with the fluoroscopy table in the erect position and ideally using a carbonated barium solution. Timing of the swallow for imaging is all important and it is of value when explaining the requirements to give the patient a trigger word such as telling them to swallow when they hear the word 'now' as in 'swallow now'.

Table 8.1 Potential causes of dysphagia

High (pharyngeal) dysphagia	Low (esophageal/gastro-esophageal) dysphagia
Neuromuscular discoordination (e.g. post CVA, Parkinson's)	Tertiary contraction/motility disorders
Zenker's pulsion diverticulum	Benign peptic stricture
Pharyngeal pouch	Barrett's esophagus
Prominence of the cricopharyngeus	Presby esophagus
Osteophyte impression	Schatzki ring
Pharyngeal web(s)	Hernia (e.g. para-esophageal, volved incarcerated, Morgagni)
Neoplasia	Neoplasia
	Achalasia
	Systemic sclerosis (scleroderma)

CVA, cerebrovascular accident

Before commencement of formal imaging, the patient is given an initial swallow of barium, and its passage to the stomach is screened to check there is no mechanical obstruction. The patient is placed in the right anterior oblique or lateral position as this projects the esophagus away from the spine and trachea. In this position, there is a better chance of differentiating barium in the trachea originating from a tracheo-esophageal fistula from that which has been aspirated. Regardless of the cause of the barium in the trachea, the patient will cough if that reflex is present. Coughing will result in the barium coating the trachea which might subsequently make it difficult to determine the cause for the barium being present.

Imaging

As an optimal minimum, imaging patients with high dysphagia should include videofluoroscopy or rapid imaging sequences of the pharynx (e.g. at least 3–4 frames per second). Videofluoroscopic assessment of swallowing disorders is expored further in Chapter 7.

The pharynx is examined in the *lateral*, the *left or right anterior oblique*, and the *anteroposterior* projection. The alternate oblique need only be considered if an abnormality is suggested. If pharyngeal imaging options are limited, the lateral projection provides the greatest breadth of information and can demonstrate aspiration and pharyngeal abnormalities such as pharyngeal pouch, webs, pharyngeal neoplasm, prominence of the cricopharyngeus (Figures 8.1, 8.2, 8.3, 8.4 and 8.5) and osteophyte impression.

Imaging of the esophagus, esophago-gastric junction and gastric fundus must always be included whether symptoms suggest high or low dysphagia. Turning the patient towards the right anterior oblique position will demonstrate the esophagus away from the spine (Figures 8.6 and 8.7).

Demonstration of the esophagus can be achieved by asking the patient to drink the barium and keep swallowing as quickly as possible. Esophageal distension is maintained by the second swallow inhibiting the first and the

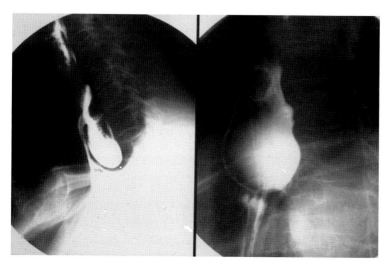

Figure 8.1 Lateral pharynx – pharyngeal pouch.

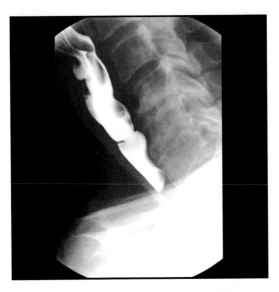

Figure 8.2 Lateral pharynx – web demonstrated.

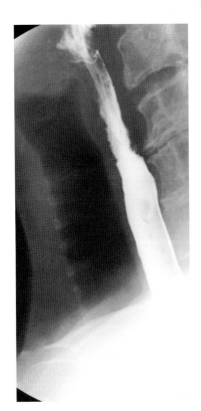

Figure 8.3 Lateral pharynx – carcinoma.

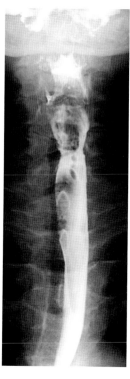

Figure 8.4 Anteroposterior pharynx.

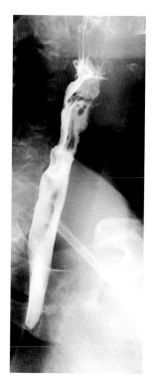

Figure 8.5 Right anterior oblique pharynx – carcinoma.

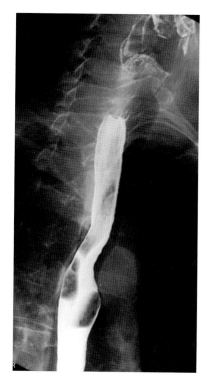

Figure 8.6 Upper esophagus.

CHAPTER 8

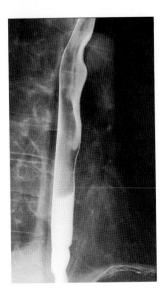

Figure 8.7 Mid esophagus.

third inhibiting the second etc. If the patient cannot cope with continuous swallowing, the alternative is to take a number of separate swallows, overlapping imaging of the distended esophagus.

The importance of obtaining full distenson of the esophagus cannot be emphasized enough as plaque lesions can be missed (Figure 8.8). *If full distension is not considered to have been achieved the swallow* must *be repeated.*

Subtle esophageal strictures may not demonstrate convincingly on a liquid barium swallow; in these instances asking the patient to swallow a small barium sulfate coated marshmallow can be effective in demonstrating the point of hold-up.

Separate images should be taken of the *esophago-gastric junction* (Figures 8.9, 8.10 and 8.11); the optimal degree of obliquity can be identified from the initial screened swallow. Additional images should be considered as appropriate if an abnormality is suggested.

Lesions in the gastric fundus can present as dysphagia and examination of this part of the stomach forms an integral part of the barium swallow. In the erect position, swallowed barium is likely to by-pass the fundus, gas from carbonated barium migrating to the fundus.

With the patient in the anteroposterior position, the table is tilted to horizontal. Coating the fundus with barium can be achieved by turning the patient to the left and then prone and finally to the right lateral position, tilting the table head up to a point that the barium drains out of the fundus to be replaced by the gas. *Lateral* (Figure 8.12) and then *left anterior oblique* (Figure 8.13) images of the upper body/lower fundus are taken at this point; reflux and motility are checked as described in the barium meal section below.

Images are taken of the fundus with the patient and table in the erect position (Table 8.2), then to complete the examination an overview can be taken of the stomach demonstrating gastric emptying. When the patient's clinical condition severely limits movement, the barium swallow can still be

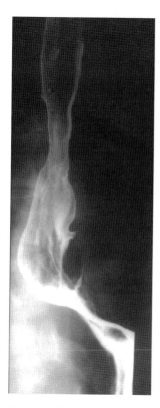

Figure 8.8 Plaque tumor above hiatus hernia.

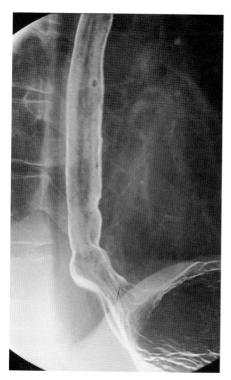

Figure 8.9 Lower esophagus and gastro-esophageal junction.

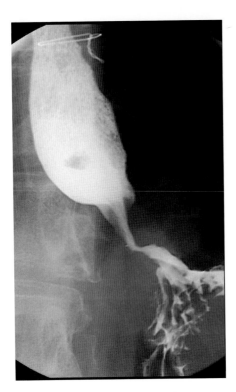

Figure 8.10 Carcinoma in lower esophagus.

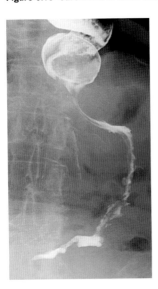

Figure 8.11 Achalasia. Distended esophagus with debris.

considered. The table need only be tilted up from the horizontal position as far as the patient will tolerate.

Where possible, turning the patient onto their side will reduce the risk of accidental aspiration should the patient expel the contrast medium.

In patients with a poor swallow or gag reflex, examination of the lower esophagus can be achieved by the trans-nasal insertion of a fine bore tube

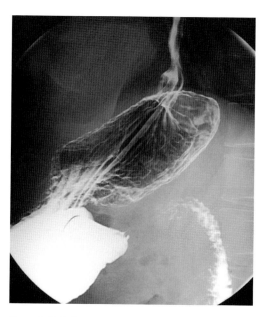

Figure 8.12 Left side raised lateral stomach.

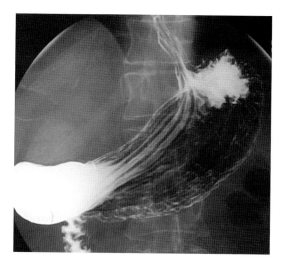

Figure 8.13 Left anterior oblique upper body/lower fundus of stomach.

into the distal esophagus or site of obstruction, followed by the infusion of a contrast medium which, if necessary, can be aspirated through the tube at the end of the examination (see Chapter 11).

The double contrast barium meal (DCBM)

The demand for the double contrast barium meal has been significantly reduced in recent years. This is mainly due to the increased use of endoscopy and availability of endoscopists. Nurses, and more recently, radiographer endoscopists have become established and widely accepted, working as independent practitioners (Swarbrick et al., 2005).

Table 8.2 A quick reference guide to a standard barium swallow technique

Pharyngeal swallow technique Erect imaging	Esophageal swallow technique Erect imaging
Right anterior oblique screen barium bolus through to esophagus Videofluoroscopy or rapid imaging series Left or right anterior oblique pharynx Anteroposterior pharynx Lateral pharynx	Anteroposterior imaging of distended esophagus Images of gastro-esophageal junction
	Table horizontal
	Turn patient – coat fundus Right lateral distended fundus Oblique fundus Check esophageal motility and gastro-esophageal reflux Erect view(s) of fundus Overview of stomach Confirm initiation of gastric emptying

Helicobacter pylori: the decline in peptic ulcer disease can be attributed to the discovery of *Helicobacter (H.) pylori* by Marshall and Warren (1984). Except in patients taking non-steroidal anti-inflammatory drugs (NSAIDs), all those with peptic ulcers have *H. pylori* infection. This can be tested for and treated if present, without the need for either endoscopy or DCBM.

For patients with dyspepsia who are seropositive, non-invasive testing for *H. pylori* in conjunction with anti-*H. pylori* therapy is considered the most cost effective management strategy (Ofman et al., 1997) and cures peptic ulcer disease (Ladabaum et al., 2002).

Makris et al., (2003) conclude that, although a management strategy based on the urea breath test (UBT) is the most costly, it is the most effective in patients over 45 years and neither endoscopy nor the double contrast barium meal were considered cost effective approaches to the managment of dyspepsia in patients under 45 years.

So where does this leave the double contrast barium meal? If gastroscopy fails or is declined by the patient, the DCBM is currently the best of the limited number of test options for the examination of the stomach and duodenum. Knowing how to undertake the DCBM will also give an insight on how to obtain the optimum imaging when the clinical condition of the patient significantly limits the examination (Levine and Rubesin, 1995).

The objective of the practitioner in performing the DCBM is to coat the gastric mucosa, and subsequently the duodenum, with a skim of barium. Turning the patient as required and using the gas double contrast enables all aspects of the stomach and duodenum to be distended and imaged.

Double contrast barium meal technique

The patient is starved for 4 hours to make sure the stomach is empty.

With a horizontal fluoroscopy table and the patient supported upon their elbow on their left side, the effervescent powder followed by the citric acid activating agent are given to the patient along with a high density barium such as 340 g EZ HD (E Z Em) diluted with 65 ml H_2O. The patient then, without sitting up, turns to lie on their back, thus keeping the barium within the gastric fundus. At this stage, an intravenous hypotonic agent is given (see Chapter 3).

Turning the patient to their right through 270 degrees enables the barium to wash over the posterior wall of the mid and distal stomach, the lesser curve and then the anterior wall with the patient prone. The greater curve is then coated with barium, ending with the patient on their left side with the barium flowing back into the fundus once again. If coating is not satisfactory, the turning should be repeated.

From the right side raised lateral position the patient is turned into the right anterior oblique position (RAO) (Figure 8.14) to demonstrate the gas filled gastric *antrum* before barium passes into the duodenum overlapping and possibly obscuring parts of the stomach.

Maintaining the barium within the fundus, the patient is placed in the *supine* position (Figure 8.15), gas will then fill the *body and upper body*, although as the antrum is projecting posteriorly in this position it is not always gas filled or seen to its fullest extent.

Turning the patient onto their right side and tilting the table head up will enable the barium to drain out of the fundus and be replaced by gas distension. A *left side raised lateral* image of the *fundus* is recorded (see Figure 8.12). The barium passes to the gastric antrum and on into the duodenum.

Controlling the patient's movement, they are then turned towards the *left anterior oblique* under fluoroscopic control. The practitioner is watching for the movement of barium and gas to demonstrate the *fundus and upper body distal to the esophago-gastric junction*. The optimum position is immediately

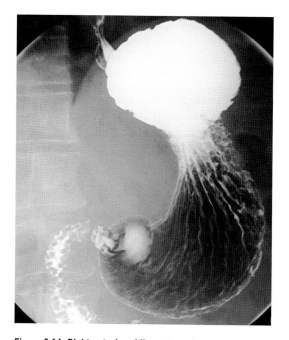

Figure 8.14 Right anterior oblique stomach.

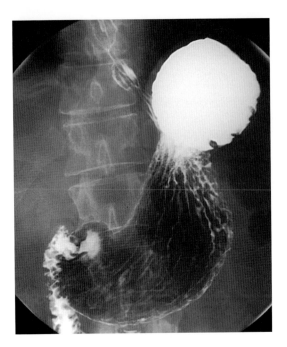

Figure 8.15 Supine stomach.

before the barium gas interchange occurs (see Figure 8.13). Depending on the shape and size of the stomach, altering the table position may or may not be of value.

With the patient supine, the table is returned to the horizontal position where barium is confirmed to be in the duodenum. Tilting the table up enough to drain barium out of the duodenal bulb, the patient is turned to the left lateral position and the table returned to the horizontal with barium in the third/fourth part of the duodenum and gas refills the antrum. With a pad held in the midline of the epigastrium, the patient is turned prone onto the pad. *Pad compression* of the stomach against the spine minimizes the passage of barium and optimizes the viewing of the *duodenal loop* (Figure 8.16).

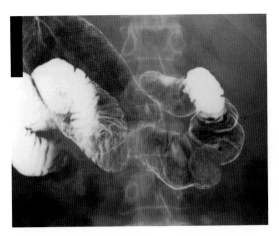

Figure 8.16 Prone duodenal loop demonstrating an adenoma.

Returning the patient onto their left side, magnified views are taken of the *duodenal bulb* in varying degrees of obliquity starting with the RAO (Figure 8.17A–D). Should the gas be expelled and the bulb collapse, it only requires turning the patient onto their left side once more to enable the bulb to reinflate.

The patient and table are tilted to the erect position, being aware that the patient may feel they are falling forwards during travel through the last few degrees to the vertical. Gas will migrate to the fundus so that an *erect image* can be acquired of stomach and, in particular, the distended dome of the *fundus* (Figure 8.18). In the erect position, an RAO is taken of the *duodenal bulb* (Figure 8.19), in particular to demonstrate the apex of the bulb. The LAO may be of value, but imaging is often limited by overlapping gastric or duodenal anatomy.

The esophagus is now imaged as described in the barium swallow section of this chapter. Once imaging of the stomach and duodenum is completed it does not matter about the additional barium entry from examining the esophagus.

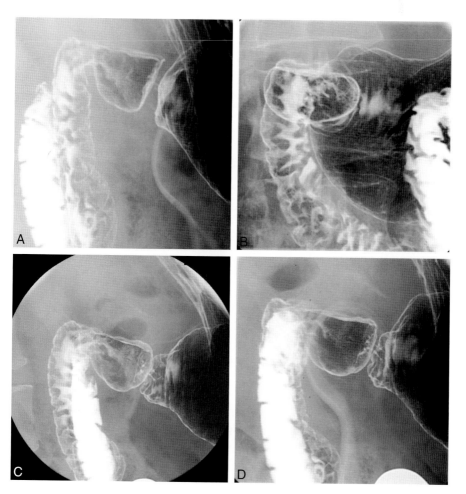

Figure 8.17 (A–D) Four views of the duodenal cap with the table horizontal.

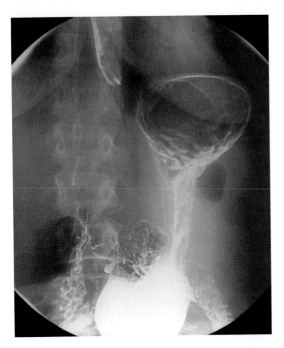

Figure 8.18 Erect stomach showing the dome of the fundus.

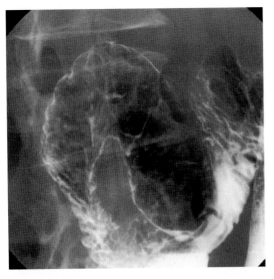

Figure 8.19 Erect right anterior oblique demonstrating the apex of the duodenal bulb.

Reflux. Anyone can be made to reflux and, in checking for its presence, it should not be forced. Options to check for reflux could include tilting the table head down with the patient slightly in the LAO position, bringing the barium in the fundus in contact with the esophago-gastric junction. Peristalsis as a result of the patient going through the act of swallowing should demonstrate reflux should it be present. An alternative method is to raise the patient's legs and ask them to cough.

Table 8.3 Quick reference guide to the double contrast barium meal

Patient lies on their left to ingest contrast	**Duodenal bulb**
Supine	RAO
	Supine
	LAO
Intravenous hypotonic agent given	**Erect**
Turn to right through 360 degrees to coat stomach	Erect fundus
RAO – antrum.	Erect whole stomach
Supine – body and upper body.	Apex of duodenal bulb
Patient on right, tilt table up to drain fundus	RAO
	LAO
Right lateral – fundus	Esophageal/esophagogastric imaging as Table 8.2
LAO – fundus and upper body.	Check for motility and gastro-
Table supine, turn patient to left, then apply pad	esophageal reflux
Prone image – duodenal loop with pad	

RAO, right anterior oblique; LAO, left anterior oblique

Motility. A simple test to assess motility is to have the patient in the prone position with their head turned to the side. Ingesting a mouthful of barium in one swallow and observing its passage will enable the stripping of the primary and secondary peristaltic wave to be observed. It is important the patient does not swallow twice in succession as the second swallow will inhibit assessment of the first. A method of inhibiting a second swallow is for the patient to open their mouth immediately after the first swallow (Table 8.3).

Hiatus hernia. If a hiatus hernia is suspected and requires evaluation, the value of the barium examination includes:

- Confirming clinical suspicion
- Identifying the point of herniation through the diaphragm (it may not be through the diaphragmatic hiatus but (for example) may be a Morgagni hernia)
- Determining the extent of gastric herniation
- Demonstrating the degree to which the stomach has turned about its axis (volved) and whether or not the herniated stomach is incarcerated (Figure 8.20)
- Identifying the cause of any possible delay of contrast passing into the intra-abdominal component of the stomach, such as compression of the stomach within the diaphragmatic hiatus or barium pooling due to the convoluted geography of the stomach
- Ascertaining whether the bowel has herniated through the diaphragm with the stomach (Figure 8.20 arrowed)
- Evaluating the esophagus as for a barium swallow.

The acute esophagus, stomach and duodenum

If an iatrogenic or pathological *esophageal perforation* is being questioned, a low-osmolar water-soluble contrast medium, such as oral Gastromiro (Bracco UK Ltd), should be used or, if infused via a fine bore tube, Ultravist

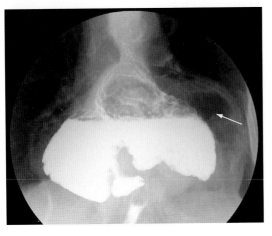

Figure 8.20 Volved incarcerated hiatus hernia bowel arrowed.

240 (Scherring Health Care Ltd). The use of the cheaper hyperosmolar contrast medium 'Gastrografin' is dangerous, particularly if the patient is at risk of aspirating, as it can possibly induce severe bronchial irritation and pulmonary edema (Morcos, 2003).

Every effort should be made to place the contrast medium dependent to all aspects of the esophageal lumen. If an anastomotic leak is being queried, post esophagectomy, imaging should first be undertaken with a low osmolar water-soluble contrast agent. If no leak is demonstrated, barium should be used (Tanomkiat and Galassi, 2000).

If *gastric or duodenal perforation* is being considered (Figures 8.21 and 8.22), barium preparations should never be used due to the risk of leakage into the abdominal cavity. Complications of barium sedimenting within the peritoneum can include peritonitis, abscess formation and barium granuloma. If a

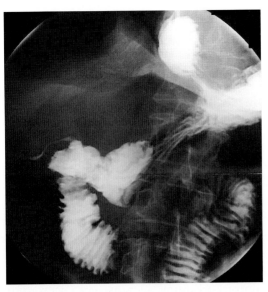

Figure 8.21 Water-soluble contrast examination, gastro-esophageal reflux, duodenal perforation.

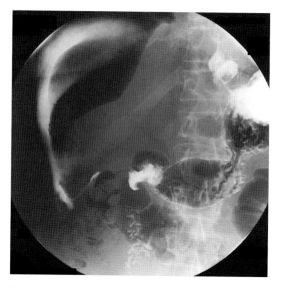

Figure 8.22 Duodenal perforation. Contrast tracking around liver.

nasogastric drainage tube is present and sited so that all the ports are in the stomach, dilute hyperosmolar contrast medium can be considered as long as there has been no evidence of the patient being at risk from aspiration.

Hypotonic duodenography

This examination can be used to identify stricturing, mucosal abnormality and filling defects. It can be performed using an 8 French gauge fine bore tube or by the ingestion of barium and an effervescent; both techniques are performed in conjunction with the injection of an intravenous hypotonic agent (see Chapter 3). In both cases, the duodenum is coated with barium and then distended with gas.

Intubation

A tube is placed in the second part of the duodenum and enough barium is infused to coat the whole of the duodenal loop. The patient may need to be turned from the supine to the left and then prone to coat the anterior wall. Returning to the supine position, air is gently infused through the tube. Images are taken in the RAO, supine and LAO and, if possible, prone position with magnified views as required. The benefit of this technique is that there will be no barium in the stomach to overlie the duodenal loop.

Oral ingestion

The technique for transmitting barium and effervescent agent to and around the duodenum is similar to that for the barium meal. The disadvantages of this technique are the barium in the stomach overlying the duodenum and the possibility of suboptimal lumen distension.

References

Esfandyari, T., Potter, J.W., Vaezi, M.F., 2002. Dysphagia: a cost analysis of the diagnostic approach. Am. J. Gastroenterol. 97 (11), 2733–2737.

Hansmann, J., Grenacher, L., 2006. Radiological imaging of the upper gastrointestinal tract, part 1. The oesophagus. Radiologe 46 (12), 1077–1088.

Ladabaum, U., Chev, W.D., Scheiman, J.M., et al., 2002. Reappraisal of non-invasive managment strategies for uninvestigated dyspepsia: a cost minimization analysis. Aliment. Pharmacol. Ther. 16 (8), 1450–1491.

Levine, M.S., Rubesin, S.E., 1995. The Helicobacter pylori revolution: radiologic perspective. Radiology 195, 593–596.

Makris, N., Barkun, A., Crott, R., et al., 2003. Cost-effectiveness of the alternative approaches in the management of dyspepsia. Int. J. Tech. Assess. Health Care 19 (3), 446–464.

Marshall, B.J., Warren, J.R., 1984. Unidentified curved bacilli in the stomach of patients with gastritis and peptic ulceration. Lancet 323 (8390), 1311–1315.

Morcos, S.K., 2003. Review article: effects of radiographic contrast media on the lung. Br. J. Radiol. 76 (905), 290–295.

Ofman, J.J., Etchason, J., Fullerton, S., et al., 1997. Management strategies for helicobacter pylori-seropositive patients with dyspepsia: clinical and economic consequences. Ann. Intern. Med. 126 (4), 280–291.

Sebastian, A., 1999. Barium swallow. A dictionary of the history of medicine, Parthenon Publishing, p. 103. Google 12th Jan 2007.

Swarbrick, E., Harnden, R., Hodson, R., et al., 2005. Non medical endoscopists. A report of the working party of the British Society of Gastroenterologists. http://www.bsg.org.uk

Tanomkiat, W., Galassi, W., 2000. Barium sulphate as a contrast medium for evaluation of postoperative anastomotic leaks. Acta Radiologica 41 (5), 482–485.

Thomas, A., 1998. An occasional newsletter, No.10 The radiology history & heritage charitable trust. http://www.rhhct.org.uk/news/10.htmlt

Further reading

Alaani, A., Vengala, S., Johnston, M.N., 2007. The role of barium swallow in the management of the globus pharyngeus. Eur. Arch. Otorhinolaryngol. 264 (9), 1095–1097.

Harar, R.P., Kumar, S., Saeed, M.A., et al., 2004. Management of globus pharyngeus: review of 699 cases. J. Laryngol. Otol. 118 (4), 507–522.

Tumors of the upper gastrointestinal tract

Nyla Nasir, Najib Haboubi, Emil Salmo

Contents

The esophagus

Benign tumors and tumor-like lesions

A diversity of benign tumors and related conditions occur in the esophagus. They are, however, mostly uncommon lesions and their main importance lies in distinction from malignant tumors (Crawford, 1999). Benign tumors are mostly *mesenchymal* in origin and lie within the esophageal wall. Clinically, they may be asymptomatic or produce dysphagia and sometimes bleeding (Choong and Meyers, 2003).

Leiomyomas

Leiomyomas are the most common benign non-epithelial tumors of the esophagus and are of *smooth muscle origin* (Postlethwait, 1983; Mutrie et al., 2005). Generally, they occur as a solitary 20–50 mm submucosal mass lesion at the lower one third of the esophagus, bulging into the lumen as a sessile intramural mass or as pedunculated polyps (Geboes, 2002). They may occur in up to 10% of adult esophagi but rarely attain a size to produce symptoms. If they are large they may ulcerate and produce pressure symptoms. Histologically, they are composed of interlacing smooth muscle fascicles with variable fibrosis and appear as a white whorled mass on gross examination (Mutrie et al., 2005).

Mesenchymal submucosal tumors

Other benign *mesenchymal submucosal tumors* include fibromas, lipomas, hemangiomas, neurofibromas and lymphangiomas; these, however, are very rare (Crawford, 1999).

Mucosal polyps

Mucosal polyps descriptively titled as *fibrovascular polyps* are composed of a combination of fibrous, vascular and adipose tissue covered by intact mucosa. They occur in the upper third of the esophagus and are often large and pedunculated (Ozcelik et al., 2004; Sultan, 2005).

Fibrous polyps

Fibrous polyps are also known as *inflammatory pseudotumors* and are considered to be reactive non-neoplastic lesions. They are located in the upper or mid esophagus as sessile or pedunculated lesions and may attain a large size. On microscopic examination, these lesions comprise myomatous fibrous tissue with thin walled blood vessels. Mucosal ulceration is present and hence mimics a malignant lesion. Biopsy is essential to distinguish between the two (Santos et al., 2004; Ozolek et al., 2004).

Inflammatory reflux polyps

Inflammatory reflux polyps are a special variant and are made up mostly of granulation tissue situated in the lower esophagus. They are thought to be related to reflux disease and hence the term reflux or gastro-esophageal polyp-fold complex. They are not pre-malignant (Geboes, 2002).

Squamous papillomas

Squamous papillomas are smooth, round, pink, sharply demonstrated, sessile lesions. They are usually single but occasionally multiple lesions with a central fibrovascular connective tissue core covered by bland hyperplastic papilliform squamous mucosa. The age range for presentation is between 17 and 78 years. These rare lesions are typically found in the lower esophagus and range over a few millimeters to 200 mm in diameter (Mosca et al., 2001; Geboes, 2002). In some cases, human papilloma virus (HPV) antigen has been identified (Woo and Yoon, 1996). The distinction between squamous papilloma and viral wart is unclear and, indeed, they may be related. There is no association with malignancy but they may recur after resection.

Malignant lesions

Most esophageal cancers are either *squamous cell carcinomas* or *adenocarcinomas*. Rare, uncommon and aggressive lesions include small cell carcinoma, adenoid cystic carcinoma, mucoepidermoid carcinoma, melanoma and carcinoma with a spindle cell component. *Metastatic tumors* can involve the esophagus by direct spread from the stomach and upper and lower respiratory tract. Rare blood-borne metastasis may occur from distant sites (Crawford, 1999).

Squamous cell carcinoma

Squamous cell carcinoma accounts for most esophageal cancers. It occurs in adults over the age of 50 with a male predominance; the male:female ratio is 4:1. There are wide geographical variations in its incidence. Areas of high rate of incidence include Puerto Rico, South Africa, Central Asia, Northern China and Eastern Europe. Low risk areas include most of Western Europe and North America (Crawford, 1999). The major *risk factors* are alcohol and tobacco (Bahmanyar and Ye, 2006; Hashibe et al., 2007). *Human papilloma virus* (HPV) has also been implicated as a probable etiological factor in the development of squamous cell carcinoma of the esophagus (Woo and Yoon 1996; Matsha et al., 2007). Dietary and environmental factors have been proposed to increase the risk and nutritional deficiencies act as promoters and potentiators of the tumorigenic effects of environmental carcinogens (Bahmanyar and Ye, 2006). Broad spectrum p53 gene point mutations present in these tumors are related to the effects of methylating nitroso compounds in the diet and in tobacco smoke (Meltzer, 1996; Mandard et al., 1997). Mutations in p16 gene and allelic loss involving other chromosomes are prevalent in these cancers as well, in keeping with the step-wise acquisition and accumulation of genetic alterations which ultimately give rise to cancer (Meltzer, 1996; Fujiki et al., 2002).

Clinically, it has an insidious onset and produces dysphagia and obstruction gradually. Weight loss and debilitation result from impaired nutrition and the effects of the tumor itself. Hemorrhage and sepsis occur with tumor ulceration (Crawford, 1999). Complications include aspiration of food through a cancerous tracheo-esophageal fistula and extension into adjacent mediastinal structures (Anderson and Lad, 1982).

Most frequently, it occurs in the lower two thirds of the esophagus. Morphologically, early lesions appear as small gray-white plaque-like thickening or mucosal elevations (Sugimachi et al., 1989). Late lesions are tumor masses which may eventually encircle the lumen and present as polypoid fungating exophytic masses (Figure 9.1), flat diffuse infiltrative forms or deeply irregular excavated ulcers with nodular margins (Mandard et al., 1984).

The microscopic appearances are similar as in squamous cell carcinoma anywhere else. The *degree of differentiation* may vary and variation within a tumor is common. The histological criteria are keratinization and intercellular bridges, which are prominent in well-differentiated carcinoma, sparse and focal in poorly differentiated tumors (Fletcher et al., 2000). *Dysplastic squamous epithelium* frequently borders invasive squamous cell carcinoma

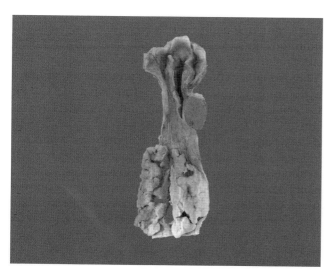

Figure 9.1 Gross appearance of an esophageal carcinoma of polypoid fungating type.

and represents the histological precursor (Sugimachi et al., 1989). This epithelium is characterized by varying degrees of altered maturation and cytoplasmic differentiation with nuclear pleomorphism, hyperchromasia, irregular chromatin and abnormal mitoses (Kuwano et al., 1987).

Five-year survival with superficial carcinoma is 75% compared with less than 25% in patients with advanced disease (Fletcher et al., 2000). Local and distant recurrence after surgery is common. The important prognostic features in a resection specimen are tumor size, depth of invasion, presence of lymph node metastasis and status of resection margins (Edwards et al., 1989; Lam et al., 1996).

Adenocarcinoma

The vast majority of primary esophageal *adenocarcinomas* arise in the lower esophagus in a background of *columnar metaplasia*, also known as *Barrett's esophagus*, and hence are associated with chronic gastro-esophageal reflux (Haggitt, 1994; Williams et al., 2006; Sayana et al., 2007; De Jonge et al., 2007). Rare adenocarcinomas arising from ectopic gastric mucosa are distinguished by their location in the upper esophagus (Christensen and Sternberg, 1987). Adenocarcinoma arising in the setting of Barrett's esophagus occurs in patients over 40 years with a median age in their 50s with an increasing incidence in the Western population (Williams et al., 2006; Sayana et al., 2007). Although the exact pathogenesis is unclear, genetic alterations in this disease are well documented.

Barrett's esophagus is a condition in which the normal stratified squamous epithelium is replaced by metaplastic columnar epithelium that predisposes to the development of esophageal adenocarcinoma (Figures 9.2, 9.3, see color insert) and Figure 9.4 (Haggitt, 1994). Neoplastic progression in Barrett's esophagus occurs by a multistep process associated with genomic instability and the development of aneuploid cell populations (Ramel et al., 1992). Molecular and immunohistochemical studies have suggested that mutations of the p53 gene accompanied by chromosome 17p allelic loss play an important role in the pathogenesis of the tumor (Fitzgerald, 2005; Sayana et al., 2007). p53 protein over-expression and allelic deletions on chromosome 17p have been shown to be present in some Barrett's adenocarcinomas (Ramel et al., 1992).

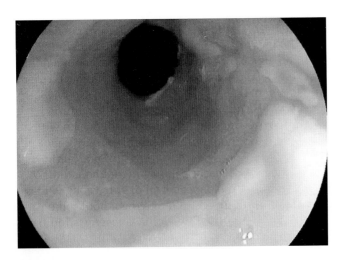

Figure 9.4 Barrett's esophagus seen at endoscopy.

Endoscopically, early cancers appear as flat lesions, while advanced cancers present as large ulcerating, fungating, polypoid or diffusely infiltrating masses (Geboes, 2002). Microscopically, these are mucin-producing glandular tumors with a tubular or papillary appearance exhibiting irregular invasive intestinal type glands lined by cytologically malignant cells (Fletcher et al., 2000). Since most cases arise in a background of Barrett's esophagus, high grade dysplasia in a background of Barrett's type metaplastic glandular epithelium is common in the adjacent mucosa (Williams et al., 2006; Sayana et al., 2007).

As with other forms of esophageal carcinoma, most patients present at an advanced stage with dysphagia, progressive weight loss, bleeding and chest pain (Crawford, 1999). The prognosis is poor; the mortality from esophageal adenocarcinoma exceeds 80% at 5 years (Fitzgerald, 2005). Resection of early cancers, limited to the mucosa and submucosa, improves the survival rate by 80% (Fletcher et al., 2000).

The stomach

Benign tumors and tumor-like lesions

Gastric polyps are clinically important lesions that are frequently encountered in routine pathology (2–3% of all gastroscopies). They may occur sporadically or in polyposis syndromes, such as familial adenomatous polyposis coli (FAP), Peutz-Jeghers syndrome, juvenile polyposis, Cowden's disease and Cronkhite-Canada syndrome. Sporadic polyps are classified as fundic gland polyps and hamartomatous and heterotopic tissue polyps; reactive polypoid lesions which include regenerative/hyperplastic polyps and inflammatory fibroid polyps (Oberhuber and Stolte, 2000; Borch et al., 2003).

Regenerative/hyperplasic polyps

Regenerative/hyperplasic polyps are one of the commonest types of gastric polyps. They are thought to arise from excessive regeneration following mucosal damage. Coexistent gastric abnormalities include chronic gastritis, partial gastrectomies, *Helicobacter pylori* and intestinal metaplasia (Gencosmanoglu et al., 2003). They are sessile or pedunculated with a smooth or lobulated surface (Figure 9.5). They are usually multiple and vary from few millimeters to 40 mm (Gencosmanoglu et al., 2003; Santos et al., 2004). Microscopically, there is hyperplasia of gastric foveolae leading to elongated and tortuous glands with cystic change and irregular branching. The stroma is edematous with infiltrated chronic inflammatory cells and contains smooth muscle fibers from the muscularis mucosa (Figure 9.6, see color insert) (Haboubi, 2002a). They are mostly benign and occasionally are complicated by carcinoma (Geboes, 2002). The incidence of synchronous or metachronous cancer elsewhere in the stomach is up to 3% of cases (Geboes, 2002). In cases of multiple hyperplastic polyps, however, there is a greater incidence of carcinoma associated with the polyps and synchronous cancers are significantly more commonly seen. Treatment for solitary polyps is polypectomy. Where multiple polyps exist, close follow up is required. They may recur after polypectomy.

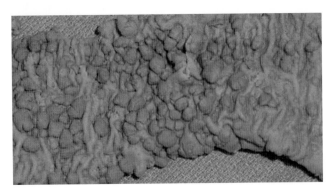

Figure 9.5 Gross appearance of hyperplastic/regenerative polyps which appear as multiple sessile polyps.

Inflammatory fibroid polyps

Inflammatory fibroid polyps are tumor-like lesions. These are rare lesions and can occur in any part of the gastrointestinal tract, but most commonly occur in the stomach (see esophagus) (Haboubi, 2002a). These are bulky growths involving mucosa and submucosa, composed of vascularized and inflamed fibromuscular tissue with a prominent eosinophilic infiltrate and covered by a thin mucosa (Harned et al., 1992; Santos et al., 2004). They are solitary lesions most commonly located in the antrum. They protrude into the lumen and may occlude the pyloric channel abruptly and present as gastric outlet obstruction (Mutrie et al., 2005). They are benign and not known to be associated with cancer. Treatment is polypectomy.

Adenomas

Adenomatous polyps are true neoplasms and contain proliferative dysplastic epithelium and thereby have malignant potential. They may be sessile without a stalk or pedunculated (stalked). The most common location is the antrum. The lesions are usually single and may grow up to 3–4 cm (Gencosmanoglu et al., 2003). Malignant transformation is related to size and is rare if the polyp is under 2 cm. Over 2 cm, malignancy is seen in 40–50% of adenomas. Polypectomy is the treatment of choice.

Malignant lesions

Gastric adenocarcinoma is the commonest malignant lesion of the stomach. Less common gastric tumours include gastric lymphomas, neuroendocrine tumors and mesenchymal tumors (Crawford, 1999).

Adenocarcinoma

Adenocarcinoma accounts for most gastric cancers. Males are affected more commonly with a male:female ratio of 2:1. High incidence areas include Japan, Central and South America and some parts of northern and eastern Europe (Crawford, 1999). From the epidemiological point of view, *environmental factors* implicated in gastric cancer include low socioeconomic status, smoking, alcohol consumption and diet, particularly high intake of salt, dried and pickled food (Lynch et al., 2005). *Precancerous conditions* include chronic

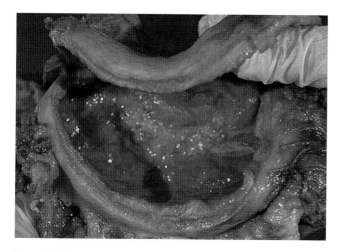

Figure 9.7 Gastric carcinoma linitis plastica type.

gastritis associated with long-standing *H. pylori* infection, atrophy and intestinal metaplasia, Menitriers disease and possibly long-standing peptic ulcer (Crawford, 1999). E-cadherin germ line mutations are seen in *familial gastric cancers* (Guilford et al., 1998; Lynch et al., 2005).

Early gastric cancer, also termed *surface or superficial carcinoma*, is confined to the mucosa and submucosa and is a potentially curable stage even if there is lymph node metastasis. Macroscopically, this may appear as an uneven mucosal surface or as a nodular, polypoid or villous form (Haboubi, 2002a).

Advanced gastric cancers may take the form of a polypoid, fungating, ulcerated or diffusely infiltrating form also known as the *linitis plastica type* (Figure 9.7) or may show a combination of these (Crawford, 1999). The diffusely infiltrating form occurs as an ill-defined, superficially ulcerating plaque accompanied by conspicuous thickening of the underlying gastric wall, or as diffuse thickening of the entire stomach (known as the leather bottle stomach). Hence the production of excess extracellular mucin gives the tumor a gelatinous appearance (Lynch et al., 2005).

Microscopically, the *Lauren classification system* classifies gastric carcinoma under two major histopathological variants, an intestinal type and a diffuse type. The *intestinal type* exhibits components of glandular, solid or intestinal architecture, as well as tubular structures. The *diffuse type (linitis plastica)* pathology is characterized by poorly cohesive clusters of signet ring cells infiltrating the gastric wall, leading to its widespread thickening and rigidity (Figure 9.8, see color insert) (Lauren, 1965). The outcome of advanced gastric cancer is usually poor and depends on accurate staging, i.e. extent and local infiltration, lymph node and extranodal metastasis.

Neuroendocrine tumors

Neuroendocrine tumors, also known as *carcinoids*, originate from the enterochromaffin cells in the gastrointestinal mucosa (Norton et al., 2004; Borch et al., 2005, Robertson et al., 2006). These lesions comprise less than 1% of gastric tumors (Haboubi, 2002a). In view of the distinct pathological behavior of gastric carcinoids, it has been proposed (Modlin et al., 1995) that they are divided into three types:

Type 1 is associated with type A chronic atrophic gastritis with or without pernicious anemia

Type 2 is associated with Zollinger Ellison syndrome (ZES) and multiple endocrine neoplasia (MEN 1)

Type 3 is sporadic.

Both types 1 and 2 represent syndromes with multiple small polyps, associated with hypergastrinemia and having low invasive or metastasizing potential. Sporadic lesions are almost always solitary; they evolve in a background of normal gastric mucosa and display a moderately aggressive behavior with the ability to metastasize (Haboubi, 2002a). Rarely, they present with clinical effects related to the hypersecretion of the peptide hormone, serotin, as *carcinoid syndrome* (Borch et al., 2005; Robertson et al., 2006).

Macroscopically, they appear as small, smooth, well-circumscribed polypoid elevations with a yellow-gray cut surface involving mucosa and submucosa. Larger tumors involve full thickness of the wall and may show central ulceration (Soga, 2005; Borch et al., 2005). Microscopically, gastric carcinoids are composed of small uniform polygonal to cuboidal cells with eosinophilic cytoplasm dispersed in the form of nests, trabeculae or cords involving mucosa and submucosa (Yu et al., 1998; Haboubi, 2002a). Malignant tumors are characterized by a more infiltrative pattern of growth, areas of necrosis, cytological atypia and mitoses (Yu et al., 1998).

Gastrointestinal stromal tumors (GISTs)

A wide variety of *mesenchymal neoplasms* may occur broadly classified under the term *gastrointestinal stromal tumors (GISTs)*. They occur most commonly in the stomach (Artigau et al., 2006). These tumors are thought to originate from mesenchymal stem cells that differentiate toward the interstitial cells of Cajal (ICCs). They express the tyrosine kinase c-kit (CD117) activity receptor. Mutations in this receptor cause neoplastic development (Artigau et al., 2006; Miettinen and Lasota, 2006a). These tumors occur in adults over 30 years of age, with males and females equally affected (Miettinen and Lasota, 2006b). Macroscopically, they may be single or multiple and vary in size from a few millimeters to 100 mm, presenting as small intramural lesions to bulky tumor masses which can occur in any part of the stomach (Geboes, 2002). Most tumors are well-circumscribed unencapsulated lesions that project into the gastric lumen as exophytic polypoid submucosal growths and are prone to surface ulceration (Figure 9.9) (Haboubi, 2002a; Alvarado-Cabrero et al., 2007). Microscopically, they are composed of interlacing bundles or whorls of uniform spindle cells or epithelioid cells (Alvarado-Cabrero et al., 2007) (Figure 9.10). Tumors over 50 mm are considered malignant. Other useful features suggestive of malignancy are increased mitoses, hypercellularity, nuclear pleomorphism and necrosis (Miettinen and Lasota, 2006a). Surgery still remains the main stay therapy but other treatment modalities are being successfully introduced.

Lymphomas

Gastric lymphomas represent 5% of all gastric malignancies. They may be primary or secondary to *systemic lymphoma* (Crawford, 1999). The great majority of primary gastric lymphomas are of B cell origin arising from *mucosa associated lymphoid tissue (MALT)* (Bacon et al., 2007). Virtually all

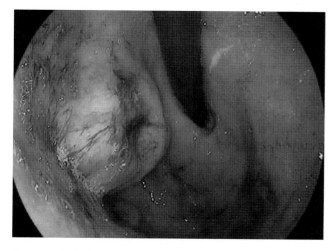

Figure 9.9 GIST. Gross appearance is of well-circumscribed unencapsulated lesions that project into the gastric lumen as an exophytic polypoid mass.

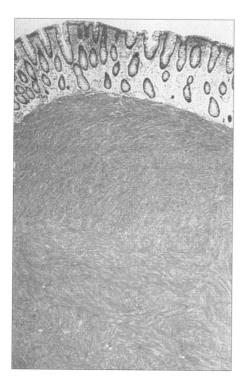

Figure 9.10 GIST. Microscopic appearances are composed of interlacing bundles or whorls of uniform spindle cells.

tumors arise in a background of *helicobacter-associated gastritis* (Moss and Malfertheiner, 2007). Macroscopically, they appear as polypoid, fungating or ulcerating tumors, most commonly located at the antrum. Microscopy shows a heavy population of polymorphous B lymphocytes infiltrating diffusely into the mucosa and invading gastric glands to form lymphoepithelial lesions with florid destruction of gastric glands (Figure 9.11, see color insert) (Bacon et al., 2007).

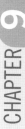

Outcome relates to the type of lymphoma; small cell type has a better prognosis than large cell type. Treatment modality includes eradication of *H. pylori* in the early stages of tumor development. In advanced disease, surgery is recommended.

The duodenum

Benign tumors and tumor-like lesions

Peutz-Jeghers polyps

Peutz-Jeghers polyps are hamartomatous lesions associated with Peutz-Jeghers syndrome and characterized by gastrointestinal polyposis, oral pigmentation and an autosomal mode of inheritance (Giardiello and Trimbath 2006; Zbuk and Eng, 2007). They are composed of coarse bands of extensively branching smooth muscle with an arborizing pattern covered by normal appearing glandular epithelium (Zbuk and Eng, 2007). Displacement of epithelium may occur within the submucosa and muscular coat (Jass, 2000).

Brunner's gland hamartoma

Other hamartomatous lesions include *Brunner's gland hamartoma*. This consists of a sessile mass composed of proliferated but otherwise normal appearing Brunner's glands with associated ducts and stroma (Bal et al., 2007).

Hyperplastic lesions

Hyperplastic lesions include lymphoid hyperplasia and Brunner's gland hyperplasia (Haboubi, 2002b).

Duodenal heterotopia

Duodenal heterotopia is comprised of heterotopic gastric mucosa which most often occurs in the first part of the duodenum as single or multiple nodules less than 10 mm, located in the submucosa or intramurally. *Heterotopic gastric mucosa* comprises an orderly collection of gastric glands, ducts and lamina propria (Spiller et al., 1982).

Pancreatic heterotopia

Pancreatic heterotopia may include an admixture of smooth muscle with both endocrine and exocrine elements or pancreatic ducts alone (Contini et al., 2003).

Adenomas

Adenomatous polyps

Duodenal adenomatous polyps are rare. The commonest site is the periampullary region suggesting there is a role for bile secretion in the genesis of the adenomas. They are usually single. They vary in size from microscopic lesions to large sessile or pedunculated lesions (Haboubi, 2002b). Multiple duodenal adenomas may occur in the setting of familial adenomatous polyposis (FAP) (Spigelman et al., 1994). Some may remain small, others progress to frank malignancy (Haboubi, 2002b).

The microscopic appearances are similar to their colonic counterparts with a tubular, villous or tubulovillous morphology displaying varying degrees of dysplasia, although absorptive type columnar cells are more prominent (Jass, 2000; Heidecke et al., 2002). However, unlike the colon, the presence of neoplastic epithelium in the lamina propria is a strong indicator of malignancy (Haboubi, 2002b). In patients with FAP, there is strong evidence to support the adenoma–carcinoma sequence (Spigelman et al., 1994).

Malignant lesions

Duodenal adenocarcinoma

Duodenal adenocarcinoma is an uncommon tumor and comprises 0.3% of all gastrointestinal tumors (Haboubi, 2002b). Carcinoma may develop in a background of familial adenomatous polyposis, celiac disease or Crohn's disease (Jass, 2000). Most cases occur in the periampullary region and present as obstructive jaundice. Macroscopically, these tumors grow in an annular ring encircling pattern or as polypoid or fungating masses (Hung et al., 2007). Microscopically, the appearances are similar to carcinoma elsewhere in the GI tract with varying degrees of differentiation. The cell population may include absorptive secretory and, to a lesser extent, Paneth and endocrine cells (Haboubi, 2002b). It is common to see an associated adenomatous component emphasizing the adenoma–carcinoma sequence (Perzin and Bridge, 1981). At the time of diagnosis, most tumors have already penetrated the bowel wall, invaded the mesentery or other segments of the gut (Hung et al., 2007).

Neuroendocrine tumors

Duodenal carcinoids are rare lesions and account for 1–2% of all *gastro-intestinal carcinoids* (Modlin et al., 2003). They may be single or multiple and vary in size from 2 to 50 mm and occur in the first and second parts of the duodenum (Haboubi, 2002b). Macroscopically, they appear as small polypoid masses with a characteristic solid yellow tan appearance (Jass, 2000). Microscopically, they are composed of small monotonous cells dispersed in an organoid pattern with granular cytoplasm and speckled nuclear chromatin (Figure 9.12, see color insert) (Bal et al., 2007). *Carcinoid tumors* produce a variety of polypeptide hormones. Some carcinoids are associated with other conditions including Zollinger Ellison syndrome, Von Recklinghausen disease, gastrinoma, pheochromocytoma and multiple endocrine neoplasia (Jass, 2000). Malignancy in carcinoids is related to a size more than 20 mm, mitoses and invasion of the muscularis propria (Haboubi, 2002b).

Gastrointestinal stromal tumors (GISTs)

Only 3–5% of GISTs occur in the duodenum and more commonly occur in the first part of the duodenum (Kwon et al., 2007). The appearances are similar to those occurring elsewhere is the gastrointestinal tract.

Lymphomas

Long-standing *celiac disease* is a predisposing factor for the development of lymphoma. These lymphomas are of *T cell origin* (Farrell and Kelly, 2001; Silano et al., 2007). They appear as multifocal ulcerating plaques with expansions of the mucosa and submucosa. The diffusely infiltrating lesions produce full thickness mural thickening with loss of mucosal folds and focal ulcerations. Others may be polypoid or fungating ulcerated masses (Jass, 2000; Haboubi, 2002b). Microscopically, these lesions are composed of a pleomorphic population of T lymphocytes (Isaacson, 2005). The adjacent mucosa shows villous atrophy with crypt hyperplasia and infiltration of the crypt epithelium with T lymphocytes (Yasuoka et al., 2007).

References

Alvarado-Cabrero, I., Vázquez, G., Sierra Santiesteban, F.I., et al., 2007. Clinicopathologic study of 275 cases of gastrointestinal stromal tumors: the experience at 3 large medical centers in Mexico. Ann. Diagn. Pathol. 11 (1), 39–45.

Anderson, L.L., Lad, T.E., 1982. Autopsy findings in squamous-cell carcinoma of the esophagus. Cancer 50 (8), 1587–1590.

Artigau, A., Luna, A., Dalmau, P., et al., 2006. Gastrointestinal stromal tumors: experience in 49 patients. Clin. Transl. Oncol. 8 (8), 594–598.

Bacon, C.M., Du, M.Q., Dogan, A., 2007. Mucosa-associated lymphoid tissue (MALT) lymphoma: a practical guide for pathologists. J. Clin. Pathol. 60 (4), 361–372. Epub 2006 Sep 1.

Bahmanyar, S., Ye, W., 2006. Dietary patterns and risk of squamous-cell carcinoma and adenocarcinoma of the esophagus and adenocarcinoma of the gastric cardia: a population-based case-control study in Sweden. Nutr. Cancer 54 (2), 171–178.

Bal, A., Joshi, K., Vaiphei, K., Wig, J.D., 2007. Primary duodenal neoplasms: a retrospective clinico-pathological analysis. World J. Gastroenterol. 13 (7), 1108–1111.

Borch, K., Ahrén, B., Ahlman, H., et al., 2005. Gastric carcinoids: biologic behavior and prognosis after differentiated treatment in relation to type. Ann. Surg. 242 (1), 64–73.

Borch, K., Skarsgård, J., Franzén, L., et al., 2003. Benign gastric polyps: morphological and functional origin. Dig. Dis. Sci. 48 (7), 1292–1297.

Choong, C.K., Meyers, B.F., 2003. Benign esophageal tumors: introduction, incidence, classification, and clinical features. Seminars in Thoracic Cardiovascular Surgery 15 (1), 3–8.

Christensen, W.N., Sternberg, S.S., 1987. Adenocarcinoma of the upper esophagus arising in ectopic gastric mucosa. Two case reports and review of the literature. Am. J. Surg. Pathol. 11 (5), 397–402.

Contini, S., Zinicola, R., Bonati, L., et al., 2003. Heterotopic pancreas in the ampulla of Vater. Minerva Chirurgie 58 (3), 405–408.

Crawford, J.M., 1999. The gastrointestinal tract. In: Kotran, R.S., Kumar, V., Collins, T. (Eds.), Robbins pathologic basis of disease. sixth ed. WB Saunders Company.

De Jonge, P.J., Wolters, L.M., Steyerbery, E.W., et al., 2007. Environmental risk factors in the development of adenocarcinoma of the oesophagus or gastric cardia: a cross-sectional study in a Dutch cohort. Aliment. Pharmacol. Ther. 26 (1), 31–39.

Edwards, J.M., Hillier, V.F., Lawson, R.A., et al., 1989. Squamous carcinoma of the oesophagus: histological criteria and their prognostic significance. Br. J. Cancer 59 (3), 429–433.

Farrell, R.J., Kelly, C.P., 2001. Diagnosis of celiac sprue. Am. J. Gastroenterol. 96 (12), 3237–3246.

Fitzgerald, R.C., 2005. Genetics and prevention of oesophageal adenocarcinoma. Recent Results Cancer Research 166, 35–46.

Fletcher, C.F., Bogomoletz, V., Williams, G.T., 2000. Tumours of the oesophagus and stomach. In: Fletcher, C.D.M. (Ed.), Diagnostic histopathology of tumours. second ed. Churchill Livingstone.

Fujiki, T., Haraoka, S., Yoshioka, S., et al., 2002. p53 gene mutation and genetic instability in superficial multifocal esophageal squamous cell carcinoma. Int. J. Oncol. 20 (4), 669–679.

Geboes, K., 2002. Polyps of the oesophagus. In: Haboubi, N., Geboes, K., Shepard, N., Talbot, I. (Eds.), Gastrointestinal polyps. Greenwich Medical Media, London, San Francisco, pp. 1–21.

Gencosmanoglu, R., Sen-Oran, E., Kurtkaya-Yapicier, O., et al., 2003. Gastric polypoid lesions: analysis of 150 endoscopic polypectomy specimens from 91 patients. World J. Gastroenterol. 9 (10), 2236–2239.

Giardiello, F.M., Trimbath, J.D., 2006. Peutz-Jeghers syndrome and management recommendations. Clin. Gastroenterol. Hepatol. 4 (4), 408–415.

Guilford, P., Hopkins, J., Harroway, J., et al., 1998. E-cadherin germline mutations in familial gastric cancer. Nature 392 (6674), 402–405.

Haboubi, N.Y., 2002a. Polyps of the stomach. In: Haboubi, N., Geboes, K., Shepard, N., Talbot, I. (Eds.), Gastrointestinal polyps. Greenwich Medical Media, London, San Francisco, pp. 23–48.

Haboubi, N.Y., 2002b. Polyps of the duodenum. In: Haboubi, N., Geboes, K., Shepard, N., Talbot, I. (Eds.), Gastrointestinal polyps. Greenwich Medical Media, London, San Francisco, pp. 53–67.

Haggitt, R.C., 1994. Barrett's esophagus, dysplasia, and adenocarcinoma. Hum. Pathol. 25 (10), 982–993.

Harned, R.K., Buck, J.L., Shekitka, K.M., 1992. Inflammatory fibroid polyps of the gastrointestinal tract: radiologic evaluation. Radiology 182 (3), 863–836.

Hashibe, M., Boffetta, P., Zaridze, D., et al., 2007. Esophageal cancer in Central and Eastern Europe: tobacco and alcohol. Int. J. Cancer 120 (7), 1518–1522.

Heidecke, C.D., Rosenberg, R., Bauer, M., et al., 2002. Impact of grade of dysplasia in villous adenomas of Vater's papilla. World J. Surg. 26 (6), 709–714.

Hung, F.C., Kuo, C.M., Chuah, S.K., et al., 2007. Clinical analysis of primary duodenal adenocarcinoma: an 11-year experience. J. Gastroenterol. Hepatol. 22 (5), 724–728.

Isaacson, P.G., 2005. Gastrointestinal lymphoma: where morphology meets molecular biology. J. Pathol. 205 (2), 255–274.

Jass, J.R., 2000. Tumours of the small and large intestine. In: Fletcher, C.D.M. (Ed.), Diagnostic histopathology of tumours. second ed. Churchill Livingstone.

Kuwano, H., Matsuda, H., Matsuoka, H., et al., 1987. Intra-epithelial carcinoma concomitant with esophageal squamous cell carcinoma. Cancer 59 (4), 783–787.

Kwon, S.H., Cha, H.J., Jung, S.W., et al., 2007. A gastrointestinal stromal tumor of the duodenum masquerading as a pancreatic head tumor. World J. Gastroenterol. 13 (24), 3396–3369.

Lam, K.Y., Ma, L.T., Wong, J., 1996. Measurement of extent of spread of oesophageal squamous carcinoma by serial sectioning. J. Clin. Pathol. 49 (2), 124–129.

Lauren, P., 1965. The two histological main types of gastric carcinoma; diffuse and so called intestinal type carcinoma. An attempt at a histoclinical classification. Acta Pathol. Microbiol. Scand. 64, 31–49.

Lynch, H.T., Grady, W., Suriano, G., et al., 2005. Gastric cancer: new genetic developments. J. Surg. Oncol. 90 (3), 114–133; discussion 133.

Mandard, A.M., Marnay, J., Gignoux, M., et al., 1984. Cancer of the esophagus and associated lesions: detailed pathologic study of 100 esophagectomy specimens. Hum. Pathol. 15 (7), 660–669.

Mandard, A.M., Marnay, J., Lebeau, C., et al., 1997. Expression of p53 in oesophageal squamous epithelium from surgical specimens resected for squamous cell carcinoma of the oesophagus, with special reference to uninvolved mucosa. J. Pathol. 185 (3), 334–335.

Matsha, T., Donninger, H., Erasmus, R.T., et al., 2007. Expression of p53 and its homolog, p73, in HPV DNA positive oesophageal squamous cell carcinomas. Virology 369 (1), 182–190. Epub 2007 Aug 29.

Meltzer, S.J., 1996. The molecular biology of esophageal carcinoma. Recent Results Cancer Research 142, 1–8.

Miettinen, M., Lasota, J., 2006a. Gastrointestinal stromal tumors: review on morphology, molecular pathology, prognosis, and differential diagnosis. Arch. Pathol. Lab. Med. 130 (10), 1466–1478.

Miettinen, M., Lasota, J., 2006b. Gastrointestinal stromal tumors: pathology and prognosis at different sites. Semin. Diagn. Pathol. 23 (2), 70–83.

Modlin, I.M., Gillian, C.J., Lawton, G.P., et al., 1995. Gastric carcinoids. The Yale experience. Arch. Surg. 130, 250–255.

Modlin, I.M., Lye, K.D., Kidd, M.A., 2003. 5-decade analysis of 13,715 carcinoid tumors. Cancer 97 (4), 934–959.

Morandi, E., Pisoni, L., Castoldi, M., et al., 2006. Gastric outlet obstruction due to inflammatory fibroid polyp. Ann. Ital. Chir. 77 (1), 59–61.

Mosca, S., Manes, G., Monaco, R., et al., 2001. Squamous papilloma of the esophagus: long-term follow up. J. Gastroenterol. Hepatol. 16 (8), 857–861.

Moss, S.F., Malfertheiner, P., 2007. Helicobacter and gastric malignancies. Helicobacter 12 (Suppl. 1), 23–30.

Mutrie, C.J., Donahue, D.M., Wain, J.C., et al., 2005. Esophageal leiomyoma: a 40-year experience. Ann. Thorac. Surg. 79 (4), 1122–1125.

Norton, J.A., Melcher, M.L., Gibril, F., et al., 2004. Gastric carcinoid tumors in multiple endocrine neoplasia-1 patients with Zollinger-Ellison syndrome can be symptomatic, demonstrate aggressive growth, and require surgical treatment. Surgery 136 (6), 1267–1274.

Oberhuber, G., Stolte, M., 2000. Gastric polyps: an update of their pathology and biological significance. Virchows Arch. 437 (6), 581–590.

Ozcelik, C., Onat, S., Dursun, M., et al., 2004. Fibrovascular polyp of the esophagus: diagnostic dilemma. Interac. Cardiovasc. Thorac. Surg. 3 (2), 260–262.

Ozolek, J.A., Sasatomi, E., Swalsky, P.A., et al., 2004. Inflammatory fibroid polyps of the gastrointestinal tract: clinical, pathologic, and molecular characteristics. Appl. Immunohistochem. Mol. Morphol. 12 (1), 59–66.

Perzin, K.H., Bridge, M.F., 1981. Adenomas of the small intestine: a clinicopathologic review of 51 cases and a study of their relationship to carcinoma. Cancer 48 (3), 799–819.

Postlethwait, R.W., 1983. Benign tumors and cysts of the esophagus. Surg. Clin. N. Am. 63 (4), 925–931.

Ramel, S., Reid, B.J., Sanchez, C.A., 1992. Evaluation of p53 protein expression in Barrett's esophagus by two-parameter flow cytometry. Gastroenterology 102 (4 Pt 1), 1220–1228.

Robertson, R.G., Geiger, W.J., Davis, N.B., 2006. Carcinoid tumors. Am. Fam. Physician 74 (3), 429–434.

Santos, G.C., Alves, V.A., Wakamatsu, A., et al., 2004. Inflammatory fibroid polyp: an immunohistochemical study. Arq. Gastroenterol. 41 (2), 104–107. Epub 2004 Oct 27.

Sayana, H., Wani, S., Sharma, P., 2007. Esophageal adenocarcinoma and Barrett's esophagus. Minerva Gastroenterol. Dietol. 53 (2), 157–169.

Silano, M., Volta, U., Vincenzi, A.D., et al., 2007. Effect of a gluten-free diet on the risk of enteropathy-associated T-cell lymphoma in celiac disease. Dig. Dis. Sci. Oct 13 [Epub ahead of print].

Soga, J., 2005. Early-stage carcinoids of the gastrointestinal tract: an analysis of 1914 reported cases. Cancer 103 (8), 1587–1595.

Spigelman, A.D., Talbot, I.C., Penna, C., 1994. Evidence for adenoma-carcinoma sequence in the duodenum of patients with familial adenomatous polyposis. The Leeds Castle Polyposis Group (Upper Gastrointestinal Committee). J. Clin. Pathol. 47 (8), 709–710.

Spiller, R.C., Shousha, S., Barrison, I.G., 1982. Heterotopic gastric tissue in the duodenum: a report of eight cases. Dig. Dis. Sci. 27 (10), 880–883.

Sugimachi, K., Ohno, S., Matsuda, H., et al., 1989. Clinicopathologic study of early stage esophageal carcinoma. Br. J. Surg. 76 (7), 759–763.

Sultan P.K., 2005. Fibrovascular polyps of the esophagus. J. Thorac. Cardiovasc. Surg. 130 (6), 1709–1710.

Williams, L.J., Guernsey, D.L., Casson, A.G., 2006. Biomarkers in the molecular pathogenesis of esophageal (Barrett) adenocarcinoma. Curr. Oncol. 13 (1), 33–43.

Woo, Y.J., Yoon, H.K., 1996. In situ hybridization study on human papillomavirus DNA expression in benign and malignant squamous lesions of the esophagus. J. Korean Med. Sci. 11 (6), 467–473.

Yasuoka, H., Masuo, T., Hashimoto, K., et al., 2007. Enteropathy-type T-cell lymphoma that was pathologically diagnosed as celiac disease. International Medicine 46 (15), 1219–1224. Epub 2007 Aug 2.

Yu, J.Y., Wang, L.P., Meng, Y.H., et al., 1998. Classification of gastric neuroendocrine tumors and its clinicopathologic significance. World J. Gastroenterol. 4 (2), 158–161.

Zbuk, K.M., Eng, C., 2007. Hamartomatous polyposis syndromes. Nat. Clin. Pract. Gastroenterol. Hepatol. 4 (9), 492–502.

Symptoms of lower gastrointestinal disease

Anne M. Pullyblank

Contents |||||||||||||||||||||||||||||||||||||||||||||||||||||||||||||||||||||||||

Introduction

Gastrointestinal symptoms are very common within the general population (Thompson et al., 2003). There is a high prevalence of rectal bleeding (Crossland and Jones, 1995; Thompson et al., 2000), change in bowel habit (Everhart et al., 1989) and abdominal pain (Sandler, 1990). Since any one of these symptoms alone can be due to benign, transient disease, symptom complexes are more useful for predicting serious pathology (Thompson et al., 2007). In the UK, this has led to the 'two week wait guidelines' for suspected cancer (Department of Health, 2000). This means that patients with symptoms most predictive of colorectal cancer (Table 10.1) must be seen within 2 weeks from the date of referral.

This chapter will explore symptoms and symptom complexes of lower gastrointestinal disease, the possible diagnosis and the investigation performed for each symptom group.

Table 10.1 Criteria for urgent referral for suspected colorectal cancer under the two-week rule

Sign, symptom or combination	Age threshold
Rectal bleeding *with* a change in bowel habit to looser stools and/or increased frequency of defecation persistent for 6 weeks	Over 40 years
A definite right-sided abdominal mass	All ages
A definite palpable rectal (not pelvic) mass	All ages
Change of bowel habit to looser stools and/or increased frequency of defecation, *without* rectal bleeding and persistent for 6 weeks	Over 60 years
Rectal bleeding persistently *without* anal symptoms	Over 60 years
Iron deficiency anemia without an obvious cause (Hb <11 g/dl in men or <10 g/dl in postmenopausal women)	No age criterion

Rectal bleeding

Bleeding from the gastrointestinal tract can be overt or occult. With *overt rectal bleeding*, the blood is recognized and is usually noticed on defecation. If this is the case, the origin of the bleeding is usually in the left colon or distal transverse colon. If the bleeding is *occult*, the blood loss is not recognized in the stool and the patient presents with anemia.

When a patient presents with rectal bleeding, there are features that can help locate the source of the bleeding, such as the color of the blood. *Bright red rectal bleeding* tends to originate from a distal source such as the rectum, whereas *dark red blood* tends to originate from a more proximal source but within the left colon or distal transverse colon. Another feature is whether the blood is separate to the stool or mixed in when it is passed. If the blood is separate to the stool, the patient notices it on the toilet paper or in the water in the toilet bowl, this usually suggests a very distal source such as hemorrhoids. If blood has had time to mix in with the stool, it suggests a more proximal source of bleeding.

Coexisting symptoms are also very important. A change in bowel habit to looser stools coupled with rectal bleeding is a symptom complex with a high predictive value for cancer (see above) or colitis. Anal pain may suggest a fissure. Change in bowel habit to constipation may merely mean that constipation has exacerbated hemorrhoids. Common combinations of symptoms associated with rectal bleeding, the possible causes and appropriate investigations are detailed below.

Bright red rectal bleeding with anal symptoms

Rectal bleeding with anal symptoms without a change in bowel habit is the lowest predictor of colorectal cancer (Thompson et al., 2007). It usually suggests *hemorrhoids* (associated with mucus, skin tags or prolapsing lumps) or an *anal fissure* (associated with anal pain on defecation). *Distal proctitis* (inflammation of the very distal rectum) may also be a cause. The exception to this is anal cancer that may present with these symptoms but is often associated with a lump or ulcer in the anal canal

Investigation: no radiological investigation may be necessary. This diagnosis can usually be made in the outpatient clinic on rigid sigmoidoscopy and/ or proctoscopy. In the case of a fissure, examination may not be possible and a painful per rectum (PR) examination may be diagnostic.

Bright red rectal bleeding without anal symptoms

This may suggest a *distal rectal cancer*, although this is often associated with change in bowel habit to looser stools, fecal leakage or a feeling of incomplete evacuation (tenesmus).

Investigation: radiological investigation may not be necessary for this symptom complex. It should be diagnosed on PR examination ± rigid sigmoidoscopy or proctoscopy. Flexible sigmoidoscopy would be appropriate in the over 40s to exclude malignancy. Should a stricture prevent the passage of the endoscope, a barium enema (Figure 10.1) or computed tomography (CT) should be considered.

Although a barium enema may exclude cancer in a patient presenting with a symptom complex associated with bright red rectal bleeding, it may not diagnose the cause. Patients with these symptoms may need a rigid sigmoidoscopy to establish the cause of their bleeding.

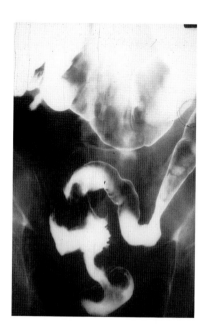

Figure 10.1 Rectal synchronous tumors.

Bright red rectal bleeding with change in bowel habit (CIBH) to looser stools

This carries the highest risk of *bowel cancer* (Thompson et al., 2007) but is also symptomatic of colitis, which may be infective, ischemic, ulcerative colitis (UC) or Crohn's disease (Figures 10.2, 10.3 and 10.4).

Investigation: since recognizable rectal bleeding usually originates in the left colon, a flexible sigmoidoscopy will diagnose the cause of this symptom complex with the advantage of obtaining a tissue diagnosis. A barium enema or CT colonography is also a reasonable test to request. However, the disadvantage is that a tissue diagnosis will still be necessary, it is possible to miss mild/moderate colitis on barium enema and, if the barium enema is normal, as discussed above, it does not exclude a very distal cause of blood loss and the patient should have a coloproctological examination.

Bright red rectal bleeding with constipation

Often the constipation has exacerbated bleeding from hemorrhoids or a fissure, rarely due to cancer.

Investigation: the clinician may request a barium enema or CT colonography to find a cause for the change in bowel habit. Constipation alone is a poor predictor of cancer. However, it is a predisposing factor for *diverticular*

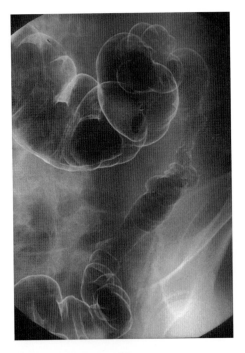

Figure 10.2 Ischemic colitis.

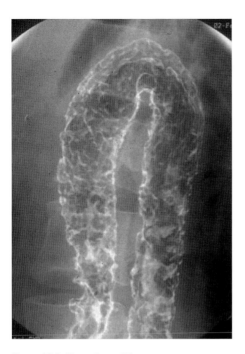

Figure 10.3 Ulcerative colitis.

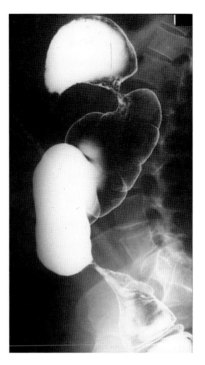

Figure 10.4 Crohn's colitis.

disease and so this is a common finding in patients with constipation. A colo-proctological referral will still be needed to assess the distal bleeding. If the constipation is long standing and an underlying functional bowel disorder is being considered, a colonic transit study (Figure 10.5) may be requested.

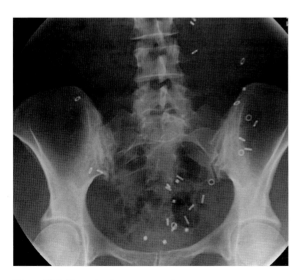

Figure 10.5 Normal colon transit study appearance.

Dark red rectal bleeding without a CIBH

Usually this presentation results from *diverticular bleeding*. This may present as a large bleed where dark blood and clots are passed with very little stool. The patient usually presents as an emergency or may give a history of a few large bleeds rather than continuing ongoing bleeding (see also Chapter 15).

Investigation: a flexible sigmoidoscopy may be useful but, in the acute situation, may be suboptimal if the colon is full of blood. A reasonable strategy is that once the bleeding has settled down, the clinician may request a barium enema, CT colonography or flexible sigmoidoscopy.

Dark red rectal bleeding with a CIBH

This may mean a more proximal tumor in the sigmoid, descending colon (Figure 10.6) or transverse colon or more proximal colitis.

Investigation: recognizing their attendant advantages and disadvantages, barium enema, CT colonography, flexible sigmoidoscopy or colonoscopy can all be considered.

Change in bowel habit alone

While CIBH with rectal bleeding is often indicative of significant pathology, CIBH alone is less predictive. This is because many of the population experience a CIBH at some point (Everhart et al., 1989) and 10–20% (Longstreth et al., 2006) have *irritable bowel syndrome*. When asking about change in bowel habit, it is essential to ascertain what the patient means. For example, does

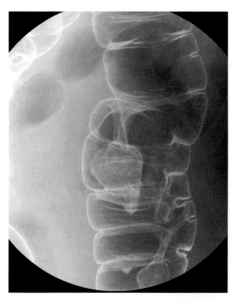

Figure 10.6 Pedunculated neoplastic polyp with two smaller pedunculated pdyps in descending colon.

diarrhea mean more frequent stools, looser stools or both? Some patients describe diarrhea as a slightly looser stool; others will only use the term if they are passing watery stools. It is the same with constipation. Some patients describe this as hard stools, some as less frequent stools and some mean they are not going at all. In fact, patients with an obstructing malignancy may describe 'constipation' and, although they may be hardly passing any stool, when they do so, it may be watery.

Constipation

True constipation is described as less than three stools per week. Patients who present with a very infrequent bowel frequency may have had problems since childhood. In these patients, a colonic transit study may be appropriate or even a rectal biopsy to exclude a late diagnosis of *Hirschsprung's disease*. If the bowel habit change is less dramatic, a barium enema or CT colonography is a reasonable request and *diverticular disease* will be a common finding.

Absolute constipation means no passage of stool *or flatus* and is a sign of *bowel obstruction*. This rarely presents in an outpatient and is more likely to be a symptom experienced by a patient admitted as an emergency. However, these patients should *not* have a prepared double contrast barium enema as the stimulant bowel preparation carries a risk of perforation. These patients should have an unprepared (Gastrografin) enema or a CT scan to elucidate the site of obstruction.

CIBH to looser stools alone

Again, the investigation chosen depends on the severity of the symptoms. A barium enema or CT colonography is a very good first choice in patients who may have a slight increase in bowel frequency. Most clinicians would expect the change to have persisted for at least 6 weeks before investigation for the reasons described above and infection to be excluded by a negative stool sample. If the diarrhea is severe, i.e. 10–20 times a day, this suggests a diagnosis of *colitis* and so a colonoscopy or flexible sigmoidoscopy is a better investigation as a tissue diagnosis can be obtained.

Irritable bowel syndrome (IBS)

It is worth mentioning this as a separate entity as it probably accounts for many of the patients with a negative barium enema who present with symptoms. It is *not* a diagnosis of exclusion and has very specific diagnostic criteria based on the Rome Criteria (Sandler, 1990). In 2008, the National Institute for Clinical Excellence (NICE) produced guidelines for the diagnosis and management of IBS.

The positive diagnostic criteria are:

Abdominal pain/discomfort either:
  Relieved by defecation
  or
  Associated with altered bowel frequency or stool form

and at least two of the following:

> altered stool passage (straining, urgency, incomplete evacuation)
> abdominal bloating
> symptoms exacerbated by eating
> passage of mucus.

Investigation: NICE has ruled that for patients who meet the positive diagnostic criteria for IBS, neither barium enema nor colonoscopy is necessary (NICE, 2008).

Iron deficiency anemia

This may be diagnosed on a routine blood test as defined above or the patient may present with shortness of breath, fatigue or fainting. It is usually related to *occult blood loss* from either the upper GI tract or the right colon where it may be associated with a mass.

Investigation: The British Society of Gastroenterology Guidelines (Goddard et al., 2005) recommend investigation of both the lower and upper GI tract in men and post-menopausal women. This can consist of a barium enema then esophagogastroduodenoscopy (OGD) or an OGD and colonoscopy at the same sitting. It is important that, if tests are done consecutively, that the lower GI tract is examined as anemia can be mistakenly attributed to mild gastritis. If the patient is frail or elderly and will not withstand bowel prep, a CT scan is a good first line test as it has good sensitivity for the diagnosis of *right-sided colonic tumors* (Figure 10.7) (Ng et al., 2002).

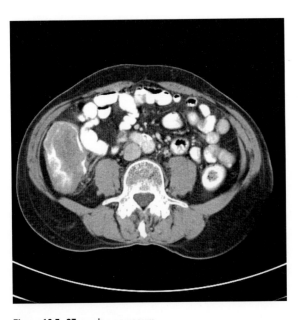

Figure 10.7 CT carcinoma cecum.

Melena

This is the passage of altered blood per rectum. Patients may describe black stools. True melena is very distinctive. It has an offensive smell and is described as black and tarry and is usually a reflection of a large bleed, most commonly due to an *upper GI source* such as a gastric or duodenal ulcer. It can be due to a *right-sided colonic tumor.*

Investigation: an OGD is essential in the acute situation to exclude a bleeding ulcer. If this is normal and a right-sided colonic tumor is suspected, the investigations are the same as for iron deficiency anemia.

Abdominal pain

Abdominal pain alone is rarely discriminatory for problems affecting the lower GI tract. In general, pain from the large bowel presents as lower abdominal pain, whereas pain from the small bowel presents as upper or central abdominal pain. Pain from an obstructing lesion is generally colicky and comes in waves, whereas pain from an inflammatory process, e.g. diverticulitis, is usually constant (see also Chapter 15). The features of the pain such as exacerbating and relieving factors, radiation (whether it spreads anywhere) and any associated symptoms also help determine the cause. In obstruction, (Figures 10.8, 10.9A and 10.9B), the pain may be exacerbated by eating and may be associated with vomiting and a change in bowel habit.

In an inflammatory process, the pain may be made worse by moving or coughing or anything that causes peritoneal irritation.

Investigation: if the pain is obviously related to the gut and associated with gastrointestinal symptoms, the investigations of the large bowel described above

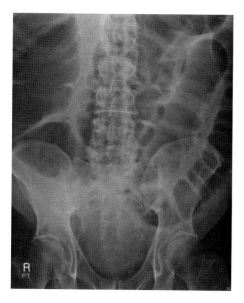

Figure 10.8 Large bowel obstruction.

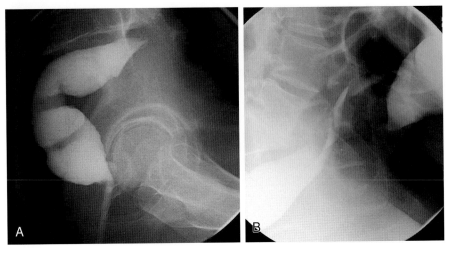

Figure 10.9 (A) Distal large bowel obstruction. (B) Obstruction caused by a twisted loop of bowel.

will be appropriate. If not obviously intestinal, an ultrasound scan or abdominal and pelvic CT with oral contrast is a good first line investigation, as it will identify common *extracolonic causes* of abdominal pain such as abscess formation or that originating from the gallbladder, pancreas or gynecological tract.

Incontinence

This is a distressing symptom, which is either due to a weak anal sphincter, a change in bowel habit to loose stools or a combination of both. If the bowels are loose, correcting the underlying cause can often improve the incontinence.

Investigation: if damage to either the internal or external sphincter is suspected, anorectal physiology tests and an endoanal ultrasound will be necessary.

Rectal prolapse

Rectal prolapse is described as 'something coming down' or protruding out from the anal canal. There are degrees of prolapse that can affect bladder, uterus, vagina and rectum and the underlying cause is a *weak pelvic floor*, commonly due to childbirth. Prolapse is thought to be a gradual condition, which may start as the rectum prolapsing within itself (intussuscepting). The symptoms of this may be tenesmus, inability to defecate (obstructed defecation), passage of blood or mucus and a heavy feeling in the rectum.

Investigation: if the prolapse is extending beyond the anal canal the diagnosis is obvious, but if it is internal, radiological investigation may be necessary. In this case, a defecating proctogram will give information on the degree of prolapse if present and give information to help plan appropriate surgery (see Chapter 13).

References

Association of Coloproctology of Great Britain and Ireland, 2007. Guidelines for the management of colorectal cancer, third ed.

Crossland, A., Jones, R., 1995. Rectal bleeding; prevalence and consultation behaviour. Br. Med. J. 311, 486–488.

Everhart, J.E., Go, V.L.W., Johannes, R.S., et al., 1989. A longitudinal survey of self reported bowel habits in the United States. Dig. Dis. Sci. 34, 1153–1162.

Department of Health, 2000. Referral guidelines for suspected cancer. Health service circular HSC 2000/013. Published 13 April 2000.

Goddard, A.F., James, M.W., McIntyre, M.S., et al., 2005. (On behalf of the British Society of Gastroenterology). Guidelines for the management of iron deficiency anaemia. British Society of Gastroenterology Guidelines.

Longstreth, G.F., Thompson, W.G., Chey, W.D., et al., 2006. Functional bowel disorders. Gastroenterology 130, 1480–1491.

Ng, C.S., Doyle, T.C., Pinto, E.M., et al., 2002. Caecal carcinomas in the elderly: useful signs in minimal preparation CT. Clin. Radiol. 57 (5), 359–364.

NICE, 2008. Clinical guideline 61. www.nice.org

Sandler, R.S., 1990. Epidemiology of irritable bowel syndrome in the United States. Gastroenterology 99, 409–415.

Thompson, J.A., Pond, C.L., Ellis, B.G., et al., 2000. Rectal bleeding in general and hospital practice 'the tip of the iceberg'. Colorectal Dis. 2, 288–293.

Thompson, M.R., Heath, I., Ellis, B.G., et al., 2003. Identifying and managing patients at low risk of bowel cancer in general practice. Br. Med. J. 327, 263–265.

Thompson, M.R., Perea, R., Senapati, A., et al., 2007. Predictive value of common symptom combinations in diagnosing colorectal cancer. Br. J. Surg. 94, 1260–1265.

Fluoroscopically guided fine bore intubation

Robert L. Law

Contents

Background

The UK National Patient Safety Agency (NPSA) has reported that approximately 500 000 fine bore feeding tubes are distributed annually within the National Health Service (NPSA, 2005). The vast majority of nasogastric intubations are uncomplicated and dealt with by suitably trained practitioners within the ward environment. Patients requiring *fine bore intubation* for nutritional support are by virtue of the requirement to be intubated, unwell and vulnerable to complications from misplaced intubations or the distress of repeated attempts.

The NPSA reported that they were aware of 11 deaths between 2002 and 2004 resulting from *misplaced nasogastric (NG) tubes* and, since that time, the NPSA Patient Safety Bulletin has reported a further five deaths and four near misses from misplaced nasogastric tubes (NPSA 2005, 2007).

Accurate information is sparse as to the nature and number of complications associated with fine bore intubation; however, from the serious complications reported to the NPSA, misreading of x-ray checks is a significant factor and it is suggested that interpretation of these images must be carried out by practitioners trained to report them (NPSA, 2005).

Checking intubation siting

There are numerous tests to check the position of the tube tip. Some, such as auscultation or the use of blue litmus paper to test acidity/alkalinity, have been discredited (NPSA, 2005).

In the ward environment, the measurement of the *pH of gastric aspirate* is currently considered the safest and easiest repeatable means of confirming the siting of a fine bore tube in the stomach. However, gastric pH can be above 5.5 in a number of circumstances, falsely suggesting that the tube might not be in the stomach, for example in patients taking proton pump inhibitors (PPIs), patients who have pernicious anemia, or who have had a recent fluid intake. The type of fluid, feeding formulae or medication is also relevant (Stroud et al., 2003; Bain, 2005).

Endoscopy can be used to insert fine bore tubes when blind intubation on the ward has failed, although local anesthesia to the pharynx and sedation may be required; additionally, the tube can be dragged back upon removal of the endoscope. In normal circumstances, *endoscopically guided fine bore tube insertion* could be considered excessive. Diagnostic upper gastrointestinal endoscopy has associated complications. Quine and Bell (1995) indicated a mortality and morbidity in the region of 1:12 000 and 1:230 respectively and, more recently, the British Society of Gastroenterology figures reported by Teague (2003) suggested little change.

In discussing the thoracic and non-thoracic complications of gastric and enteric intubation, Pillai et al. (2005) refer to the radiographic check of tube placement as continuing to be the 'gold standard'.

Radiography provides a snapshot of the fine bore tube position at the time of the x-ray, accurately identifying the site of misplaced tube tips (Figures 11.1, 11.2, 11.3 and 11.4).

However, inexperience in image interpretation can lead to the misreading of tube siting. The benefits of fluoroscopy are shown in a case where misinterpretation of chest radiographs on an unconscious patient in a high dependency unit led to a number of failed blind and endoscopic intubations. The tube was considered repeatedly to be sited in the right side of the chest (Figure 11.5). *Fluoroscopic tube guidance* and the careful infusion of a water-soluble contrast medium demonstrated a redundant loop of colon and a strictured cologastric anastomosis. The appearance is of a late onset complication from a previous colonic interposition for esophageal atresia of which the clinical team were unaware (Figure 11.6) (Law, 2006).

Radiographer and radiologic technologist involvement

Imaging departments are a focal point for ward patients within a hospital. The health, safety and comfort of patients who attend for a check x-ray on the siting of a fine bore tube tip are best served if mispositioned tubes are correctly placed before the patient returns to the ward.

Price and Le Masurier (2007) suggest that 80% of District General Hospitals in the UK have radiographers performing DCBE examinations. Radiography provides an accurate snapshot of the fine bore tube position at the time of the x-ray. As long as the tube is radiopaque, a skilled practitioner can provide

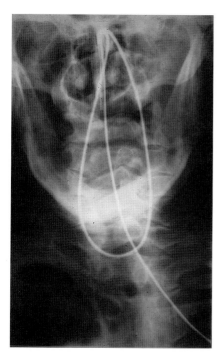

Figure 11.1 Tube coiled in pharynx.

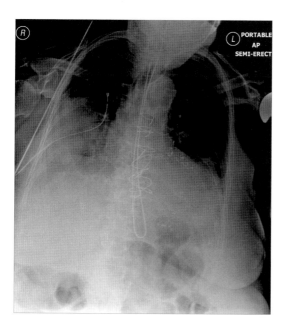

Figure 11.2 Tube tip in pharynx, loop in distal esophagus.

accurate information as to whether the tube is in the stomach or not. However, this raises the question of what should happen when an x-ray shows the tube is not correctly placed: should patients return to wards for tube resiting?

Radiographers skilled in GI fluoroscopy are ideally positioned to provide an *intubation service* and can quickly and easily acquire expertise in

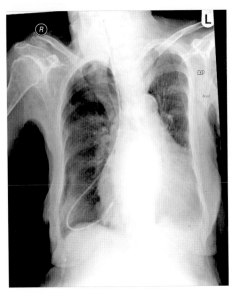

Figure 11.3 Tube tip passed via right bronchus penetrating the pleural cavity – associated pneumothorax.

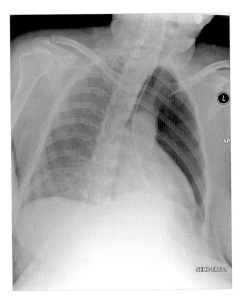

Figure 11.4 Tube tip passing via the left bronchus penetrating the pleural cavity – pneumothorax.

nasogastric/enteric intubation. With the wide potential for gaining experience, radiographers may well succeed with nasogastric intubating without recourse to fluoroscopy even if blind intubation on the ward has been unsuccessful.

The expertise acquired will also make this group of radiographers ideally suited to extend their role to *'hot reporting' of check images*. By the time the patient returns to the ward, an expert assessment of tube position could be provided, tube resiting undertaken if required and a report generated.

A protocol to enable nutritional support to be given at the earliest opportunity might include the following:

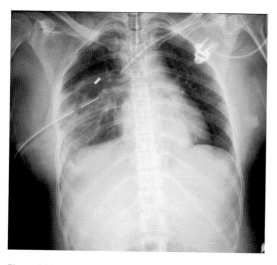

Figure 11.5 Gastric tube mistakenly considered to be in the right lung.

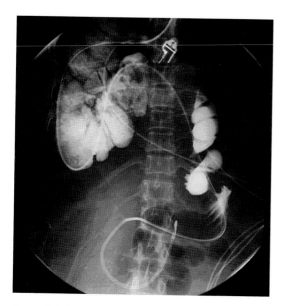

Figure 11.6 Redundant loop of colon and a strictured cologastric anastomosis, late onset complications post colonic interposition for esophageal atresia.

For correctly positioned tubes:

- The named nurse on the ward is informed by telephone
- If the notes are with the patient a notation is made of the report
- The hot reporting of images
- As in normal circumstances the image is penetrated to include the mediastinum and upper abdomen, as a routine, the generated report should only give details pertinent to the position of the nasogastric tube
- A rider in the report states that the clinical state of the chest has not been evaluated.

For incorrectly placed tubes:
The role of the clinical radiographer might include:

- Confirm the guide wire has been left in situ
- Decide whether the existing position can be adjusted or whether the tube needs to be removed for reintubation
- Decide whether blind or fluoroscopic intubation is appropriate
- Reintubate
- If intubation is blind, reimage; if fluoroscopically guided, save the last fluoroscopy image
- Inform the ward and referring clinician as for a correctly placed tube but also add:
  - the initial placement of the tube
  - whether a contrast medium was used
  - any observed stricturing or deviation to the normal anatomy
- So that no confusion can occur with the original image of the misplaced tube, it should have an annotation on it to the effect that 'the demonstrated mispositioned tube has been resited to its appropriate location and a repeat image taken'
- If iatrogenic trauma, such as a pneumothorax, is suggested, radiological advice should be sought as to further imaging and the referring clinical team informed.

Fluoroscopically guided intubation of nasoenteric fine bore tubes is a safe and effective technique (Prager et al., 1986; Law, 1990). A core team of radiographers or radiologic technologists skilled in GI fluoroscopy developing expertise in siting problematic fine bore tubes, have the potential to offer major positive changes regarding intubation and to offer the development of a more flexible service.

Tube wire requirements

Fundamental to any intubation, problematic or otherwise, is the design of the *fine bore (FB) tube* (Law and Longstaff, 1992). The following features should be considered when selecting an FB tube (Box 11.1):

- A streamlined shape to the tip that omits any pill shape. The perceived benefit of an expanded shape of the tube tip is compromised by the significant discomfort of its passage through the nasal cavity

---

BOX 11.1 The tube

- Streamlined tip with no pill shaping
- No ridge at tip attachment to tube
- Tube should be unweighted
- Tube/wire rigidity should be enough to minimize propensity to coil
- Should be of suitable length and lumen size for purpose
- 40% barium (or equivalent) tube tip density
- Hydrophilic coating to the tube lumen

- There should be no ridge at the attachment point between tip and tube. Upon egress of the tube, ridges can readily catch on the nasal concha and at best cause discomfort, at worse require removal through the mouth
- The tube should be unweighted
- The degree of rigidity of the tube and wire combination should be such that there is not a propensity to coil in the pharynx on insertion
- The tube should be of suitable length and lumen size for its function
- A 40% barium density of the tube tip is required to allow easy visualization whether on an x-ray check or on fluoroscopy
- There must be ease of egress and insertion of the wire guide even if the tube is looped in the stomach; this requires the lumen to have a hydrophilic coating.

Nasopharyngeal intubation

If the patient cannot say which nostril is the easiest to breathe through, proceed with caution. Deviation to the nasal septum from a past trauma often means that one nasal passage is significantly easier than the other. Unless there are contraindications, a nostril is anesthetized with a *lidocaine spray*.

There is no need for the patient either to sit up or swallow water to assist with intubation (in many cases neither is possible due to the patient's condition). Rather than supporting the head, which might make the patient feel trapped, the pillow when laid flat will provide its own support.

- A fine bore (FB) tube with a hydrophilic coating to its lumen is of significant benefit.
- Flush the tube and wet the tip, additional KY jelly will be required.
- Removing the stilette approximately 3 cm, the tube is passed over the ridge of the anterior nasal spine of the maxilla then passes downwards in a slightly medial line through the nasal vestibule, along the line of the hard palate. The patient's head may be tilted back to reduce the acute nature of the angle between the nasal passage and the oropharynx.
- Gentle forward pressure may be required on the tube to pass it over the fibrous lamella and out of the nasopharynx. The fibrous lamella (the palatine aponeurosis), supports muscles including the tensor and levator palatini muscles.
- Feel for resistance in the nasopharynx.
- Watch and use volitional or involitional swallowing.
- Watch for any change in the patient that night suggest misintubation:
  - Color
  - Cough
  - Distress
  - Try and sense tube movement and picture what is happening and where.

If pharyngeal intubation is not achieved or the patient demonstrates distress, it might be due to the tube passing into the middle nasal meatus or prominence of the superior aspect of the palatine aponeurosis directing the tube superiorly towards the basilar part of the occipital bone.

> **BOX 11.2** Pharyngeal complications that might require lateral fluoroscopy to guide naso- and oropharyngeal intubation
>
> - Difficulty in determining nasal passage
> - Post faciomaxillary trauma
> - Prominent cricopharyngeus
> - Cervical osteophyte impression
> - Loss of swallowing and gag reflex
> - Presence of an endotracheal tube
> - Post cervical spine surgery
> - Presence of a pharyngeal pouch

Intubation of a critically ill patient (for example, one who has a serious base of skull fracture) will be aided by the use of a 'C' arm to enable horizontal beam lateral screening. This enables the passage of the tube across the posterior border of the nasopharynx to be observed.

Conventional fluoroscopy can be used in the majority of cases. Where the patient is able to turn, lateral imaging can assist when blind naso- or oropharyngeal intubation has been problematic and direct guidance is required (Box 11.2).

With *complicated intubations*, it is important that the tube should be as streamlined as possible and as small a size as possible (i.e. 8 Fg for adults, 6 Fg for children). A *hydrophilic coating* to the lumen allows easy movement of the stylet. It is the skill the practitioner acquires in understanding the feel and interplay between the tube and stylet that is all important. Generally, withdrawing the stylet a relevant distance will provide flexibility to the tube, allowing it to find its own way with a degree of forward guidance, inserting the stylet when the distal end of the tube requires either straightening or else when more direct forward pressure is necessary.

There is always a chance of *pharyngeal pathology*, such as a pouch, which can be intubated, with the attendant risk of rupture by the tube (Stroud et al., 2003). However, with care, the pouch can often be by-passed. Large pouches can impress on the esophagus. This can be confirmed with the patient swallowing a water-soluble contrast medium and, if necessary, occluding the pouch neck with a Foley balloon which also helps deviate the tube into the esophagus (Birchall and Law, 1987) (Figures 11.7 and 11.8).

It is an important part of the underpinning knowledge required of anyone developing fluoroscopically guided intubation as a skill to understand the nature and potential hazards of transgressing pathological, traumatic or surgical deviations to the normal anatomical pathway.

The vast majority of trans-naso-esophageal intubations are straightforward and able to be dealt with within the ward environment. Contraindications or occasions where caution must be applied should be considered whether intubation is blind or fluoroscopically guided (Box 11.3).

Trans-esophageal intubation

Normally, once the esophagus has been intubated, onward passage into the stomach occurs without incident; however, the normal gastric fundus can produce a prominent posterior ballooning. A fine bore tube can loop in the

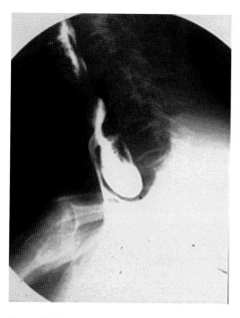

Figure 11.7 Barium in a pharyngeal pouch.

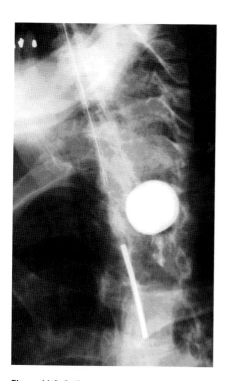

Figure 11.8 Balloon occluding pharyngeal pouch showing a tube passing directly into the esophagus.

fundus. If the tube does not have a hydrophilic coating, looping can make it difficult to remove the stylet. Even if a tube has a hydrophilic coating, ballooning of the fundus can cause problems in passing the tube into the gastric antrum.

BOX 11.3 Cautions and contraindications of pathological, surgical or traumatic origin

- Deviation or occlusion to the nasal septum
- Compression of the pharynx
- Loss of swallow or gag reflex
- Pharyngeal pouch or diverticulum
- Hemangioma
- Perforation
- Fistula
- Benign or malignant stricturing
- Esophageal varices
- Ulceration
- Hiatus hernia
- Post upper gastrointestional resection
- Anastomotic leaks

With the patient supine, withdraw the stylet to the gastro-esophageal (GO) junction, advance the tube until a long loop is passed into the gastric antrum. It does not matter that the tube tip is still lodged and looped in the fundus. Maintaining the stylet at the GO junction, gently withdraw the tube until the looping in the fundus is uncoiled. Advance the stylet to the apex of the loop in the antrum, then, using a paradoxical movement, gently withdraw the tube back over the stiletto until the tip flicks forward, then advance both together.

If the patient is mobile, it may assist in the passage of the tube tip from gastric fundus to body by having the patient lying on their right side and infuse air through the tube to distend the fundus, reducing the risk of the tube tip lodging. With the stylet maintained at the GO junction, even if a loop occurs, onward passage into the gastric body can be achieved. Maintaining tube tip position, the loop can now be uncoiled before advancing the stylet.

Perforation

Using a non-ionic hypo-osmolar *water-soluble contrast medium* (such as Ultravist 240) to identify the location of the lesion, the patient may require turning so that the side of the lesion is raised and the tube lies on the dependent wall as it passes the site of the leak (Figure 11.9).

Hemangioma and esophageal varices

Inserting a tube past lesions that have the propensity to bleed profusely should only be undertaken following considered discussion and then with great care (Stroud et al., 2003).

Hiatus hernia

A hiatus hernia is not an uncommon occurence; slightly less common is when the hernia is volved and incarcerated. To circumvent this type of hernia with

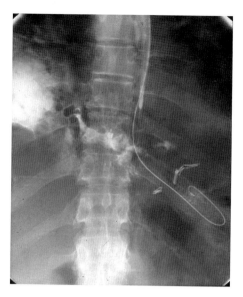

Figure 11.9 Wire guided intubation bypassing an iatrogenic perforation at the esophagogastric junction.

an FB tube, it may be of value for a contrast agent, such as dilute barium or Gastromiro, to be swallowed by the patient or infused to outline the intrathoracic stomach.

Turning the patient may be required to enable the barium to be passed around the gastric loop. The tube is passed around the initial gastric curve, adjusting the stylet as required, then further advanced to the diaphragmatic hiatus. With a final advancement of the stylet, the tube is passed through the diaphragmatic hiatus (Figure 11.10).

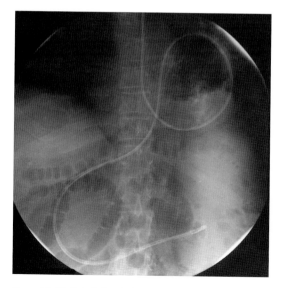

Figure 11.10 Enteric intubation via an incarcerated hiatus hernia.

Benign stricturing

Examples include achalasia, fibrotic and postoperative stricturing. As much the complication to intubation in these circumstances as passage through the stricture is tube coiling within the distended esophagus or stomach.

Malignant stricturing

It is important to have full knowledge of the tract through a malignant stricture whether intubation is for fine bore feeding or as a part of a stent (SEMS) deployment (Law, 2008). The patient either swallows a mouthful of barium or it is infused through the tube when sited at the proximal end of the lesion. The lumen through a neoplastic stricture can often be tortuous and there is always the concern as to the presence of fistulous tracts.

Often, an *8 Fg fine bore tube* can be passed into and through a stricture. If passage proves problematic, maintain the tube at the proximal end of the stricture and advance a *260 cm 0.35 'Jag' wire* which may be fine and soft enough to be fed through the stricture. Subsequently, railroad the tube over the wire. A *Lunderquist torque control wire* might be considered, replacing the stylet within the NG tube to improve manipulative capability. Open ended tubes, such as the 5 Fg Van Andel exchange cannula or straight or angled Cordis type catheter, can allow tube access through a particularly problematic stricure. Use a stiff guide wire exchange if a tube is required to be passed beyond the lesion (Figure 11.11).

Anastomotic leaks. Perforated duodenal ulceration

Fluoroscopic visualization of an anastomotic leak or perforation should be undertaken using a water-soluble contrast agent, as this will aid tube guidance past the area of concern (Law, 1990). It is important that the tube is directed

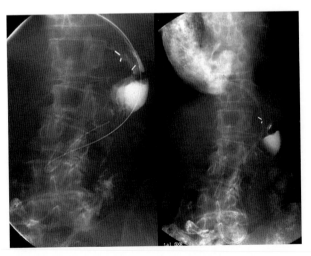

Figure 11.11 Previous esophagectomy for carcinoma. Wire guided intubation demonstrated via a neoplastic stricture in the gastric antrum.

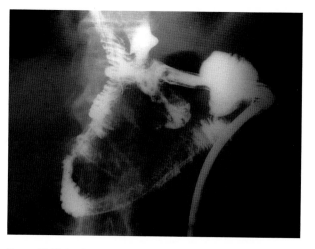

Figure 11.12 Intubation bypassing post gastrectomy anastomotic leak.

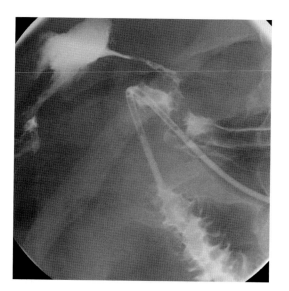

Figure 11.13 Intubation distal to postoperative duodenal leak.

away from the leak or perforation. A soft tipped wire, such as the angled 'Jag', will assist in directing the passage of the tube (Figures 11.12 and 11.13).

Gastro-duodenal intubation

Fluoroscopically guided enteral intubation has a high success rate. Law et al. (2004) reported a success rate of 98% in a series of 1011 attempted intubations for enteroclysis.

Technique

Nasogastric intubation has already been discussed; subsequent small bowel access may be achieved with gentle forward probing, with the stylet withdrawn, in the region of the pylorus. If the tube appears to loop across the origin of the pylorus, insert the wire to put some spring tension on the tube and draw it back: it can 'flip' into the canal.

The main problem with intubation of the duodenum is that the line of the pylorus and duodenal bulb is not necessarily that which might be suggested from schematic representations of anatomy. Without over distending the stomach, the *infusion of air* will act as a contrast agent to outline the gastric lumen, pylorus and duodenum. It will also reduce the chance of the tube tip lodging in a ruggal folds. With air in the stomach and the stylet withdrawn approximately 10 cm, the more flexible distal end of the tube may be advanced and effectively 'surfed' on a gastric wave to the pyloric origin and, in many instances, on through into the duodenal bulb. The best viewing of the pylorus and air distended duodenal bulb may require the patient to turn into the right anterior oblique position (Figure 11.14).

An alternative approach is with the patient turned towards their right side and infusing barium or a water-soluble contrast agent (depending on the clinical history) into the gastric antrum. The contrast pool at the pylorus offers viewing of its passage into the duodenum.

Duodenal obstruction may require intubation for diagnostic, nutritional or interventional purposes.

With the patient turned towards their right side, the liquid contrast agent has a greater chance of remaining in the second part of the duodenum. If the stricture is too tight for easy transgression, it would be worth considering a fine soft wire such as the 'Jag' via an open ended Law II tube. Once the passage of a wire has been achieved, the tube can be fed over the wire. If intubation were oro-enteric as a precursor to stenting, an 'extra stiff' or 'super stiff' wire can subsequently be introduced via the tube (Figures 11.15, 11.16, 11.17 and 11.18).

Gastroduodenal obstruction will often result in fluid distending the stomach. The viscous nature of the gastric fluid will make tube manipulation more difficult and a likelihood of tube coiling. If intubation for diagnostic or nutritional purposes is required, a nasogastric drain should be considered. If a drainage tube is already in situ, it should be ascertained if it is likely to

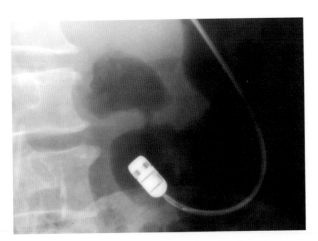

Figure 11.14 Early image of a wire guided Crosby capsule showing the use of air contrast to outline the pylorus and duodenal bulb.

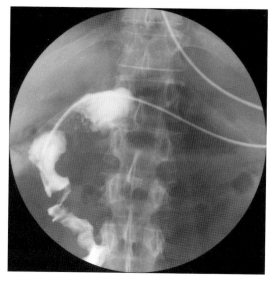

Figure 11.15 Contrast infused via a tube sited immediately proximal to duodenal stricture.

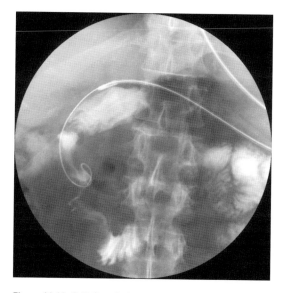

Figure 11.16 Soft tipped wire advanced and manipulated across stricture.

be removed, or whether endoscopy is to be undertaken in the near future. The removal of the drainage tube or endoscope is likely to extract the in situ fine bore tube. If stenting is to be undertaken through a fluid distended stomach, an endoscopic technique will most likely be required.

Complications associated with trans-nasal extubation

Although complications associated with extubation of fine bore tubes are uncommon, two that may occur are the *knotting of an enteral tube* that has migrated back into the stomach, or a *tube tip that (due to its size and shape)*

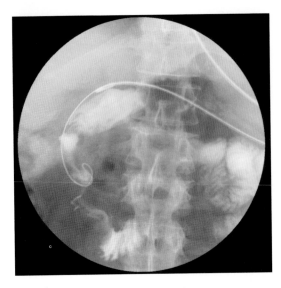

Figure 11.17 Tube advanced over the wire.

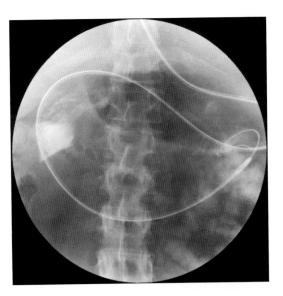

Figure 11.18 Tube sited at the duodenal/jejunal flexure.

lodges in the nasal concha. In both cases, extubation should not be forced. In the case of the tube lodging in the concha, it should be advanced on into the esophagus. A tube recovery can be undertaken with the patient placed on their side (with suction immediately available). A tongue depressor and pen torch are used to enable the tube to be viewed in the oropharynx. The tube is then grasped with long handled forceps, drawn out of the mouth and cut (while maintaining hold of the loop). The proximal end of the tube is then withdrawn through the nose and the distal length of tube can be removed transorally.

Cannulation via stoma, fistula and per rectum

Retrograde intubation can be of value for both diagnostic and therapeutic purposes (Law, 2005). With retrograde intubation, a hypotonic agent is of value to relax peristalsis as well as allow contrast distension of the lumen. Use of retrograde intubation would include:

- Intubating fistulae as a means of identifying their internal point of connection
- Replacing long-standing jejunostomy tubes that are blocked or have fallen out
- Ileostomy intubation to undertake a retrograde fluoroscopic examination of the small bowel
- Colostomy or rectal fine bore intubation, either as part of a diagnostic contrast examination or as part of a therapeutic procedure.

The patient experience

Lidocaine can produce an unpleasant taste as it passes through the nasal cavity and trickles into the oropharynx, and the transient smarting can make the eyes water. However, the local anesthetic does reduce the discomfort of the most unpleasant part of the procedure, the trans-nasal passage into the oropharynx.

There can be the desire to retch as the tube passes through the pharynx and also the stomach. There is also the risk of intubation causing the patient to vomit and potentially to aspirate.

References

Birchall, I.W.J., Law, R.L., 1987. Balloon occlusion of pharyngeal pouch as aid to naso-enteric intubation. Br. Med. J. 294, 1464.

Bain, T., 2005. (September) Testing nasogastric tube position: audit of three adult intensive care units, National Patient Safety Agency, London.

Law, R.L., 1990. The value of fluoroscopy as an aid to problematic intubation of fine bore feeding tubes. J. Interven. Radiol. 5, 171–173.

Law, R.L., 2005. Abscess drainage as a part of a gastrografin enema. Radiography 11 (4), 286–289.

Law, R.L., 2006. A surprise case of colonic interposition. Radiography 12 (1), 31–33.

Law, R.L., 2008. Radiographer involvement with stent insertion to palliate symptomatic dysphagia resulting from neoplastic obstruction. Radiography 14, 39–44.

Law, R.L., Longstaff, A.J., 1992. Technical report: a 'new' tube providing rapid insertion for the small bowel enema. Clin. Radiol. 45 (1), 35–36.

Law, R.L., Slack, N.F., Harvey, R.F., 2004. Single contrast small bowel enteroclysis: the province of the radiographer? Clin. Radiol. 59 (7), 642.

Law, R.L., Slack, N.F., Harvey, R.F., 2005. Radiographer performed single contrast small bowel enteroclysis. Radiography 11 (1), 11–15.

National Patient Safety Agency, 2005 (February). Reduced harm caused by misplaced feeding tubes. National Patient Safety Agency. Newsline: www.npsa.nhs.uk

National Patient Safety Agency, 2007 (April). Nasogastric tube incidents: update. Patient Safety Bulletin 3. www.npsa.uk/pso

Pillai, J.B., Vegar, A., Brister, S., 2005. Thoracic complications of nasogastric tube: review of safe practice. Interac. Cardiovasc. Thorac. Surg. 4, 429–433.

Prager, R., Laboy, V., Venus, B., 1986. Value of fluoroscopic assistance during transpyloric intubation. Crit. Care Med. 14 (2), 151–152.

Price, R.C., Le Masurier, S.B., 2007. Longitudinal changes in extended roles in radiography: a new perspective. Radiography 13 (1), 18–29.

Quine, M.A., Bell, G.D., 1995. Prospective audit of upper gastrointestinal endoscopy in two regions of England: safety, staffing, and sedation methods. Gut 36, 462–467.

Stroud, M., Duncan, H., Nightingale, J., 2003. Guidelines for enteral feeding in adult hospital patients. Gut 52 (7), 1–12.

Teague, R., 2003. Clinical practice guidelines update: safety and sedation during endoscopic procedures. British Society of Gastroenterology. <http://www.bsg.org.uk>

Fluoroscopic investigations of the small bowel

Robert L. Law

Contents |||||||||||||||||||||||||||||||||||||||||||||||||||||||||||||||||||||||

Introduction

When compared with the high technical standards expected of barium radiology of the upper gastrointestinal tract and the double contrast barium enema, small bowel imaging could be considered to be the poor relation. Maglinte et al. (1996) suggest that small bowel imaging has been 'performed casually without attention to detail', 'for the sake of completeness'. That said, the strengths and weaknesses of barium examinations of the small bowel have all been thoroughly examined in the past and have stood the test of time. Although many of the papers on the subject were published in the 1990s, 1980s or even the 1970s, their conclusions are still relevant today.

Antes (2003) raised the concern that, with the decrease in frequency of barium examinations, 'the art of performance and interpretation (of these examinations) might get lost'. The development of computed tomography (CT) and magnetic resonance (MR) software has enabled cross-sectional imaging to establish a number of techniques to demonstrate the small bowel, but alternative modalities should only replace tried and tested techniques with caution.

Barium examinations of the small bowel using the *enteroclysis technique* are now often used as a benchmark comparator to define the capabilities of the newer and more 'high tech' small bowel imaging techniques. However, with non-medical practitioners developing a role in the performing and diagnosis of examinations previously the remit of the radiologist, the whole concept of time/cost efficiency and effectiveness of barium fluoroscopy for examining the small bowel could be revisited.

Price and Le Masurier (2007) suggest that, in the UK, 80% of District General Hospitals now have radiographers performing barium fluoroscopy, predominantly the double contrast barium enema. Historically, small bowel radiology has been the province of radiologists, but Law et al. (2005) demonstrated that radiographer performance and reporting of small bowel enteroclysis (SBE) has a sensitivity and specificity comparable to published standards.

The barium follow through (BaFT) and the small bowel enteroclysis (SBE) examination have strengths and weaknesses that need to be considered when deciding what investigation to use and when. In this chapter, we will be comparing and contrasting the various techniques for imaging the small bowel including the BaFT, SBE, ileostomy enema (IE) and Gastrografin follow-through.

Unlike upper and lower GI tract investigations, the radiological approach to investigating the small bowel is not well defined and local preference and expediency is more closely involved in the equation to determine what is considered acceptable and best practice. Departments that routinely perform small bowel enteroclysis are still in the minority (Ha et al., 2004).

Bowel preparation

To optimize small bowel barium examinations, the stomach, small bowel and right colon should be empty. Gastric fluid might precipitate vomiting and, if gastric residue is excessive, its viscous nature might also inhibit manipulation of an enteral tube.

It is not necessary to have the right colon as clear as you might wish for a double contrast barium enema, although marked fecal residue in the ascending colon can inhibit the passage of barium through the distal small bowel and ileocecal valve. A degree of clearance might also enable gross pathology affecting the iliocecal valve or proximal colon to be identified (Law, 1983; Nolan and Traill, 1997).

Certain drugs, such as sedatives, tranquillizers and antispasmodic agents, inhibit peristalsis and consideration should be given to stop these medications. Additionally, antidiarrhea medications should ideally be curtailed approximately 48 hours prior to initiating any bowel preparation.

Bowel preparation for small bowel examinations in the presence of a subacute obstruction or iliostomy should not include any purgation.

Flocculation

To maintain barium in suspension, manufacturers provide the barium particles with a protective coating, maintaining them in a separate state from one another. Muco-proteins generated in the GI tract are absorbed by the barium particles and, if prolonged exposure occurs, the absorption breaks down the protective coating of the particles allowing them to clump together. This is known as flocculation.

Flocculated barium is incapable of coating the bowel wall, reducing the diagnostic potential of the examination. The severity of flocculation will depend upon the number of particles affected.

In normal instances, there is a greater likelihood of flocculation occurring with the BaFT due to the slower transit of barium through the small bowel. Its occurrence is non-specific, but should flocculation occur during the more rapid transit of enteroclysis, there is a greater likelihood of flocculation being relevant to the diagnosis (Lomoschitz et al., 2003).

The per oral barium follow through (BaFT)

The BaFT examination is far more widely used to image the small bowel than enteroclysis. Toms et al. (2001) offered a number of reasons why the BaFT might be advocated:

- It is considered by some to be a quicker technique than the SBE suggesting that more examinations can be performed per list. Depending upon the selected technique, the time spent in the fluoroscopy room can be almost half that of the SBE (a median of 24.5 min as compared to 45 min for the SBE).
- The BaFT is better tolerated, predominantly due to the lack of intubation.

Ha et al. (2004), in reviewing radiographic examinations of the small bowel and practice patterns in the USA, stated that the BaFT is the dominant small bowel examination in the USA. The main examination technique consists of *over-couch radiographs* (of the whole abdomen), which should be coupled with *fluoroscopic spot images* of the terminal ileum. However, the paper also states the BaFT technique advocated by the American College of Roentgenologists is fluoroscopy-dependent, with *palpation* of all accessible small bowel loops including the terminal ileum, with appropriate images to demonstrate any abnormality or representative images if no abnormality is demonstrated. The technique that is advocated can result in a more time-consuming examination. Maglinte et al. (1996) state that the BaFT as 'conventionally performed has no place in the practice of cost effective medicine'. The use of the *fluoroscopy-dependent BaFT* technique is well supported (Maglinte et al., 1987, 1996; Ha et al., 2004).

The BaFT might be considered 'safer' and less invasive than the SBE and preferred by most patients as it does not require enteral intubation. Some practitioners consider the BaFT the examination of choice in known Crohn's disease. In its simplest form, the least advocated BaFT technique requires minimal fluoroscopy room occupation and might thus be considered less labour intensive (Maglinte et al., 1987, 1996; Bernstein et al., 1997; Nolan and Traill, 1997; Toms et al., 2001).

Barium follow through technique

A considered barium solution might comprise 300 ml Baritop 100 (Sanochemia UK), diluted with 400 ml water (75% w/v), 10 ml Gastrografin and 6 sachets of Carbex granules. The combined use of the hyperosmolar Gastrografin and the effervescent agent Carbex can significantly reduce *small bowel transit time* without affecting the examination quality (Summers et al., 2007); 600 ml of solution is ingested in as short a time as the patient finds comfortable.

Laying the patient on their right side for 15 minutes assists with barium passage into the duodenum. The practitioner places the patient supine for fluoroscopy, palpation and imaging when appropriate. If the stomach is seen to empty of contrast, sit the patient up to ingest a further 100 ml of barium solution before returning them to the right lateral position.

Once barium is in the colon, relaxing the bowel muscle by using an *intravenous hypotonic agent* has been reported as being of value (Bernstein et al., 1997). *Focal images* are taken of the terminal ileum and any identified abnormality as well as fluoroscopic or over-couch images taken to demonstrate an overview of the whole small bowel (Box 12.1).

Limitations of the barium follow through

Nolan and Traill (1997) and Toms et al. (2001) suggest that because of the nature of the technique, a higher number of BaFT examinations require further investigation to confirm normality or otherwise. Good distension is not usually achieved therefore early strictures, subtle appearances and fine nodules are more likely to be missed.

Maglinte et al. (1987, 1996) report that the sensitivity and specificity of the BaFT is technique and operator dependent, although Maglinte et al. (1982) refer to diagnostic errors being more of a technical nature than perceptual.

BOX 12.1 Single contrast barium follow through technique

- A solution of 300 ml of 100% barium (Baritop 100), 400 ml of water, 10 ml Gastrografin and 6 sachets of Carbex granules (23% w/v)
- Initially, the patient ingests 600 ml of barium solution
- Lay the patient on the right side to aid barium passage out of the stomach
- If barium appears to be delayed, it may be due to air trapped within the small bowel; in these instances, it is worth considering intermittently turning the patient into the prone position to aid onward passage
- Observe, palpate and image (magnify as appropriate)
- Give the patient more barium solution if the stomach is seen to be devoid of contrast
- Injection of an IV hypotonic agent (1 mg in 1 ml Buscopan or 10 mg in 1 ml glucagon) will halt peristalsis when barium reaches the colon
- Thoroughly palpate and image the terminal ileum
- Provide an overview image of the whole small bowel

Small bowel enema or enteroclysis (SBE)

The word *enteroclysis* derives from the Greek words 'enteron' meaning 'intestine' and 'klysis' meaning 'a high enema'. Its use in the context of this examination is of uncertain origin but might be to disassociate from the word enema and the perception that rectal intubation will be required.

Despite advances in other imaging techniques and the limited popularity of *small bowel enteroclysis*, the SBE is widely accepted as currently being the optimum technique for examining the small bowel. The SBE is also commonly used as the reference point for other small bowel imaging methods (Maglinte et al., 1987, 1992; Nolan and Traill, 1997; Nolan, 1997; Antes, 2003).

The techniques of performing small bowel enteroclysis have evolved over 80 years. Pesquera (1929) published a technique using duodenal intubation as a means of infusing a barium, acacia and water mixture that enabled the demonstration of the whole small bowel. Sellink (1976) mentions Gershon-Cohen and Shay (1939), Scott-Harden et al. (1961) and Bilbao et al. (1967) who, among others, over the intervening years, advanced the development of techniques to examine the small bowel. In the 1970s, single contrast enteroclysis re-emerged, gaining popularity through the distillation of ideas and publications of advocates such as Sellink (1974) who consider the mitigating features of the SBE outweigh the arguments that are put forward against its use.

The patient experience

- Local anesthetic spray causes a transient cold sting to the affected nasal mucosa and has an unpleasant taste when it trickles into the oropharynx
- Initial passage of the tube is uncomfortable, this can be more marked if transit through the nasal passage is problematic but, in normal instances, discomfort is reduced once the tube is in the esophagus
- Some patients have a low tolerance to oropharyngeal irritation resulting in retching and the patient becoming distressed (this must be taken into account when considering continuing intubation or converting to a BaFT)
- Once in situ the tube will be felt as a minor irritant in the throat
- Barium passage through the tube will feel cool, the patient might also feel bloated with barium infusion, particularly if there is delay in passage through the small bowel
- The justification of using an intubation technique should be considered where transit is known to be slow, such as in the presence of known motility disorders.

Principle of the single contrast SBE technique

The SBE can be performed by a radiologist, radiographer or radiologic technologist. It involves the *trans-nasal insertion* of a *fine bore tube* (commonly 10 Fg) as far as the duodenal jejunal flexure.

A *low density barium suspension* of around 20% w/v (such as 300 ml Baritop 100 diluted with 1500 ml water) is infused through the tube at a rate that

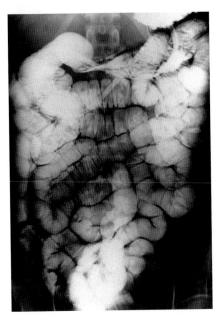

Figure 12.1 The single contrast small bowel enema.

allows a single column of barium to distend and pass through the small bowel to the colon (Figure 12.1).

Barium transit to the colon is reported as often being less than 35 minutes. Optimum results are best achieved by:

- The operator being in attendance throughout the examination
- Obtaining good small bowel distension
- The frequent intermittent observation of the barium column
- Thorough *small bowel palpation*. (With the use of a palpating spoon overlapping small bowel loops can be compressed and separated to demonstrate pliability or to assist in demonstrating abnormalities such as adhesions (Figures 12.2 and 12.3), terminal ileal Crohn's disease (Figure 12.4), fistulae (Figure 12.5) or polypoid lesions (e.g. malignant melanoma) (Figure 12.6A&B).

Spot images should be taken at appropriate times to record the whole of the distended small bowel and, in particular, the terminal ilium. More focused images should be taken to record any abnormality. If barium is in the colon, a cursory examination of the demonstrated large bowel can be of value (Figure 12.7) (Maglinte et al., 1982, 1996; Goei et al., 1988; Bessette et al., 1989; Nolan, 2000).

Advantages of the SBE

The SBE is widely reported as having a high sensitivity, specificity and positive predictive value for small bowel stricturing and mucosal abnormalities (Barloon et al., 1994; Nolan, 2000). The SBE has also been reported as having a sensitivity of between 93% and 100% for Crohn's disease (Maglinte et al., 1980, 1982, 1985, 1987, 1992, 1996; Bessette et al., 1989;

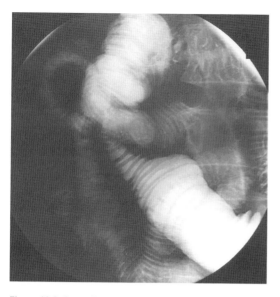

Figure 12.2 Star adheson without palpation.

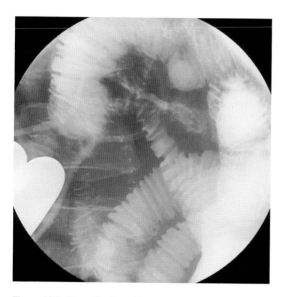

Figure 12.3 Star adhesion with palpation.

Chen et al., 1991; Chernish et al., 1992; Link et al., 1993; Nolan, 1997; Nolan and Traill, 1997; Lappas and Maglinte, 1990; Cirillo et al., 2000; Mako et al., 2000; Reiber et al., 2000; Toms et al., 2001; Law et al., 2005).

The high negative predictive value of the SBE is also important in the exclusion of pathology. If the presence of small bowel Crohn's disease is being questioned, further imaging is considered unnecessary in light of an SBE reported as normal by an experienced reviewer (Law et al., 2005).

Enteroclysis remains a primary investigation if clinically a Meckel's diverticulum is suspected. Observing the flow of barium through the small bowel in conjunction with palpation can enable Meckel's diverticulum to be identified (Figure 12.8).

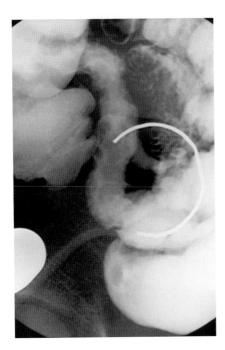

Figure 12.4 Palpation of Crohn's disease with cobblestone ulceration.

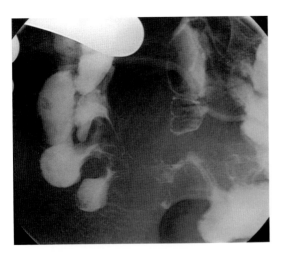

Figure 12.5 Terminal ileal Crohn's disease with enterocolic fistulae and incidental Meckel's diverticulum.

Partial small bowel obstruction (SBO) is well demonstrated by enteroclysis. With high SBO, intubation is of value as fluid in the stomach or small bowel can be aspirated prior to barium infusion.

Critically ill or symptomatic, frail, elderly patients may well be unable to tolerate swallowing the volume of barium required for a BaFT, but can often tolerate barium infused through a tube. The SBE requires minimal movement and only one visit to the fluoroscopy room; additional confirmatory imaging is not normally required. The main clinical indications for the SBE are given in Box 12.2. The value of the SBE is tabulated in Box 12.3.

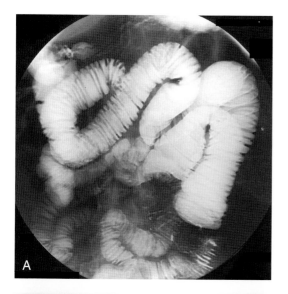

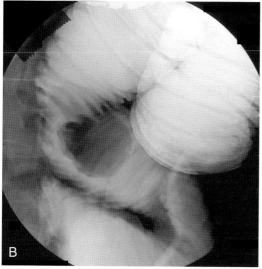

Figure 12.6 (A)&(B) Malignant melanoma causing partial small bowel obstruction.

The enteroclysis tube

Intubation requires patient consent and compliance. The psychological preparation of the patient is important if maximum cooperation and a successful examination is to be obtained. An explanation of what is involved should be given by someone accredited to undertake the procedure. It has been suggested that poor patient tolerance is related to lack of operator experience not the technique (Maglinte et al., 1987, 1996).

The size of the tube lumen can affect patient comfort, ease of intubation and flow rate. Over the last twenty years, enteroclysis tube styles and dimensions have changed; in the 1990s tubes of 14 French gauge (Fg) were often

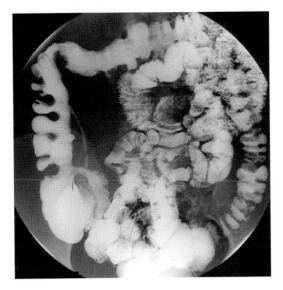

Figure 12.7   Normal small bowel, colonic Crohn's disease.

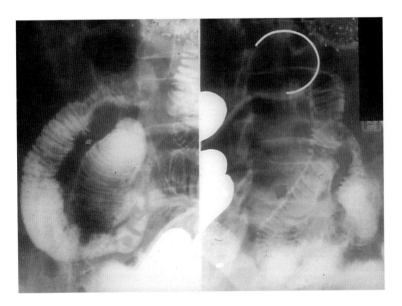

Figure 12.8   Two examples of Meckel's diverticulum.

employed, however, these sizes are now considered both uncomfortable and unnecessary. Tubes with tungsten weighted tips are also unnecessary, increasing patient discomfort and having a limited manipulative capability. *Unweighted 10 Fg polyurethane tubes* are considered to have a high intubation success rate with the minimum of discomfort (Goei et al., 1988; Nolan and Traill, 1997; Toms et al., 2001; Law et al., 2005).

BOX 12.2 Clinical indications for small bowel enteroclysis

- Abdominal pain
- Clinical suspicion of inflammatory bowel disease
- Exacerbation of known small bowel Crohn's disease
- Diarrhea
- Subacute small bowel obstruction
- Malabsorption
- Unexplained GI bleeding (upper and lower GI endoscopy normal)
- Post surgical evaluation
- Continued high suspicion of abnormality despite negative or inconclusive BaFT

BOX 12.3 Benefits of small bowel enteroclysis

- Widely considered the reference point for other SB imaging techniques
- High sensitivity and specificity
- High negative predictive value
- High positive predictive value
- High sensitivity and specificity for Crohn's disease
- Good demonstration of fistula
- Number and extent of adhesive subacute obstructions
- Of value where, via oral ingestion, a significant volume of barium would not be tolerated (i.e. acutely ill and frail patients)
- Of value for unexplained GI bleeding, Meckel's and small bowel neoplasia
- Transit time often 20–35 minutes
- Can be performed by radiographers/radiologic technologists

If a patient has *an indwelling gastric drainage tube,* there is nothing to preclude an enteroclysis tube being inserted through the other nostril. Enteroclysis techniques can also be adapted to use a *pre-existing enteral tube,* the in situ tube negating the need to pass a specific enteroclysis tube. However, the practitioner must be aware of the type of tube in situ – if the tube has numerous side ports, barium might be infused into the stomach and not the small bowel. During extubation, attaching a 20 ml syringe with which to apply gentle suction will prevent barium in the lumen from draining into the nose or pharynx.

Contraindications

There are few absolute contraindications to intubation; these would include:

- Lack of, or withdrawal of, consent to intubate
- Previous failure to intubate by a competent practitioner due to patient distress
- High risk comorbidity, such as poorly controlled angina
- The known presence of hemangioma or esophageal varices where there would be a risk of a significant bleed.

There are some relative contraindications to *nasoenteric intubation* and careful consideration should be given as to the justification, nature and approach to intubation (i.e. nasal or oral route); these would include:

- Patients prone to severe nose bleeds
- Where there is a known active ulceration, particularly of the pyloric canal or duodenal bulb (there is a risk of perforating through the ulcer crater in attempting passage of the tube tip)
- Patients with sinusitis
- Where there has been recent trauma or surgical deviation to the nasal septum.

Intubation

Check with the patient for any contraindications to intubation. To provide a degree of *local anesthesia*, the selected nostril is sprayed with 2% lidocaine prior to the insertion of a naso-enteric tube. The patient should be warned that the lidocaine has an unpleasant taste as it passes into the oropharynx and might smart, bringing tears to the eyes. Nasal intubation is to be preferred as it is normally easier. Once intubated the discomfort for the patient should subside (Halligan et al., 1994).

Care has to be taken that the tube tip follows the line along the roof of the hard palate as it can so easily rise into the nasal concha through which passage will be difficult and uncomfortable despite local anesthesia. Although the patient might feel the tube in the back of the throat, the direct downwards passage of the tube reduces gagging and the patient cannot bite the tube. Should the patient retch or vomit, the tube is less likely to be expelled (Dixon et al., 1993) and there is little hindrance to the patient swallowing and talking.

During intubation, the patient lies on their right side, both for comfort as well as safety should they vomit. If the tube tip is repeatedly directed upwards into the nasopharynx, tilting the patient's head back can help make the angle between the hard palate and oropharynx less acute. The subsequent tilting of the head down can reduce the curvature of the cervical spine making onward passage towards the esophagus more direct. Fluoroscopy (ideally pulsed) can greatly assist in guiding the tube if blind passage proves problematic. Also of value is observing the patient swallow, either directly or fluoroscopically and then using the force of the swallow to propel the tube into the esophagus.

It is important that the intubator is aware of the potential presence of previously undiagnosed pathology that might cause a deviation to the normal anatomy, such as prominence of the cricopharyngeus muscle, pharyngeal diverticulum or, more distally, a hiatus hernia.

With the patient in the *right lateral position*, gas in the stomach will migrate into the fundus of the stomach making it significantly easier to pass the tip of the tube into the gastric body. If the stomach is devoid of air, try infusing 100 ml of air using a syringe. If there is a problem extricating the tube from the bowl of the gastric fundus, withdraw the wire as far as the gastro-esophaeal junction and advance the tube. The tip becomes lodged against the wall and a tube loop extends into the distal body or antrum. Passing the wire to the

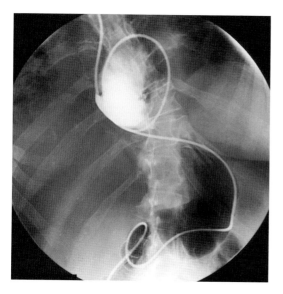

Figure 12.9 Naso-enteral intubation via a volved incarcerated hiatus hernia.

apex of the formed tube loop and using a paradoxical movement, while keeping the wire in position, gradually withdraw the tube over the wire until the tip flips forward.

The lumen of some tubes, such as the one described by Law and Longstaff (1992), has the advantage of a *hydrophilic coating* that allows ease of interplay between the tube and its guide wire. Tube length is also important as it should be enough to enable passage through complex anatomy such as a volved incarcerated hiatus hernia (Figure 12.9) or a distensile stomach.

With the tube in the gastric body, turn the patient supine and then to the right anterior oblique; air will now migrate towards the pylorus. With interplay between the tube and guide wire, the tube tip can 'ride' a peristaltic wave to the pylorus. The direction of the pyloric canal and duodenal bulb can alter significantly in position and it is worth observing air passage through the pylorus. If visualization is difficult, with the patient supine and the guide wire fully inserted, infuse 20 ml of dilute barium instead. If during passage the tube tip lodges in a small bowel fold or against the aortic impression, or as it passes through the third part of the duodenum, a 20 ml bolus of air will distend the lumen and, in most cases, dislodge the tube tip, enabling it to migrate to the duodenal-jejunal flexure. Should intubation still be unsuccessful, it may be because of occluding pathology (Figures 12.10, 12.11A, 12.11B) (see Chapter 11 for a detailed look at fine bore intubation).

Infusion techniques

Three methods are commonly used to infuse barium (Sellink, 1974; Maglinte et al., 1987; Goei et al., 1988).

Hydrostatic infusion: a bag of barium on a drip stand is connected to the naso-enteric tube. Raising and lowering the drip stand increases and reduces

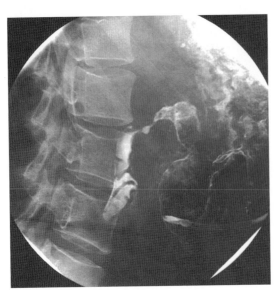

Figure 12.10 Failed intubation: duodenal ulcer and inflammatory stricture.

the infusion rate. If necessary, improved infusion pressure can be achieved by attaching a pressure cuff to the bag.

Syringing infusion: using two 50 ml syringes alternately to infuse barium through an 8 French gauge enteral tube, the potential jet effect can be controlled. The jet effect is where the pressure of the expelled barium forces a retrograde migration of the tip of the tube. Although it may not always be possible to obtain a continuous column, small bowel distension can be achieved. The operator needs to make sure the whole small bowel is observed and recorded in a distended form.

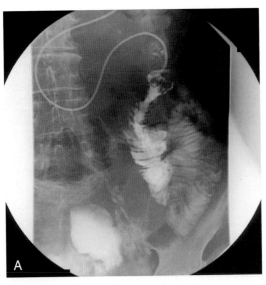

Figure 12.11 (A) Failed intubation: malignant small bowel stricture at site of gastroenterostomy;

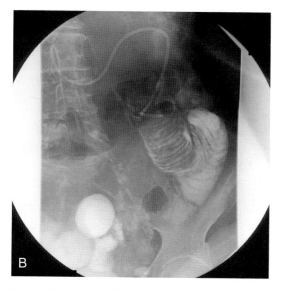

Figure 12.11—cont'd (B) intussusception at stricture site.

Infusion pumps: using an enteroclysis infusion pump, such as the one marketed by 'Guerbet' (Figure 12.12), barium can be infused through a 10 Fg tube enabling a continuous column of barium to distend and pass through the small bowel with no untoward jet effect. Flow can be optimized enabling immediate and measured adjustment of flow rate to adapt and respond to the peristaltic action and barium passage through the small bowel (Maglinte et al., 1987; Goei et al., 1988; Halligan et al., 1994; Nolan and Traill, 1997; Toms et al., 2001; Law et al., 2005).

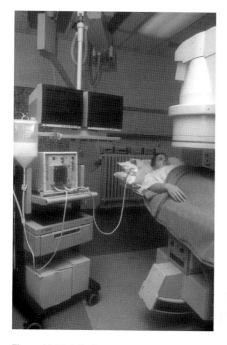

Figure 12.12 Infusion pump.

When using syringe infusion, the rate of flow is not usually a problem unless the bowel is obstructed. Hydrostatic and pump infusion should start slowly (50–60 ml/min) until peristalsis has initiated antegrade barium passage, at which point flow rate can be increased as appropriate to provide a distended single column. Flow rates in excess of 100 ml/min are not uncommon. If the flow rate is too high, the bowel lumen will become hypotonic. If hypotonia should occur, the barium infusion must be halted until peristalsis recommences.

If regular enteroclysis lists are undertaken, an infusion pump reduces labor intensity, particularly as infusion rates are easily adjusted leaving hands free for fluoroscopy and palpation.

Small bowel enteroclysis using methyl cellulose

Nolan and Traill (1997) describe a technique popularized by Herlinger (1978) in which an *ultra low density double contrast effect* can be produced by the infusion of 160–200 ml of 80–100% w/v barium sulfate, followed by up to 2000 ml of 0.5% aqueous solution of methyl cellulose (MC). Maglinte et al. (1987) also suggest a 'biphasic technique' variation for using MC; this involves infusing 400–500 ml of 50% w/v barium, performing a single contrast SBE followed by up to 2000 ml of MC.

The advantages offered by advocates of this technique include good mucosal detail offered by MC and, at the same time, the ability to view, palpate and image any abnormal segments demonstrated in single contrast by the header column. It has also been reported that MC aids in the evacuation of the contrast (Maglinte et al., 1987; Nolan and Traill, 1997).

Disadvantages of techniques using MC include the fluoroscopy and room time required to 'double view' the small bowel, initially in single then in double contrast. If MC gets ahead of the column of barium, from that point on, the diagnostic quality of the examination is compromised. This is particularly relevant when considering the frequency of distal ileal pathology such as Crohn's disease. There is no strong evidence that the use of MC greatly increases the diagnostic capability of the examination over that of the single contrast SBE. An oral version associated with the BaFT has been reported in which the ingestion of 200 ml of 70% w/v barium is followed by 600 ml of 0.5% MC (Ha et al., 1998).

Ileostomy enteroclysis

On occasion, the small bowel needs to be assessed in a patient with an ileostomy. If there is no known disruption to the small bowel, conventional enteroclysis can be performed. Bowel preparation for enteroclysis in the presence of an ileostomy should not include any purgation. With the patient in the supine position, it can assist with identifying the location of the ileostomy by taping a paperclip over the stoma site (Figure 12.13). The stoma and prestomal bowel is best viewed tangentially with the patient turned towards the right; in this way, prestomal strictures or parastomal hernia can best be identified (Figure 12.14). Inflammation in the prestomal small bowel is best seen with ileoscopy.

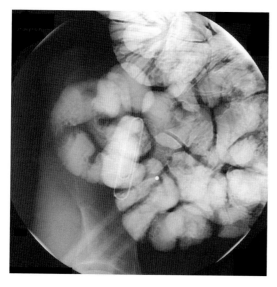

Figure 12.13 Antegrade small bowel enema to ileostomy (underlying paper clip).

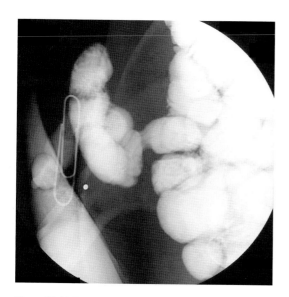

Figure 12.14 Tangential view demonstrating parastomal hernia.

If there is surgical or pathological disruption to the small bowel prevent-ing the imaging of the more distal bowel, *retrograde imaging* can be under-taken (Zagoria et al., 1986) (Figures 12.15 and 12.16).

With the patient supine, a small slit is made in the ileostomy bag towards the midline side (so that any expelled barium is contained). An unweighted 8 Fg 140 cm fine bore tube with a hydrophilic coated lumen is inserted into the stoma lumen and advanced as far as possible. Partially withdrawing the guide wire and using an interplay between tube and wire will enable the tip of the tube to be advanced. Intermittent pulsed fluoroscopy will identify tube site; dilute barium can be infused to demonstrate the direction of the small

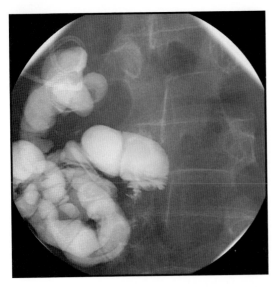

Figure 12.15 Retrograde ileostomy enema demonstrating metastatic stricture.

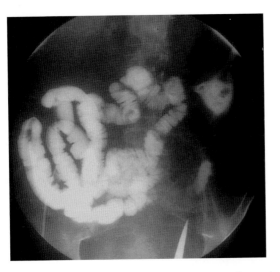

Figure 12.16 Retrograde ileostomy: fistula to psoas abscess located at 90 cm.

bowel lumen. Both intubation and enteroclysis are markedly assisted by the use of an intravenous hypotonic agent, not only does it ease retrograde infusion of barium but it also limits the risk of barium expulsion. If needed, suction can be used to remove any barium draining into the bag.

The use of air double contrast in the small bowel

With both *antegrade and retrograde air insufflation*, the patient may experience colicky abdominal pain and require analgesia. Because of the numerous over-lapping small bowel loops, the quality standards associated with the double contrast barium enema cannot be applied to the small bowel. Although it has

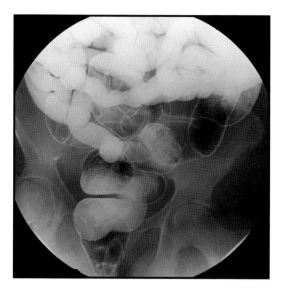

Figure 12.17 Retrograde transrectal small bowel enema.

been reported that air contrast can highlight aphthous ulcers, strictures can be missed with the use of air contrast (Nolan and Traill, 1997; Ha et al., 2004).

Antegrade: the introduction of air following barium as part of enteroclysis can provide good demonstration of the jejunum, although imaging of the mid/distal ileum may be inadequate, with poor demonstration of the clinically more problematic terminal ileum (Maglinte et al., 1987).

Retrograde: when a BaFT offers poor visualization of the terminal ileum, improved imaging is possible by the retrograde introduction of air after injecting a hypotonic agent such as Buscopan or glucagon. A rectal tube is inserted and the colon insufflated with air. Turning the patient allows air to migrate to the right colon and, in many instances, reflux through the ileocecal valve. A clean colon is desirable both to ease the passage of gas around the colon as well as reduce fecal reflux into the ileum (Nolan and Traill, 1997; Ha et al., 2004).

Post colectomy and ileorectal anastomosis: retrograde SBE is of particular benefit if pelvic small bowel adhesions are suspected following an ileorectal anastomosis. The examination requires the introduction of a double contrast enema tip and the IV injection of a hypotonic agent. A low density barium is hydrostatically infused per rectum. The subsequent introduction of air can be of value within the limits of patient comfort (Figure 12.17); however, retrograde imaging of the complete small bowel is not to be routinely advocated.

Gastrografin follow through

Due to the poor coating produced by water-soluble contrast media, this technique does not provide mucosal detail; however, it can be used to differentiate between complete and incomplete *adhesional obstruction* of the small bowel. The information gained by this technique significantly supports the decision either to operate or treat the patient conservatively.

One hundred milliliters of the hyperosmolar contrast medium 'Gastrografin' is given to the patient (orally or via a nasogastric tube), with an initial check abdominal x-ray being taken most commonly at 4–6 hours. If contrast has reached the colon within 24 hours, the patient is considered to have an incomplete (subacute) obstruction. The technique is safe and was found to reduce the need for surgical intervention in several studies (Choi et al., 2005, 2006; Al Salamah et al., 2006).

Complications associated with the SBE

Complications associated with naso-enteric intubation are covered in Chapter 11. Additional complications associated with barium infusion are likely to be vomiting and colic. Vomiting can occur if the infusion rate of the contrast is greater than the ability of peristalsis to initiate its onward passage into the small bowel, resulting in gastric reflux. Barium reflux can be overcome by reducing the infusion rate and, if necessary, turning the patient onto their right side to facilitate gastric drainage.

Pain can result from a number of complications, although it may be an aspect of the patient's clinical history. If pain is reported by the patient, then palpation should be undertaken with care and attempts made to identify the cause.

References

Al Salamah, S.M., Fahim, F., Mirza, S.M., 2006. Value of water soluble contrast (meglumine amidotrizoate) in the diagnosis and management of small bowel obstruction. World J. Surg. 30 (7), 1290–1294.

Antes, G., 2003. Barium examinations of the small intestine and colon in inflammatory bowel disease. Radiologe 43 (1), 9–16.

Barloon, T.J., Lu, C.C., Honda, H., et al., 1994. Does a normal small-bowel enteroclysis exclude small-bowel disease? A long-term follow-up of consecutive normal studies. Abdom. Imaging 134 (5), 925–932.

Bernstein, C.N., Boult, I.F., Greenberg, H.M., et al., 1997. A prospective randomized comparison between small bowel enteroclysis and small bowel follow-through in Crohn's disease. Gastroenterology 113 (2), 390–398.

Bessette, J.R., Maglinte, D.D., Kelvin, F.M., et al., 1989. Primary malignant tumors in the small bowel: a comparison of enema and conventional follow through examination. Am. J. Roentgenol. 153, 741–744.

Bilbao, M.K., Frische, L.H., Dotter, C.T., et al., 1967. Hypotonic duodenography. Radiology 89 (3), 438–443.

Chen, M.Y., Ott, D.J., Kelley, T.F., et al., 1991. Impact of the small bowel study on patients' management. Gastrointest. Radiol. 16 (3), 189–192.

Chernish, S.M., Maglinte, D.D., O'Connor, K., 1992. Evaluation of the small bowel by enteroclysis for Crohn's disease. Am. J. Gastroenterol. 87, 696–701.

Choi, H.K., Chu, K.W., Law, W.L., 2006. Therapeutic value of Gastrografin in adhesive small bowel obstruction after unsuccessful conservative treatment: a prospective randomised trial. Ann. Surg. 236 (1), 1–6.

Choi, H.K., Law, W.L., Ho, J.W., et al., 2005. Value of Gastrografin in adhesive small bowel obstruction after unsuccessful conservative treatment: a prospective evaluation. World J. Gastroenterol. 11 (24), 3742–3745.

Cirillo, L.C., Camera, L., Della Noce, M., et al., 2000. Accuracy of enteroclysis in Crohn's disease of the small bowel: a retrospective study. Eur. Radiol. 10 (12), 1894–1898.

Dixon, P.M., Roulston, M.E., Nolan, D.J., 1993. The small bowel enema: a ten year review. Clin. Radiol. 47 (1), 46–48.

Gershon-Cohen, J., Shay, H., 1939. Barium enteroclysis: a method for the direct immediate examination of the small intestine by single and double contrast technique. Am. J. Roentgenol. 82, 965.

Goei, R., Lamers, R.J., Lamers, J.J., 1988. Enteroclysis: improved performance using a flow inducer. Acta Radiol. 29 (6), 665–668.

Ha, H.K., Park, K.B., Kim, P.N., et al., 1998. Use of methyl cellulose in small bowel follow-through examination: comparison with conventional series in normal subjects. Abdom. Imaging 23 (3), 281–285.

Ha, A.S., Levine, M.S., Rubesin, S.E., et al., 2004. Radiographic examination of the small bowel: survey of practice patterns in the United States. Radiology 231 (2), 407–412.

Halligan, M.S., Jobling, J.C., Bartram, C.I., 1994. Benefits of intravenous muscle relaxants during barium follow through. Clin. Radiol. 49, 179–182.

Herlinger, H., 1978. A modified technique for the double-contrast small bowel enema. Gastrointest. Radiol. 3 (2), 201–207.

Lappas, J.C., Maglinte, D.D., 1990. Enteroclysis – a technique for examining the small bowel. CRC Crit. Rev. Diagn. Imaging 30 (2), 183–217.

Law, R.L., 1983. The small bowel enema. Radiography 49, 91–95.

Law, R.L., Longstaff, A.J., 1992. Technical report: a 'new' tube providing rapid insertion for the small bowel enema. Clin. Radiol. 45 (1), 35–36.

Law, R.L., Slack, N., Harvey, R.F., 2005. Radiographer performed single contrast small bowel enteroclysis. Radiography 11, 11–15.

Link, T.M., Koc, F., Peters, P.E., 1993. State of the art of selective small bowel enema. (Indications and results). Radiologe 33 (6), 343–346.

Lomoschitz, F., Schima, W., Schober, E., et al., 2003. Enteroclysis in adult celiac disease: diagnostic value of specific radiographic features. Eur. Radiol. 13 (4), 890–896.

Maglinte, D.D., Burney, B.T., Miller, R.E., 1982. Lesions missed on small bowel follow through. Radiology 144 (4), 737–739.

Maglinte, D.D., Chernish, S.M., Kelvin, S.M., et al., 1992. Crohn's disease of the small intestine: accuracy and relevance of enteroclysis. Radiology 184, 541–545.

Maglinte, D.D., Elmore, M.F., Chernish, S.M., et al., 1985. Enteroclysis in the diagnosis of chronic unexplained gastrointestinal bleeding. Dis. Colon Rectum 28 (6), 403–405.

Maglinte, D.D., Elmore, M.F., Isenberg, M., et al., 1980. Meckel diverticulum: radiological demonstration by enteroclysis. Am. J. Roentgenol. 134 (5), 925–932.

Maglinte, D.D., Kelvin, F.M., O'Connor, K., et al., 1996. Current status of small bowel radiography. Abdom. Imaging 3, 247–257.

Maglinte, D.D., Lappas, J.C., Kelvin, F.M., et al., 1987. Small bowel radiography: how, when, why? Radiology 163, 297–305.

Mako, E.K., Mester, A.R., Tarjan, Z., et al., 2000. Enteroclysis and spiral CT in diagnosis and evaluation of small bowel Crohn's disease. Eur. J. Radiol. 35, 168–175.

Nolan, D.J., 1997. The true yield of the small intestine barium study. Endoscopy 29, 447–453.

Nolan, D.J., 2000. Enteroclysis of non-neoplastic disorders of the small intestine. Eur. Radiol. 10, 342–353.

Nolan, D.J., Traill, Z.C., 1997. The current role of the barium examination of the small intestine. Clin. Radiol. 52, 809–820.

Pesquera, G.S., 1929. Method for direct visualisation of lesions in small intestine. Am. J. Roentgenol. 22 (3), 254–257.

Price, R.C., le Masurier, S.B., 2007. Longitudinal changes in extended roles in radiography: a new perspective. Radiography 13 (1), 18–29.

Reiber, A., Wruk, D., Potthast, S., et al., 2000. Diagnostic imaging in Crohn's disease: comparison of magnetic resonance imaging and conventional imaging methods. Int. J. Colorectal Dis. 15, 176–181.

Scott-Harden, W.G., Hamilton, H.A., Smith, S.M., 1961. Radiological investigation of the small bowel. Gut 2, 316–322.

Sellink, J.L., 1974. Radiological examinations of the small intestine. Acta Radiol. 15, 318.

Sellink, J.L., 1976. Radiological atlas of common diseases of the small bowel. Stenfert Kroese, pp. 59–61.

Summers, D.S., Roger, M.D., Allan, P.L., et al., 2007. Accelerating the transit time of barium sulphate suspensions in small bowel examinations. Eur. J. Radiol. 62 (1), 122–125.

Toms, A.P., Barltrop, A., Freeman, A.H., 2001. A prospective randomised study comparing enteroclysis with small bowel follow-through examinations in 244 patients. Eur. Radiol. 11, 1150–1160.

Zagoria, R.J., Gelfand, D.W., Ott, D.J., 1986. Retrograde examination of the small bowel in patients with an ileostomy. Gastrointest. Radiol. 11 (1), 97–101.

Fluoroscopic investigations of the large bowel

Robert L. Law
Helen Carter (proctography section)

Contents

Introduction

Halligan et al. (2003) and Halligan (2004) have suggested that 'a barium enema list is not the attractive proposition it once was' and that 'radiologists, both trainees and consultants, are less inclined to take an interest' in barium enema; in addition, the lack of interest is compounded by the perception that the examination is 'old fashioned and behind the cutting edge of imaging'. The belief that the sensitivity of the double contrast barium enema (DCBE) for colorectal cancer (CRC) is poor at only about 85% adds to the lukewarm view of the examination. Indeed, Shorvon (2003) implied that there is no room for improving the DCBE and that it is 'on a developmental plateau'.

It has been suggested by Glick (1997) that there has been a bias against the DCBE associated with a number of studies in which 75–95% of missed cancers were perceptive errors rather than technical error. This finding would suggest that many of the possible shortcomings of the DCBE examination could be overcome by double reading.

However, it is possible to achieve a very high sensitivity if appropriate attention is given to technique. It may be the case that the image sequence of the DCBE has been optimized, but fluoroscopy equipment continues to improve and is now producing higher quality images at a fraction of the radiation dose required just a few years ago.

In the USA, the DCBE was considered to detect the majority of clinically important lesions and was therefore deemed to be an appropriate method for *colorectal cancer screening* (Winawer et al., 1997). These considerations were supported by the American College of Gastroenterology, The American Association of Colon and Rectal Surgeons and the American Society of Gastrointestinal Endoscopy. A survey of US radiologists, published in 2002, indicated that 75% believe the DCBE to be a 'very effective' colorectal cancer screening procedure and, at that time, Medicare approved DCBE as a CRC screening modality in the USA (Klabunde et al., 2002). Ciatto and Castiglione (2002), in reviewing the use of the DCBE within a screening program, also concluded that DCBE was a useful adjunct to screening colonoscopy.

Complications

Vora and Chapman (2004) reviewed 348 000 barium enemas performed by 59 radiographers; 89 complications were reported (1:3900) including five deaths (a mortality rate of 1:70 000). Culpan and Chapman (2002) reported on 54 complications in a review of 134 700 barium enema examinations performed over a 3-year period by 250 radiographers who had attended the Leeds barium enema training course. The complication rate was 1:2500; three deaths indicated a mortality rate of 1:44 900.

The complication and mortality rates for radiographers are not dissimilar to those reported by Blakeborough et al. (1997a) in reviewing the responses of 756 UK consultant radiologists who had performed 738 216 barium enemas in a 3-year period. A total of 82 complications were reported by 77 radiologists (1:9000) including three deaths (a mortality rate of 1:56 786).

Complications associated with the barium enema include perforations, cardiac events and cerebrovascular accidents. In reviewing *rectal perforation* after a barium enema, de Freiter et al. (2006) report that the most catastrophic course with a high mortality rate develops from sepsis and peritonitis resulting from intraperitoneal perforation. Also reported as prognostically unfavorable is the *venous intravasation of barium*.

Comment was also made in this paper regarding the introduction of excessive intracolonic pressures, excessive colonic distension and also concern regarding the use of rectal balloon catheters. These results compare favorably with colonoscopy (de Freiter et al., 2006). Updating the British Society of Gastroenterology guidelines, Teague (2003) refered to previous audits including one by Quine et al. (1995) (in which the 30 day mortality was found to be 1:2000) and he indicated there was no evidence to suggest that mortality rates had improved significantly since the 1990s.

Radiologic technologist and radiographer involvement

Price and Le Masurier (2007) reported results of a study that suggest radiographers are performing barium enema examinations in as many as 80% of district general hospitals (DGHs) in the UK. In the USA, Thompson et al. (2006) reported that, with training, radiologic technologists can perform and interpret fluoroscopic images as effectively as radiologists with a similar sensitivity, specificity, positive and negative predictive value. These results are also supported by Culpan et al. (2002) as well as Booth and Mannion (2005). A review on radiographer DCBE reporting by Law et al. (2008), demonstrating a 98% sensitivity to CRC, also strongly supports the view that examinations by radiographers can have a sensitivity and specificity similar to those carried out by radiologists.

Using smooth muscle relaxants

Hypotonia of the colon and rectum has a number of beneficial effects:
- Lack of peristalsis provides greater ease of barium flow
- Reduced prominence of haustral folds reduces the pooling of barium, resulting in greater ease of barium manipulation
- Due to luminal relaxation and distension there is a greater surface area visible
- Colonic spasm and discomfort are reduced.

The rectal infusion of agents such as 30 ml of *peppermint oil solution* has been demonstrated to have an antispasmodic effect (Asao et al., 2003). The most commonly used hypotonic agents are 20 mg in 1 ml *hyoscine butylbromide (Buscopan)* or 1 mg in 1 ml *glucagon* (Fink and Aylward, 1995; Goei et al., 1996). The IV injection of Buscopan is likely to have no effect on the diagnostic quality of the examination whether it is given before or after the infusion of barium (Elson et al., 2000).

It is not uncommon practice to avoid giving Buscopan in patients who have *glaucoma*, however, it has been reported by Fink and Aylward (1995) that the risk only relates to patients with undiagnosed (therefore untreated) angle closure glaucoma. The recommendation is to abandon the question about the presence of glaucoma and advise instead that patients should seek urgent medical advice should eye pain and visual loss develop. However, the authors did recommend caution in the presence of heart disease as this was considered of significant importance (Fink and Aylward, 1995).

The benefits and contraindications of Buscopan (from the Boehringer Ingelheim professional leaflet on 20 mg/1 ml solution 'Buscopan') and glucagon (from Novo Nordisk professional leaflet on glucagen 1 mg hypokit) are given in Table 13.1.

The double contrast barium enema

Good bowel preparation is an important precursor to a successful DCBE (see Chapter 3). Poor coating or residue can mask or mimic pathology and should be reported as such and an alternative strategy should be suggested (e.g. a limited repeat examination following further bowel preparation, to review those areas not well demonstrated).

Prior to commencement of the examination, talking to the patient can determine the success of the bowel preparation as well as contraindications to the use of hypotonic agents. The practitioner can also identify any limitations of mobility and the nature and degree of any comorbidities, as this might have a bearing on the approach to the examination.

Table 13.1 Hyascine butylbromide (Buscopan) versus glucagon (Glucagen)

Hypotonic agent	Buscopan	Glucagen
Benefits	Good hypotonia achieved Good colonic distension Good active duration lasting for most of the examination Significantly cheaper	Can be used in the presence of narrow angled glaucoma
Side effects	Temporary tachycardia Blurred vision Dizziness Drying of the mouth	Can cause nausea Shorter acting Poorer colonic distension
Contraindications	Myasthenia gravis Megacolon Narrow angle glaucoma Tachycardia Prostatic enlargement with urinary retention GI stenosis or paralytic ileus Poorly controlled angina	Insulin dependent diabetes (glucagon has the opposite effect to insulin)
Relative contraindications		Elderly patient with a heart condition Pheochromocytoma Insulinoma Glucagonoma

The predominant difference in *rectal tube* types is related to whether or not they have a balloon cuff. There is limited advantage to having a cuff, as it can assist with contrast retention in a patient with poor sphincter control. However, significant complications can occur, such as perforation, following inadvertent cuff insufflation and barium infusion within the vagina due to incorrect tube placement. Colonic perforation following cuff insufflation in the rectum is associated with high, artificially induced, intraluminal pressure. It has been advised that balloon cuffs should be avoided (Blakeborough et al., 1997b; Chapman and Blakeborough, 1998; Culpan and Chapman, 2002).

The objective standard of all DCBE techniques should be the same:

> To provide a collective series of images that demonstrate the whole of the distended colon and rectum in double contrast (with a record of the appendix, terminal ileum or ileocecal valve to confirm arrival at the cecal pole).

If the standard has not been met, the examination, although it may be considered diagnostic is, by definition, technically suboptimal.

The technique described below using 'C' arm fluoroscopy is only one of a number of approaches to the DCBE. As long as the objective standards are met and there is consistency of approach, local variances need not be of any consequence.

Air or CO_2 double contrast

Air or carbon dioxide (CO_2) can be given to insufflate the bowel. Although practitioners need to be aware of the risks associated with over distension of the colon, if the bowel is collapsed in any view, consideration should be given to increasing gas input.

There are numerous papers discussing the benefits of air and CO_2. CO_2 dissolves faster and, although the mucosal coating is the same, the discomfort of CO_2 is reported as less. However, air is considered to provide better distension and this might outweigh the advantages in patient acceptability that CO_2 provides. Should colic result from air distension or should the effect of the chosen hypotonic agent wear off, maintaining rectal intubation will allow colonic decompression at any time but, particularly, as a routine at the end of the examination (Scullion et al., 1995; Holemans et al., 1998). One example of a DCBE protocol follows:

- With the patient supine for the injection of an IV smooth muscle relaxant, they are then turned into the *left lateral position* whereupon a rectal catheter is inserted. Care must be given to guard against vaginal intubation. If intubation is problematic (from, for example, prostatic enlargement), *digital examination of the rectum* can give guidance in directing the tube. The tube is left in situ for the duration of the examination to allow barium to be drained and replaced with air/CO_2 at any time as well as draining and decompressing the bowel upon completion of the examination.
- The intubated patient is turned prone and the tube taped low to the legs to help with any subsequent barium drainage. A solution such as 567 g EZ EM barium diluted with 550 ml H_2O (103% w/v) is infused with the table tilted a few degrees head down. *Intermittent fluoroscopy* is of value to confirm flow of barium and that no obstruction is present, in addition a pedunculated polyp, if present, may be seen oscillating within the barium flow. Occasional direct inspection of the tube will help identify if there is any barium seepage.
- Contrast should not be allowed to pass beyond the mid transverse colon. If barium is allowed to reach the right colon, it may well superimpose and denigrate subsequent imaging of the sigmoid colon. The patient is turned from the prone position via their left side to the supine, then to a position turned 45 degrees to the right to coat the rectum and sigmoid. Reversing the patient's direction the patient is turned prone once more.
- Focusing now only on the colon and rectum, a couple of puffs of air are passed into the rectum to break up the barium column and raise the rectal pressure, and the rectum is then drained of barium.
- Gently puffing air into the rectum, the patient is turned via their left side to the *right anterior oblique (RAO)* position (Figure 13.1). Depending on the field size capability of the fluoroscopy unit, an RAO of the rectum and sigmoid can be followed by an RAO image of the proximal sigmoid/distal descending colon.
- The patient is now turned via their left side into the prone position and any pooled barium is drained from the rectum and then re-inflated with

CHAPTER 13

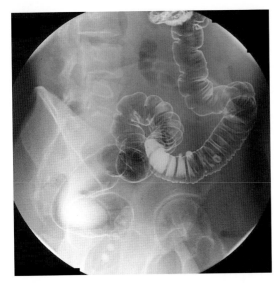

Figure 13.1 Right anterior oblique rectum and sigmoid.

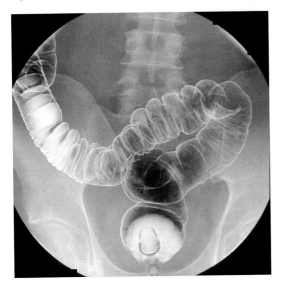

Figure 13.2 Prone rectum and sigmoid.

air. A *prone* image is taken of the rectum and sigmoid (Figure 13.2) and, if using the 'C' arm, a view is also taken of this region with optimum *caudal angulation* (Figure 13.3) suggestive of Hampton's view.

- Continuing turning the patient towards the left, the *left posterior oblique (LPO)* (Figure 13.4) is a mirror image of the RAO and, as such, barium pooling in any loop in one view will be replaced by air in the mirrored image.
- Rotating the patient in the same direction a *right lateral* image (Figure 13.5) is acquired, making sure the hips are super imposed. This view not only gives a good view of the rectum but is the best view to demonstrate the pre-sacral space. This completes the standard views of the rectosigmoid.

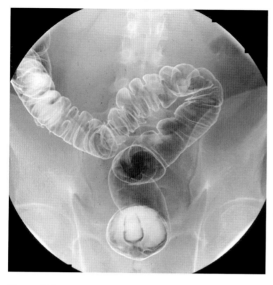

Figure 13.3 Prone with caudal angulation.

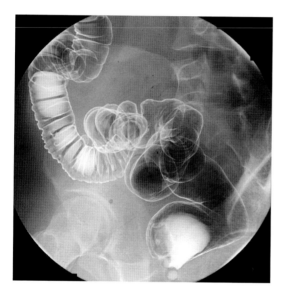

Figure 13.4 Left posterior oblique rectum and sigmoid.

As imaging of the sigmoid colon has been completed, we are not worried at this point that the direction of the patient rotation has been aiding the passage of barium into and over the hepatic flexure. Turning the patient towards the left anterior oblique (LAO), the colon is screened both to make sure there is enough barium to demonstrate the right colon and to identify where barium is pooling in the region of the splenic flexure and descending colon. To remove the pooled barium in the left colon, the table is tilted head up (it is not normally necessary to stand the table erect both from the view point of patient comfort and to reduce the risk of them becoming hypotensive and possibly fainting (Roach et al., 2001)).

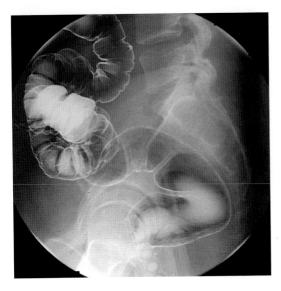

Figure 13.5 Right lateral rectum.

- The patient is turned to assist the barium to drain; the direction the patient is turned will depend on the direction the bowel is looping. It no longer matters if drained barium now returns to the sigmoid region. In the *left anterior oblique* (Figure 13.6) position, insufflating with air as required, an image is taken of the descending colon, splenic flexure and distal transverse colon.

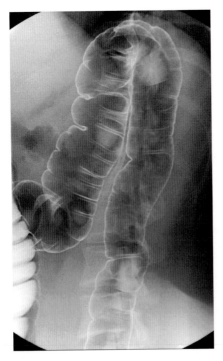

Figure 13.6 Left anterior oblique distal transverse colon, splenic flexure and descending colon.

- The hepatic loop may be exaggerated or have a redundant element to it, trapping barium. To advance barium through the hepatic flexure into the ascending colon, it may help to have the table horizontal, turn the patient a few degrees to the left for a moment then onto their back again. Tilt the table head up; this allows the barium to spill into and around the hepatic flexure then down into the ascending colon to the cecum. Imaging of the *transverse colon* (Figure 13.7) may be optimized at this time.
- With the barium in the cecal pole, coating of the right colon is achieved with the table horizontal and turning the patient onto their left side allowing the barium to coat the medial aspect. Continuing the turn until the patient is prone will enable the barium to coat the anterior aspect of the right colon and hepatic flexure as the barium spills into it. With the patient prone, as well as draining the barium out of the right colon, this position enables air to spill into this region.
- As the patient turns back onto their left side, the *right lateral decubitus* (Figure 13.8) image can be obtained. It may be necessary to take two images to cover the whole abdomen.
- To obtain views of the hepatic flexure, tilt the table head up and turn the patient so that residual barium falls to the cecal pole then into the RAO for the *hepatic flexure* (Figure 13.9).
- The *cecal pole* will often demonstrate a marked posterior cupping and can lie laterally or medially. Emptying barium from the cecum may require turning the patient either to the left or right depending on barium pooling then tilting the table head down. Occasionally, with pronounced cupping, it may be necessary to image the cecum with the patient in the prone position to obtain double contrast imaging

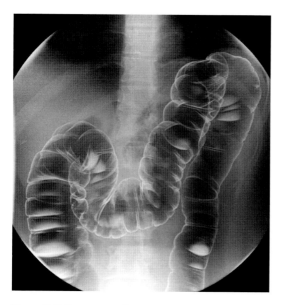

Figure 13.7 Transverse colon.

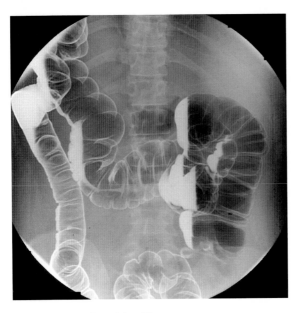

Figure 13.8 Right lateral decubitus.

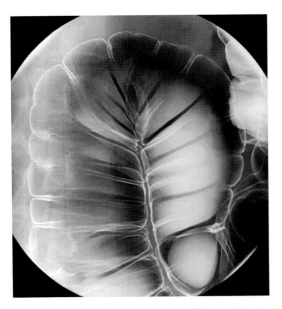

Figure 13.9 Right anterior oblique hepatic flexure and ascending colon.

of the pole. Except where clinically contraindicated, the cecum should always be palpated and two oblique views imaged (Figures 13.10 and 13.11) with additional views if aspects of the cecum are obscured by the terminal ileum. It must always be borne in mind that, however good the technique, pathology may be subtle (Figures 13.12A, 13.12B).

- Reflux into the terminal ileum not only confirms arrival at the cecal pole but may show itself to be the site of abnormality (Figure 13.13).

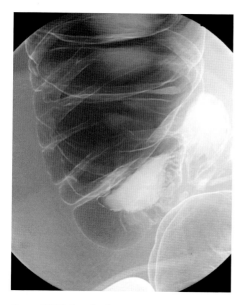

Figure 13.10 Cecal pole.

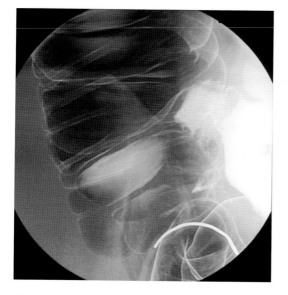

Figure 13.11 Compression view of cecal pole.

- With 'C' arm fluoroscopy it may be the case that a *whole abdomen* might not be possible on a single image, in which case, the lower abdomen can be taken with the table supine, the upper abdomen taken with the table tilted head up to allow air (or CO_2) to migrate to the upper abdomen (see Figure 13.7 and 13.14).
- The last image(s) is the *left lateral decubitus* (Figures 13.15A, 13.15B). Turning the patient to the right, lay the table horizontal, draining barium from the left colon. Consideration should always be given to replacing expelled gas (Table 13.2).

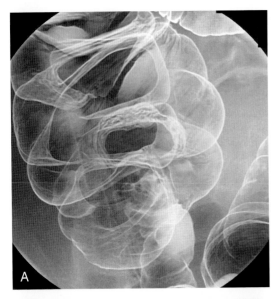

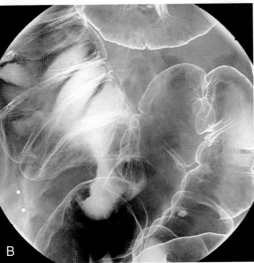

Figure 13.12 (A) Apparently normal cecal pole; (B) the same cecum, tumor clearly visible.

Single contrast enema (SCE)

Historically, an SCE was undertaken on patients with large bowel obstruction that had not perforated to confirm the degree of obstruction and its location. These patients are now better served having a less invasive CT scan (Jacob et al., 2007).

However, the suggestion by Boardman and Nolan (1994) that there are occasions when an SCE examination can be employed is still true today despite the increasing use of CT. The SCE is still of value for patients who are referred for a DCBE but, due to infirmity and immobility, cannot lie prone or turn in a manner required to achieve a full DCBE examination. In these

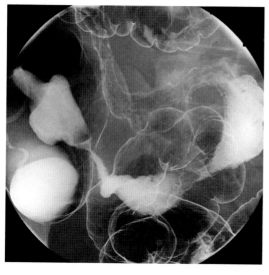

Figure 13.13 Normal colon, terminal ileal Crohn's disease.

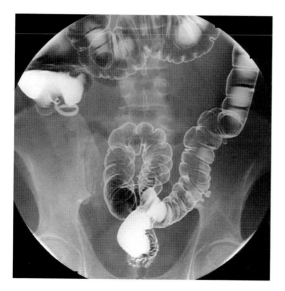

Figure 13.14 Supine view lower abdomen.

instances, infusing a dilute low density single contrast barium solution can still provide useful information. Following the injection of a hypotonic agent, the patient is turned onto their left side and the barium is infused as far as the hepatic flexure. Patient position and imaging can follow the flow of barium:

- Lateral rectum
- Descending colon
- RAO, rectum and sigmoid colon
- Supine rectosigmoid
- Supine, rectosigmoid with cranial angulation
- LAO splenic flexure and distal transverse colon.

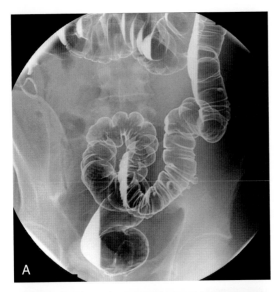

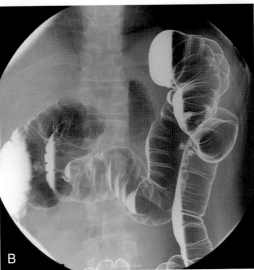

Figure 13.15 (A) Left lateral decubitus, lower abdomen; (B) left lateral decubitus, upper abdomen.

At this stage, rather than infusing more barium, draining the rectum and applying a few puffs of air will, in most instances, assist with the filling of the right colon.

- RAO proximal transverse colon, hepatic flexure and ascending colon
- Supine and oblique of the cecal pole (with compression)
- Overview images to cover the whole abdomen.

Water-soluble contrast enema (Gastrografin enema)

The most common reason for performing a water-soluble contrast enema (WSEN) is as a *postoperative check* on the integrity and patency of anastomoses following anterior resection (Figure 13.16), total proctocolectomy and ileal

Table 13.2 Double contrast barium enema positioning and imaging

Activity	Image	Example figure
Patient supine – inject hypotonic agent		
Left lateral position – intubate		
Turn patient prone		
Infuse barium just over the splenic flexure		
Turn patient to left then supine		
Turn left – prone		
Air insufflate, drain barium, air insufflate, turn patient onto left side:		
Image 1	Right anterior oblique	Figure 13.1
Turn towards left then prone		
Image 2	Prone	Figure 13.2
Image 3	Prone with caudal tube angulation	Figure 13.3
Image 4	Left posterior oblique	Figure 13.4
Image 5	Left lateral	Figure 13.5
Check barium has reached right colon		
Drain barium from left side		
Image 6	Left anterior oblique of descending colon and splenic flexure	Figure 13.6
Barium to cecal pole		
Image 7	Supine transverse colon	Figure 13.7
Turn left then prone to coat medial and anterior wall of ascending colon while draining barium from right colon		
Image 8	Right lateral decubitus	Figure 13.8
Image 9	Right anterior oblique hepatic flexure	Figure 13.9
Image 10	Supine mid ascending (if needed)	Figure 13.10
Image 11	Supine and oblique of cecum with compression	Figure 13.11
Image 12	Supine abdominal overview(s)	Figure 13.12
Image 13	Left lateral decubitus	Figure 13.13

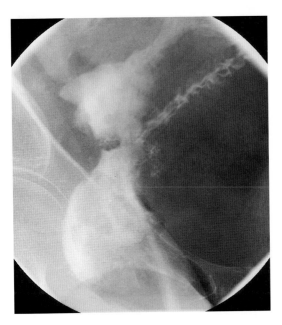

Figure 13.16 Post anterior resection: leak at the stapled anastomotic margin.

pouch-anal anastomosis prior to reversing a defunctioning ileostomy (Dolinsky et al., 2007).

Even if defunctioned, a smooth muscle relaxant is of value to relax the bowel. The patient is turned onto their left side for intubation and infusion of contrast. Gastrografin (if used) can be diluted 2:1 water to Gastrografin.

The standard barium enema tips should not be used as they are too rigid and could disrupt the surgical staples (see Figure 13.16). A soft tube such as the 16 Fg Jacques catheter is a safer option, inserting it only as far as it will freely pass. With *low anterior resections* in particular, over insertion is counter-productive as the contrast is required at the anastomotic margins. Patient positioning is aimed at putting contrast on the respective walls of the bowel (Table 13.3); however, prone imaging is to be avoided if at all possible due to patient discomfort that could be caused from the defunctioning stoma.

The WSEN can be of value in determining a *mechanical obstruction* from an ileus, assessing the level and extent of an obstructive stricture and identifying if a known malignant stricture is suitable for stenting.

Colostomy enema

The difficulty regarding a colostomy enema is the lack of a sphincter to retain the barium. A number of devices and techniques have been designed to allow barium infusion via a colostomy (Kushner et al., 1988; Williams and Scott, 2003).

Examination of the colon may be required following the formation of a colostomy (i.e. post anterior peroneal resection). To retain the barium, a 2 cm

Table 13.3 Water-soluble contrast enema image projections to review anastomosis

Activity	Function	Imaging of anastomosis
Left lateral position	Intubation with soft catheter	
	Initial infusion of contrast	
	Image left lateral dependent wall	Left lateral
Depending on stoma site, turn left and pronate as much as possible	Image left anterolateral wall	Left posterior oblique
Right anterior oblique	Image left posterolateral dependent wall	Right anterior oblique
Place supine	Image posterior dependent wall	Supine
Turn towards right	Image right posterolateral dependent wall	Left anterior oblique
Right lateral	Image right dependent wall	Right lateral
Depending on stoma site, pronate as much as possible	Image right anterolateral wall	Right posterior oblique

slit is made in the colostomy bag on the medial side of the stoma bag and a 10Fg Law II tube inserted. Depending on the site of the stoma, it is possible to pass the tube over the splenic flexure without too much difficulty (Figures 13.17 and 13.18). Following the injection of a hypotonic agent with the patient lying on their right side, barium can be infused to fill the right colon. Should barium be ejected, it will be contained within the bag which, if needed, can be drained using a suction catheter. Turning the patient supine and then towards the left allows the barium to fill the transverse colon before being aspirated.

With the patient on their left side, air can now be infused through the tube. In the left lateral position the air will migrate to, and distend, the right colon (see Figure 13.18). Imaging starts in the right lateral position with the ascending colon. Images can then be taken as required as the patient is turned onto their back (Figure 13.19).

The patient experience

Subjectively, many patients are reticent about going to see their family doctor about symptoms associated with their 'bottom'. In talking to the patient and explaining the procedure, it helps to be aware of the examination from their perspective and let them know you are aware. Many referred patients

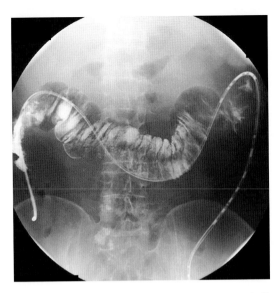

Figure 13.17 Colostomy enema: tube passed over hepatic flexure.

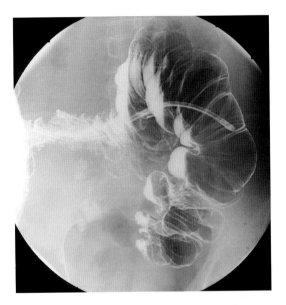

Figure 13.18 Colostomy enema: right lateral decubitus.

are of an age where comorbidities are likely to be a limiting factor and, in a number of cases, only by talking to the patient before the examination can this be properly assessed. The bowel preparation can leave the external anal margin feeling raw making intubation uncomfortable. Rectal intubation and the desire to evacuate is embarrassing and undignified. Careful control of the rate of barium infusion or gas insufflation can minimize the rectal discomfort.

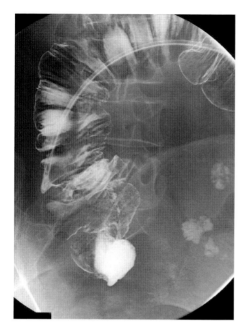

Figure 13.19 Colostomy enema: ascending colon.

Proctography

Defecation proctography provides *dynamic imaging of the pelvic floor* to assess the anatomy and dynamics of defecation (Hare et al., 2001). It can provide considerable weight to clinical decision making, such as whether surgery or conservative therapy would be more appropriate (Jones et al., 1998; Harvey et al., 1999).

Current defecation proctography methods range from utilizing rectal and small bowel contrast (Harvey et al., 1999) to what Kelvin and Maglinte (2001) and Altringer et al. (1995) describe as an extended examination incorporating bladder, small bowel, vaginal and rectal contrast. The standard examination described here can be performed and reported by a suitably trained radiographer.

Patients are predominantly female with symptoms of *obstructed defecation syndrome* (ODS) where individuals have difficulty in emptying their bowels. Symptoms of ODS often develop following injury during childbirth (Halligan, 2001). Proctography during pregnancy is contraindicated, not only because of the use of ionizing radiation, but also because the pregnancy and birth will have an effect on the pelvic floor, possibly altering the pelvic configuration and functionality (Halligan et al., 1996).

A number of *alternative examinations* complement defecating proctography (Dvorkin et al., 2005). These include:

- Colonic transit study
- Anorectal physiology/manometry
- Endoanal ultrasound
- MRI proctography (Roos et al., 2002; Dvorkin et al., 2003).

Preparation specific to defecation proctography

The patient

Defecation proctography, by its very nature, is an embarrassing and undignified procedure that requires the trust and cooperation of the patient. Practitioner guidance on performing intimate examinations is provided by the Royal College of Radiologists (RCR, 1998).

To gain informed consent and the confidence of the patient, pre-examination time and privacy must be available to discuss the procedure. Reassurance must be given with respect to their dignity and emphasis made that maximum privacy will be assured during the examination (Kelvin and Maglinte, 2001). Any discussion at this stage must involve the patient's symptoms including whether digitation or other patient-developed 'methods' to assist defecation are required on a regular basis. This allows for modifications of the standard procedure to be considered (Halligan et al., 1996).

The fluoroscopy room

The room used must provide complete privacy and have an en suite washroom facility. Patient privacy can be enhanced by using the distance between operator and subject provided by the remote control capability of a unit such as the Polystar Fluorospot unit with C-arm (Siemens), and by using a mobile lead screen beside the patient. Accessory equipment and contrast is prepared in advance of the session (Table 13.4). A specially adapted bedpan is placed so that it is readily available when required.

Proctography technique

One hour before imaging the patient drinks 100 ml Baritop diluted with 200 ml water. Ingested contrast will demonstrate the pelvic small bowel during the examination to identify a possible enterocele. The examination begins with the patient supine on the table and the technique as outlined in Box 13.1 is followed.

As well as *small bowel contrast*, rectal and vaginal contrast is also used (Kelvin and Maglinte, 2001) (Figure 13.20). The separate use of small bowel contrast once an enterocele had been indicated at defecating proctography has been reported in a study (Kelvin et al., 1992), however, it was recognized that this would increase the resultant dose of the examination.

In assessing *pelvic prolapse*, *vaginal contrast* will demonstrate during evacuation any displacement of the bladder or widening of the rectovaginal space (Low et al., 1999). To minimize the risk of extravasation (Blakeborough et al., 1997a, Chapman and Blakeborough, 1998), only 2–3 ml of barium need be used to identify the vaginal apex and whether it has prolapsed below the pubococcygeal line.

Bladder contrast (Altringer et al., 1995; Kelvin and Maglinte, 2001) can be administered intravenously or by catheterization; however, it need not and should not be used in all cases, and risk/benefit considerations should be given before the administration of intravenous contrast agent (Bettmann, 2005; Namasivayam et al., 2006).

Table 13.4 Proctography: accessory equipment and contrast preparation

Accessory equipment	Contrast	Preparation (per patient)
Specially adapted bedpan Mobile screen Measuring cup Measuring scoop Bowl Blue tray stocked with: 5 ml syringe (female patients only) 4 × 50 ml bladder syringe 24 g rectal catheter Lubricant jelly Gauze Inco sheets Large and small clear bag Blue roll Tissue paper Pad and pants Draw sheet/blanket	Baritop Packet mash/potato starch	100 ml Baritop: 200 ml water in a beaker Mix packet mash as per instructions, adding Baritop (300 ml water: 3–4 scoops powder: 60 ml Baritop should suffice 2 patients) Put this paste into 3 bladder syringes, placing on blue tray Fill fourth bladder syringe with 50 ml Baritop, placing on tray Female patients only – fill 5 ml syringe with 2–3 ml Baritop, placing on tray

---

BOX 13.1 Proctography technique and imaging

- Vaginal contrast administered
- Left lateral position – intubate, infuse barium and 'barium paste'
- Right lateral position – images taken while resting, squeezing and straining; all of which must include the pubic symphysis and coccyx
- Patient takes a seat while equipment changes to vertical position – specially adapted bedpan placed on footrest
- Right lateral position sat on bedpan – mobile screen positioned to provide some seclusion for patient
- Images taken at one frame per second while patient defecates as fast and completely as they can, again including the pubic symphysis and coccyx
- When empty, take spot films of resting, squeezing and straining
- Examination completed

Delayed, post complete rectal evacuation images are recommended as *enteroceles* often only become evident at the end of evacuation. If not almost or fully empty, re-screen following attempted evacuation in the toilet for a further 5 minutes – an anismus may prevent herniation of the small bowel (Kelvin et al., 1999; Kelvin and Maglinte, 2001).

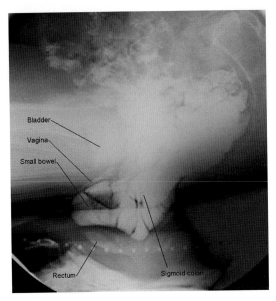

Labels on image: Bladder, Vagina, Small bowel, Rectum, Sigmoid colon

Figure 13.20 Defecating proctogram: demonstrating cystocele, enterocele, sigmoidocele, rectocele and rectoanal intussusception. Image by Helen Carter.

Aftercare

Information would include warning of the whitish colored motions for a couple of days and that if they find they get constipated to take a mild laxative.

Complications

No documented complications specific to the use of barium in defecation proctography have been identified, however, the technical similarities of contrast administration with the barium enema might suggest similar complications.

Risks such as infection or urethral trauma are associated with bladder catheterization however brief (Wong and Hooton, 1981; Colley, 1998; Pratt et al., 2007).

Interpretation of images

Interpretation of images considers the alterations in anorectal angle and position of anorectal junction in addition to the ability rapidly and completely to evacuate the contrast (Halligan, 2001). Prolapse of pelvic organs is considered in relation to the position of the pubococcygeal line and the extent of prolapse can be noted (Figures 13.21A, 13.21B).

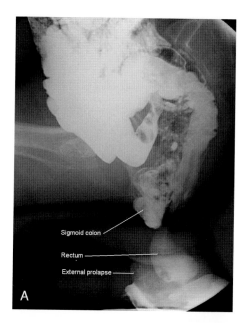

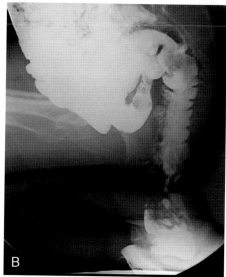

Figure 13.21 (A) Defecating proctogram: demonstrating external prolapse sac containing prolapsed rectum. (B) Same patient following straining; additionally demonstrates prolapse of sigmoid colon. Images by Helen Carter.

References

Altringer, W.E., Saclarides, T.J., Dominguez, J.M., Brubaker, L.T., Smith, C.S., 1995. Four-contrast defecography: pelvic 'fluoroscopy'. Dis. Colon Rectum 38, 695–699.

Asao, T., Kuwano, H., Ide, M., et al., 2003. Spasmolytic effect of peppermint oil in barium during double contrast barium enema compared with Buscopan. Clin. Radiol. 58 (4), 301–305.

Bettmann, M.A., 2005. Contrast media: safety, viscosity, and volume. Eur. Radiol. 159 (Suppl. 4), D62–D64.

Blakeborough, A., Sheridan, M.B., Chapman, A.H., 1997a. Complications of barium enema examinations: a survey of UK consultant radiologists 1992 to 1994. Clin. Radiol. 52 (2), 142–148.

Blakeborough, A., Sheridan, M.B., Chapman, A.H., 1997b. Retention balloon catheters and barium enemas: attitudes, current practice and relative safety in the UK. Clin. Radiol. 52 (1), 62–64.

Boardman, P., Nolan, D., 1994. Computer tomography of the colon in elderly people. (Letters) Single contrast barium study is adequate. Br. Med. J. 308 (6944), 1639.

Booth, A.M., Mannion, R.A.J., 2005. Radiographer and radiologist perception error in reporting double contrast barium enemas: a pilot study. Radiography 11, 249–254.

Chapman, A.H., Blakeborough, A., 1998. Complications from inflation of a retention rectal balloon catheter in the vagina at barium enema. Clin. Radiol. 53 (10), 768–770.

Ciatto, S., Castiglione, G., 2002. Role of double-contrast barium enema in colorectal cancer screening based on faecal occult blood. Tumori 88 (2), 95–98.

Colley, W., 1998. Female catheterisation. Nurs. Times 94 (21), 33A–33B.

Culpan, D.G., Chapman, A.H., 2002. Complications of radiographer performed double contrast barium enema examinations. Radiography 8 (2), 91–95.

Culpan, D.G., Mitchell, A.J., Hughes, S., et al., 2002. Double contrast barium enema sensitivity: a comparison of studies by radiographers and radiologists. Clin. Radiol. 57 (7), 604–607.

de Freiter, P.W., Soeters, P.B., Dejong, C.H., 2006. Rectal perforation after barium enema: a review. Dis. Colon Rectum 49 (2), 261–271.

Dolinsky, D., Levine, M.S., Rubesin, S.E., et al., 2007. Utility of contrast enema for detecting anastomotic strictures after total proctocolectomy and ileal pouch-anal anastomosis. Am. J. Roentgenol. 189 (1), 25–29.

Dvorkin, L.S., Hetzer, F., Scott, S.M., Williams, N.S., Gedroyc, W., Lunniss, P.J., 2003. Open-magnet MR defaecography compared with evacuation proctography in the diagnosis and management of patients with rectal intussusception. Colorectal Dis. 6, 45–53.

Dvorkin, L.S., et al., 2005. Rectal intussusception in symptomatic patients is different from that in asymptomatic volunteers. Br. J. Surg. 92, 866–872.

Elson, E.M., Campbell, D.M., Halligan, S., et al., 2000. The effect of timing of intravenous muscle relaxant on the quality of double contrast barium enema. Clin. Radiol. 55 (5), 395–397.

Fink, A.M., Aylward, G.W., 1995. Buscopan and glaucoma: a survey of current practice. Clin. Radiol. 50 (3), 160–164.

Glick, S.N., 1997. Colonoscopy versus barium enema: a reappraisal of the facts and issues. Gastroenterology 113, 1048–1053.

Goei, R., Nix, M., Kessels, A.H., et al., 1996. Use of antispasmodic drugs in double contrast barium enema examination: glucagon or Buscopan? Clin. Radiol. 51 (4), 305.

Halligan, S., 2004. Observer variation in the detection of colorectal neoplasia on double contrast barium enema: implications for colorectal cancer screening and training. Clin. Radiol. 59, 762–776.

Halligan, S., 2001. Introduction to functional pelvic floor imaging. Imaging 13, 435–439.

Halligan, S., Marshall, M., Taylor, S., et al., 2003. Observer variation in the detection of colorectal neoplasia on double contrast barium enema: implications for colorectal cancer screening and training. Clin. Radiol. 58, 948–954.

Halligan, S., Spence-Jones, C., Kamm, M.A., et al., 1996. Dynamic cystoproctography and physiological testing in women with urinary stress incontinence and urogenital prolapse. Clin. Radiol. 51, 785–790.

Hare, C., Halligan, S., Bartram, C.I., et al., 2001. Dose reduction in evacuation proctography. Eur. J. Radiol. 11, 432–434.

Harvey, C., Halligan, S., Bartram, C.I., et al., 1999. Evacuation proctography: a prospective study of diagnostic and therapeutic impact. Radiology 211, 223–227.

Holemans, J.A., Matson, M.B., Hughes, J.A., et al., 1998. A comparison of air, CO2 and an air/CO2 mixture as insufflation agents for double contrast barium enema. Eur. Radiol. 8 (2), 274–276.

Jacob, S.E., Lee, S.H., Hill, J., 2007. The demise of the instant/unprepared contrast enema in large bowel obstruction. Colorectal Dis. (on epub ahead of print).

Jones, H.J., Swift, R.I., Blake, H., 1998. A prospective audit of the usefulness of evacuating proctography. Ann. R. Coll. Surg. Engl. 80 (1), 40–45.

Kelvin, F.M., Maglinte, D.D.T., 2001. Extended proctography. Imaging 13, 448–457.

Kelvin, F.M., Hale, D.S., Maglinte, D.D.T., et al., 1999. Female pelvic organ prolapse: diagnostic contribution of dynamic cystoproctography and comparison with physical examination. Am. J. Roentgenol. 173, 31–37.

Kelvin, F.M., Maglinte, D.D.T., Horback, J.A., et al., 1992. Pelvic prolapse: assessment with evacuation proctography (defecography). Radiology 184, 547–551.

Klabunde, C.N., Jones, E., Brown, M., et al., 2002. Colorectal cancer screening with double-contrast barium enema: a national survey of diagnostic radiologists. Am. J. Roentgenol. 179, 1419–1427.

Kushner, D.C., Cleveland, R.H., Herman, T.E., et al., 1988. Retrograde colostomy and iliostomy enemas in neonates and infants: a simple combination of techniques. Gastrointest. Radiol. 13 (2), 180–182.

Law, R.L., Slack, N., Harvey, R.F., 2008. An evaluation of a radiographer-led barium enema service in the diagnosis of colorectal cancer. Radiography 14 (2), 105–110.

Low, V.H., Ho, L.M., Freed, K.S., 1999. Vaginal opacification during defecography: direction of vaginal migration aids in diagnosis of pelvic floor pathology. Abdom. Imaging 24 (6), 5665–6568.

Namasivayam, S., Kalra, M.K., Torres, W.E., et al., 2006. Adverse reactions to intravenous iodinated contrast media: a primer for radiologists. Emerg. Radiol. 12, 210–215.

Pratt, R.J., Pellowe, C.M., Wilson, J.A., 2007. National evidence-based guidelines for preventing healthcare-associated infections in NHS hospitals in England. J. Hosp. Infect. 65 (Suppl. 1), S1–S64.

Price, R.C., le Masurier, S.B., 2007. Longitudinal changes in extended roles in radiography: a new perspective. Radiography 13 (1), 18–29.

Quine, M.A., Bell, G.D., McCloy, R.F., et al., 1995. Prospective audit of upper gastrointestinal endoscopy in two regions of England: safety, staffing, and sedation methods. Gut 36 (3), 462–465.

Roach, S.C., Martin, D.J., Owen, A., et al., 2001. Blood pressure changes during barium enema. Clin. Radiol. 56 (5), 393–396.

Roos, J.E., Weishaupt, D., Wildermuth, S., et al., 2002. Experience of 4 years with open MR defecography: pictorial review of anorectal anatomy and disease. Radiographics 22, 817–832.

Royal College of Radiologists, 1998. Intimate examination: guidance for members and fellows. Royal College of Radiologists, London.

Scullion, D.A., Wetton, C.W.N., Davies, C., et al., 1995. The use of air or CO2 as insufflation agents for double contrast barium enema (DCBE): is there a qualitative difference? Clin. Radiol. 50 (8), 558–561.

Shorvon, P.J., 2003. Commentary on: observer variation in the detection of colorectal neoplasia on double contrast barium enema: implications for colorectal cancer screening and training. Clin. Radiol. 58, 945–947.

Teague, R., 2003. Clinical practice guidelines update: safety and sedation during endoscopic procedures. British Society of Gastroenterology. <http://www.bsg.org.uk>

Thompson, W.M., Foster, W.L., Paulson, E.K., et al., 2006. Comparison of radiologist and technologists in the performance of air contrast barium enema. Am. J. Roentgenol. 187, 706–709.

Vora, P., Chapman, A., 2004. Complications from radiographer-performed double contrast *barium enemas*. Clin. Radiol. 59 (4), 364–368.

Williams, J.T., Scott, R.L., 2003. A new universal colostomy tip for barium enemas of the colon. Am. J. Roentgenol. 180 (5), 1330–1331.

Winawer, S.J., Fletcher, R.H., Miller, L., et al., 1997. Colorectal cancer screening: clinical guidelines and rationale. Gastroenterology 112, 594–642.

Wong, E.S., Hooton, T.M., 1981. Guideline for prevention of catheter-associated urinary tract infections [last modified 2005]. Centers for Disease Control and Prevention. <http://www.cdc.gov/ncidod/dhqp/gl_catheter_assoc.html> Accessed 17/11/2007.

Further reading

Dench, J.E. Scott, S.M. Luniss, P.J., et al., 2006. External pelvic rectal suspension (the express procedure) for internal rectal prolapse, with or without concomitant rectocele repair: a video demonstration. Dis. Colon Rectum 49, 1922–1926.

Halligan, S., et al., 2001. Predictive value of impaired evacuation at proctography in diagnosing anismus. Am. J. Roentgenol. 177, 633–636.

Jayne, D.G., Finan, P.J., 2005. Stapled transanal rectal resection for obstructed defecation and evidence-based practice. Br. J. Surg. 92, 793–794.

Low, V.H., Ho, L.M., Freed, K.S., 1999. Vaginal opacification during defecography: direction of vaginal migration aids in diagnosis of pelvic floor pathology. Abdom. Imaging 24 (6), 5665–6568.

Mahieu, P., Pringot, J., Bodart, P., 1984. Defecography: I. Description of a new procedure and results in normal patients. Gastrointest. Radiol. 9 (3), 247–251.

Marshall, M., Halligan, S., 2001. Evacuation proctography. Imaging 13, 440–447.

Persson, P.B., 2005. Contrast-induced nephropathy. Eur. Radiol. 15 (Suppl. 4), D65–D69.

Satsih, S.C., Kimberly, D., Welcher, B.S., et al., 1997. Effects of biofeedback therapy on anorectal function in obstructive defecation. Dig. Dis. Sci. 42 (11), 2197–2205.

Stoker, J., Halligan, S., Bartram, C.I., 2001. Pelvic floor imaging. Radiology 218, 621–641.

14

Tumors of the small and large intestine

Emil Salmo, Najib Haboubi

Contents ||||||||||||||||||||||||||||||||||||||||||||||||||||||||||||||||||||||||||||||||

Introduction

Small and large intestinal tumors are broadly classified into non-neoplastic (or tumor-like lesions) and neoplastic tumors (Table 14.1) most of which are epithelial (arise from the surface epithelium) and the minority are non-epithelial tumors (stromal). *Non-neoplastic lesions* are those which follow a benign course and do not have a tendency for malignant transformation as opposed to *neoplastic tumors*, which are pre-malignant from which carcinoma arises (Kumar et al., 2004; Robertson and Levison, 2006).

Colorectal cancer is a major cause of morbidity and mortality worldwide (Geboes et al., 2005). Around 100 new cases of colorectal cancer are diagnosed each day in the UK and it is the third most common cancer after breast and lung (Cancer Research UK, 2007). *Epithelial tumors* of the small intestine are rare compared to the large intestine.

Both neoplastic and non-neoplastic lesions of the small and large intestines commonly present in the form of a *polyp*, which is defined as a raised lesion above the mucosa that protrudes into the lumen of the digestive tract (Geboes et al., 2005).

Table 14.1 Classification of tumors of small and large intestines

Non-neoplastic/tumor-like lesions
Hyperplastic polyp
Juvenile polyps
Peutz-Jeghers polyps
Inflammatory polyps
Lymphoid polyps

Neoplastic
Epithelial tumors
Benign:
Adenoma
Malignant:
Adenocarcinoma
Carcinoid tumor
Non-epithelial tumors
Gastrointestinal stromal tumors
Lipoma/liposarcoma
Neuroma
Angioma/angiosarcoma
Lymphoma

Non-neoplastic/tumor-like lesions

Hyperplastic/metaplastic polyps and serrated adenomas

Hyperplastic polyps are benign epithelial lesions that are usually small and less than 5 mm in maximum diameter. By definition, they do not display *dysplasia* (see glossary for definition) and, in most instances, they are not pre-neoplastic in nature. They are usually asymptomatic and can be multiple and they mainly involve the large intestine rather than the small intestine (Robertson and Levison, 2006). Histologically, they are composed of well-formed glands lined by non-neoplastic epithelial cells, most of which show maturation with small, regular nuclei located in the base of the cells (Geboes et al., 2005). They are found in approximately 40% of rectal specimens in people younger than 40 years and in 75% of older persons (Rubin and Strayer, 2007). They are usually limited to the large bowel and are believed to arise due to a defect in proliferation and maturation of normal mucosal epithelium (Geboes et al., 2005). Typically, the luminal epithelium shows *hyperplastic change* with the typical intraluminal infoldings resulting in a saw-toothed appearance (Rosai, 2004; Geboes et al., 2005). By definition, hyperplastic polyps have no malignant potential; however, this stance has recently been challenged and, in some cases, adenocarcinomas of the colon have been found to contain residual adenomatous and hyperplastic epithelium (Robertson and Levison, 2006). In patients with *hyperplastic polyposis syndrome*, the polyps tend to be large and sometimes associated with adenocarcinoma (Leggett et al., 2001). Recently, on the genetic level, these polyps are shown to contain *K-ras mutation* which is a mutation commonly associated with colorectal cancer (CRC) (Day et al., 2003).

In recent years, there has been growing evidence that there is a subgroup of hyperplastic polyps that are not homogeneous and are termed *serrated adenomas*. They are polyps showing both hyperplastic and adenomatous change (Longacre and Fenoglio-Preiser, 1990) and have a higher incidence of *microsatellite instability* (see glossary for definition) and increased risk of development of carcinoma (Day et al., 2003).

Hyperplastic polyposis encompasses a large number of hyperplastic polyps, which are distributed throughout the large bowel and are usually more than 1 cm in size (Williams et al., 1980). This disease is associated with increased risk of malignancy and usually associated with adenomatous polyps.

In conclusion, pure hyperplastic polyps are benign with no malignant potential, but there are subgroups (serrated adenomas and hyperplastic polyposis) differing in their biological behavior from pure forms. They are thought to be neoplastic with an increased risk of malignancy.

Juvenile polyps

These represent focal hamartomatous non-neoplastic malformations of the mucosal epithelium and the vast majority occur in children less than 5 years of age (Robertson and Levison, 2006). Most involve the rectum with an equal male and female distribution and gastrointestinal bleeding is the most common presentation (Day et al., 2003).

Histologically, the lamina propria is usually abundant and encloses cystically dilated glands together with abundant inflammation and frequent ulceration. They have no malignant potential (Nugent et al., 1993). However, when they occur in the setting of *juvenile polyposis syndrome* (a rare autosomal dominant disease), they do carry a higher risk of malignancy and, in this setting, most cancers occur between the age of 20 and 40 years (Robertson and Levison, 2006).

Peutz-Jeghers (PJ) polyps

These are also a *hamartomatous* type of lesion that involve the upper and lower gastrointestinal tract and are more frequently found in the small bowel rather than the large bowel. They usually occur in the setting of *Peutz-Jeghers (PJ) syndrome*, which is an autosomal dominant hereditary condition that is associated with mucosal and cutaneous pigmentation around the lips, oral mucosa, face and other parts of the body (Haggitt and Reid, 1986). Histologically, they are composed of arborizing connective tissue with well-developed smooth muscle fibers that extend into the surrounding mucosa and the lamina propria to surround the crypts (Fulcheri et al., 1991). Patients with PJ polyps commonly present with gastrointestinal hemorrhage and anemia, recurrent colicky abdominal pain and sometimes with recurring intussusceptions, especially after a meal in younger patients (Day et al., 2003). Patients with PJ syndrome have a higher risk of developing gastrointestinal and non-gastrointestinal tumors such as breast and ovarian malignancies (Trau et al., 1982).

Inflammatory polyps

These benign polyps can complicate any inflammatory/infectious disease of the gastrointestinal tract and commonly occur in the setting of *inflammatory bowel disease* (ulcerative colitis and Crohn's disease), mucosal ulceration and in the mucosal prolapse syndrome. They can complicate certain infectious conditions of the bowel, for example schistosomiasis and amebiasis (Robertson and Levison, 2006). They are usually multiple and occur as a non-neoplastic proliferation of either mucosa or granulation tissue due to various injuries to colorectal epithelium. Histologically, they are composed of a pedunculated mucosal growth that is composed of inflammation and commonly associated with surface ulceration and granulation tissue formation. They are benign polyps and have no propensity for malignant transformation (Robertson and Levison, 2006).

Benign lymphoid polyps

These are usually sessile solitary lesions associated with abundant lymphoid tissue forming follicles with active germinal centers. They commonly occur more in the small bowel rather than large bowel with no evidence of malignant transformation (Robertson and Levison, 2006).

Benign neoplastic epithelial tumors

Adenomatous polyps

Adenomas are *benign neoplastic polyps* derived from the surface epithelium and occur in both small and large intestines, involving the latter more frequently (Perzin and Bridge, 1981). *Adenomas*, by definition, are pre-malignant lesions with increased risk of malignant transformation (Leslie et al., 2002). In the small bowel, most benign adenomas occur in the region of the ampulla of Vater and generally they occur most frequently in the region of the duodenum and jejunum and less frequently in the ileum (Rubin and Isaacson, 1990; Cooperman et al., 1978).

Macroscopically, adenomas can be classified as either sessile or pedunculated. *Sessile polyps* are attached to the mucosa without a stalk and are usually raised, while *peduculated polyps* have a stalk (usually composed of normal mucosa) of variable length attached by a narrow base (Figures 14.1 and 14.2) (Robertson and Levison, 2006; Rubin and Strayer, 2007).

Microscopically, they are composed of closely packed and branching glands and can be classified as either *tubular*, *villous* or *tubulovillous* (Geboes et al., 2005). All adenomas, by definition, show disordered cytological differentiation called *dysplasia* (Geboes et al., 2005; Rubin and Strayer, 2007). Dysplasia is derived from the Greek word, which means 'dys' (bad or wrong) and 'plasis' (form) (Rubin and Strayer, 2007). Dysplasia in general is defined as 'unequivocal', non-invasive neoplastic transformation that is confined within the basement membrane of the glands (Riddell et al., 1983). These changes are pre-neoplastic and can lead to malignant transformation. The cytological features that define dysplasia include nuclear enlargement and hyperchromasia with abnormal chromatin pattern. It also includes nuclear

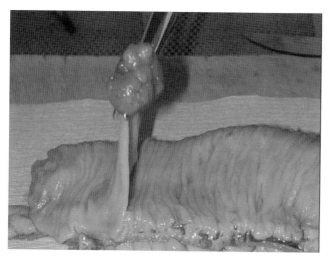

Figure 14.1 A benign colonic polyp attached to the mucosa by a long stalk (pedunculated polyp).

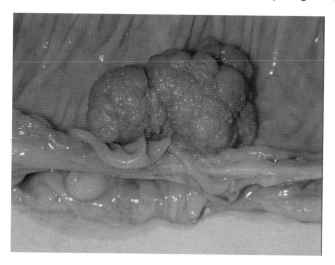

Figure 14.2 A benign colonic polyp attached directly to the mucosa without a stalk (sessile polyp).

crowding and stratification with increased mitotic figures (Figure 14.3, see color insert) (Riddell et al., 1983). These changes may deviate minimally from normal (*low grade dysplasia*) or severely from normal (*high grade dysplasia*). This classification depends upon the histological examination of the degree of cellular immaturity and nuclear features together with the architectural distortion of the glands. Adenomas displaying high-grade epithelial dysplasia have a higher risk of developing adenocarcinoma.

In the large bowel, 40% of adenomatous polyps are found in the right side, 40% in the left side and 20% involve the rectum (Konishi and Morson, 1982) with their frequency rising with age and being uncommon before the age of 30. Most polyps are asymptomatic, but the most common presentation is gastrointestinal bleeding and vague abdominal pain (Sobin, 1985). The risk factors for developing adenomas are the same for colorectal cancer, which include a low fiber and high fat diet and alcohol consumption (Martinez et al., 1996).

The malignant risk of an adenoma if left untreated has been reported to be 2.5%, 8% and 24% after 5, 10 and 20 years. The risk of malignant transformation is very much increased if there is severe dysplasia, villous configuration of the polyp and size over 2 cm (Stryker et al., 1987; Brenner et al., 2007).

Malignant epithelial tumors

Malignant tumors of the small and large intestine can be of *epithelial, mesenchymal* or *lymphoid origin*. The most common malignant tumors involving the bowel are of epithelial origin and comprising epithelial derived adenocarcinomas. *Adenocarcinoma* of the small bowel is 40 to 60 times less common than large bowel carcinoma (Rosai, 2004) with approximately 40–60% occurring in the region of the ampulla of Vater in the duodenum (Rudan et al., 1984).

Colorectal cancer (CRC)

CRC is the third most common cancer and the fourth most frequent cause of cancer deaths worldwide (Robertson and Levison, 2006). At present, in the UK, colorectal cancer is the third most common cancer after breast and lung (Cancer Research UK, 2007). The left side of the colon is affected more than the right and the rectosigmoid junction accounts for over half of all cases (Cancer Research UK, 2007). Eighty-three percent of cases arise in people who are 60 years or older. The disease is more common in North America and Northern Europe and relatively uncommon in Africa (Day et al., 2003). The 5-year survival in developed countries exceeds 60% due to better access to specialist treatment, while it is less than 40% in developing countries (Weitz et al., 2005).

Etiology and risk factors of CRC

Sporadic CRC

Most colorectal cancers are sporadic in which genetic and environmental factors are important in the etiology (Weitz et al., 2005). Some of the *risk factors* associated with the development of colorectal cancer include older age, male sex, cholecystectomy and hormonal factors in women (nulliparity and early menopause). Some *environmental factors* are also known to increase the risk of developing colorectal cancer including a diet rich in meat and fat and poor in fiber, folate and calcium (Weitz et al., 2005). Such a diet is associated with slower transit of fecal contents through the colon and permits longer exposure of the mucosa to possibly toxic substances in the stool. There is a close relationship between per capita meat intake and colorectal cancer incidence (Drasar and Irving, 1973). High intake of fruit, vegetables and fiber is associated with reduced risk of developing CRC (Weitz et al., 2005; Wickam and Lassere, 2007).

Other factors are also known to be associated with an increased risk of developing colorectal cancer including obesity, diabetes mellitus, smoking, previous radiation therapy and high alcohol intake (Weitz et al., 2005). People reporting long-term (at least ten years) regular use of non-steroidal anti-inflammatory drugs or taking at least two tablets a day have a significantly reduced risk of bowel cancer (Chan, 2005).

Colorectal cancer may arise in patients affected by inflammatory bowel disease. This risk depends on the disease duration (at least after 8 years), extent of inflammation, family history of CRC and presence of primary sclerosing cholangitis (Weitz et al., 2005), hence regular surveillance in these patients is recommended for early detection of this complication.

Hereditary CRC

Approximately 5–10% of all colorectal cancers develop in the setting of hereditary cancer syndromes. The two main syndromes associated with an increased risk of developing colorectal cancers are *familial adenomatous polyposis* (FAP) and *hereditary non-polyposis colorectal cancer* (HNPCC) (Lynch, 2003).

FAP is an autosomal dominant disease with a mutation in the adenomatous polyposis coli (APC) gene on chromosome 5 (Chan, 2005). Patients with FAP can develop hundreds of mucosal adenomatous polyps that carpet the mucosa and, if left untreated, almost all patients develop cancer by the age of 40 (Weitz et al., 2005). These patients can also have adenomatous polyps elsewhere in the bowel, such as the duodenum and the stomach, from which carcinoma can arise (Bulow et al., 2004).

HNPCC (also known as *Lynch syndrome*) is an autosomal dominant disorder caused by mutation of the mismatch repair genes. Microsatellite (which are short repeated DNA sequences) instability is considered to be the main etiology of the disease (Grady, 2003). Patients with this syndrome also have increased risk of developing tumors elsewhere, such as the genitourinary system particularly of the endometrium, as well as the pancreas and the biliary system. Interestingly, increased risk of developing brain tumors is present with both FAP and HNPCC with medulloblastomas common in the former and gliomas in the latter (Vasen et al., 1996).

Pathology and pathogenesis of colorectal cancer

Almost 95% of colonic tumors are of epithelial origin and arise from the *glandular epithelium* (Drasar and Irving, 1973; Robertson and Levison, 2006). *Adenomatous polyps* precede colorectal cancer in 70–90% of patients and 50% of large polyps (more than 2 cm in diameter) become malignant while the risk is smaller with smaller polyps (less than 5 mm) (Drasar and Irving, 1973). Adenomatous polyps are up to six times more common in colonic specimens with cancer (Day et al., 2003).

This strong link between adenomas and colorectal cancer led to the development of the *multistep theory of colorectal carcinogenesis*. This is a well-documented pathway and involves multistep progression from normal mucosa to dysplastic epithelium to invasive carcinoma (Bulow et al., 2004; Robertson and Levison, 2006; Leslie et al., 2002). This multistep model, developed by Fearon and Vogelstein (1990), involves certain oncogenes and tumor suppressor genes with accumulation of multiple genetic alterations and mutations. Mutations of normal oncogenes inhibit the deregularity effect of these genes and promote cancer growth, whereas mutations in the normal tumor suppressor genes (e.g. p53) inhibit the tumor suppressor activity of these genes and subsequently promote the development of cancer cells (Vasen et al., 1996).

The most common first step in the development of colorectal cancer is the mutation of the *adenomatous polyposis coli gene*, which leads to cellular deregulation and the development of adenomatous polyps (Drasar and Irving, 1973).

The most common next step is the mutation of the *K-ras oncogene* and *deleted in colorectal cancer gene*, which leads to an increase in the size of an established adenoma. The final step is the loss or mutation of *p53 tumor suppressor gene* (Robertson and Levison, 2006) that leads to the development of carcinoma.

Another suggested pathway occurs through microsatellite instability that involves *DNA mismatch repair genes*. Microsatellites are small regions of deoxyribonucleic acid (DNA), one to five base pairs long, that are repeated multiple times. They are widely dispersed throughout the genome and are susceptible to errors during DNA replication. In health, the DNA mismatch repair proteins are responsible for correcting replication errors. However, if this repair mechanism is faulty or absent, numerous replication errors remain uncorrected and, if present at a significant level, the term '*microsatellite instability*' is used. Microsatellite instability is responsible for the development of adenocarcinomas with a predilection for the right side of the colon, poor histological differentiation, but a relatively favorable prognosis (Robertson and Levison, 2006). However, the exact sequence of development of adenocarcinoma is not always known, as colorectal cancers are usually heterogeneous (Syngal et al., 2006).

Adenocarcinoma of the large bowel (Figure 14.4) is more commonly found in the left side of the colon than the right side, in which the rectosigmoid region is involved in approximately 55% of cases and the cecum and ascending colon in 22% of cases (Robertson and Levison, 2006). Right-sided tumors tend to be more polypoidal and present as exophytic masses projecting into the lumen, while left-sided tumors tend to be more circumferential, causing strictures and tumors in this region which are more liable to cause large bowel obstruction.

Histological examination is of utmost importance in establishing the diagnosis of carcinoma. By definition, invasion of malignant glands into the submucosa establishes the diagnosis of carcinoma. Depending on the degree of differentiation, adenocarcinoma can be divided into well, moderate and poorly differentiated depending on the amount of well-formed glands that constitute the tumor and their similarity to the normal epithelium. The *degree of differentiation*, together with other factors, affects the prognosis of the patient with the disease (Rosai, 2004). Other factors likely to be associated with worse

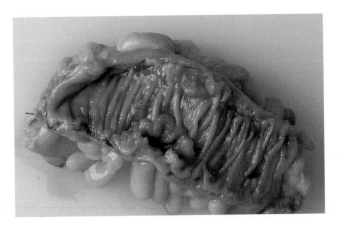

Figure 14.4 Colonic adenocarcinoma presents as a raised and centrally ulcerated tumor.

Table 14.2 Dukes staging system for CRC

Dukes stage	Definition
A	Tumor limited to wall (not beyond muscularis propria), nodes negative
B	Tumor invading beyond muscularis propria, nodes negative
C	Tumors with metastasis to regional lymph nodes (apical node negative 'C1'; apical node positive 'C2')
D	Distant metastases present

prognosis include very young and very old age, tumor perforation, vascular invasion and lymph node involvement. However, the most influential factor which affects the prognosis of patients with CRC is the *stage of the disease*, which is the degree of tumor spread or extension.

Several *staging systems* have been used for colorectal cancer. The most common staging system is the *Dukes stage* (Table 14.2) (Dukes, 1932). The Dukes stage depends on the depth of tumor invasion and lymph node involvement. The *TNM (tumor, node and metastasis) staging system* is also used increasingly for colorectal cancers (Table 14.3). The prognosis and hence survival of patients with CRC mainly depends on the stage. For patients with Dukes stage 'A' (tumor limited to the wall), the *5-year survival* is 95–100% while with Dukes 'C' (tumor with lymph node involvement) the prognosis is poor and the *5-year survival* is between 10 and 35% (Day et al., 2003; Robertson and Levison, 2006).

Neuro-endocrine tumors

The most common neuro-endocrine tumor is the *carcinoid tumor*. They arise from the neuro-endocrine cells of the surface mucosal epithelium and can be divided into non-functioning and functioning (Robertson and Levison, 2006). *Functioning tumors* release peptide hormones such as gastrin, somatostatin and serotonin and they are usually associated with the so-called *carcinoid syndrome*. The appendix is the commonest site to be involved (Kumar et al., 2004).

Mesenchymal tumors

Gastrointestinal stromal tumors (GIST) are the most common non-epithelial tumors of the gastrointestinal tract and, until recently, they were thought to be of smooth muscle origin. However, recently, it has been demonstrated that they originate from the interstitial cells of Cajal which are the cells involved in the innervation of the gut (Fletcher et al., 2002). Macroscopically, these are usually well-circumscribed tumors, exophytic and protruding into the lumen of the gut with frequent surface ulceration. They most commonly occur in the stomach (approximately 60%) and approximately 25–40% arise in the small bowel. These tumors can be divided into benign, malignant and of indeterminate behavior according to the tumor size, number of mitoses and the presence or absence of cellular atypia. These tumors contain a protein, which is usually detected on immunohistochemistry (CD117). This finding has a

Table 14.3 TNM staging system for CRC

Tumor	Definition
Tx	Primary tumor cannot be assessed
T0	No evidence of primary tumor
Tis	Carcinoma in situ: intraepithelial or invasion into the lamina propria with no extension through muscularis mucosae into submucosa
T1	Tumor invades into submucosa, but not the muscularis propria
T2	Tumor invades into but not through the muscularis propria
T3	Tumor invades through bowel wall into subserosa or non-peritonealized pericolic/perirectal tissues
T4	Tumor invades other organs and structures and/or perforates visceral peritoneum
Nodes	
Nx	Regional lymph nodes cannot be assessed
N0	No regional lymph node metastases
N1	1–3 regional lymph node(s)
N2	4 or more regional lymph nodes
Metastases	
Mx	Metastatic disease cannot be assessed
M0	No evidence of metastatic disease
M1	Distant metastases present

therapeutic benefit to patients because these patients are usually responsive to the drug Imatinib (Robertson and Levison, 2006).

Lipomas

These are benign tumors of *fatty tissue* and are infrequently found to involve the intestine. However, they can arise near the area of the ileocecal valve within the submucosa causing narrowing of the lumen and, in some cases, obstruction (Robertson and Levison, 2006). *Liposarcomas*, the malignant counterparts of lipomas rarely involve the small and large intestine.

Angiomas

Angiomas are benign tumors of *vascular origin* and are infrequently found within the gastrointestinal tract. Histologically, they can appear as either a *cavernous* or *capillary hemangioma* and they can sometimes bleed and lead to melena and anemia (Robertson and Levison, 2006).

Lymphomas

These are of *lymphoid origin* and are more common in the small bowel than the large bowel. It is one of the commonest tumors to involve the small bowel and accounts for 17% of tumors at this site, whereas it accounts for only 0.2% of tumors of the large bowel. Most intestinal lymphomas are of *B-cell non-Hodgkin's type*, but *T-cell type* also occurs and these are commonly associated with and complicate celiac disease (Rooney and Dogan, 2004), termed *enteropathy associated T-cell lymphoma*.

Glossary

Benign tumors: tumors which grow slowly and are usually treatable (by surgery) and are not life threatening.

Dysplasia: is an abnormal growth and differentiation of cells where the cells grow in a disordered manner with abnormal maturation. It is a pre-neoplastic process.

Epithelium: the covering of the internal and external organs of the body and also the lining of vessels, body cavities, glands and organs.

Hamartoma: a hamartoma is a peculiar benign neoplasm, which is a localized but haphazard growth of tissues normally found at a given site (pulmonary hamartoma has jumbled cartilage, bronchial epithelium and connective tissue).

Hyperplasia: is an increase in the size of a tissue or organ due to an increase in the number of constituent cells. It is not considered to be a pre-neoplastic process.

Malignant tumors: they grow fast and are liable to metastasize to distant body sites and are usually life-threatening neoplasms.

Mesenchymal tumors: they are connective tissue tumors such as fibromas, lipomas or osteomas and their malignant counterparts.

Microsatellite: microsatellites are small regions of deoxyribonucleic acid (DNA), one to five base pairs long, that are repeated multiple times.

Neoplasm (tumor): is an abnormal mass of tissue, the growth of which exceeds and is uncoordinated with that of normal tissue and persists in the same excessive way after cessation of the stimuli which evoke the change.

References

Brenner, H., Hoffmeister, M., Stegmaier, C., et al., 2007. Risk of progression of advanced adenomas to colorectal cancer by age and sex: estimates based on 840 149 screening colonoscopies. Gut 56 (11), 1585–1589.

Bulow, S., Bjork, J., Christensen, I., et al., 2004. Duodenal adenomatosis in familial adenomatous polyposis. Gut 53 (3), 381–386.

Cancer Research UK, 2007. Colorectal cancer statistics. <http://www.cancerresearchuk.org> Accessed 10 August, 2007.

Chan, A., 2005. Long-term use of aspirin and nonsteroidal anti-inflammatory drugs and risk of colorectal cancer. J. Am. Med. Assoc. 294 (8), 914–923.

Day, D., Jass, J., Price, A., et al., 2003. Morson and Dawson's gastrointestinal pathology. fourth ed. Blackwell Publishing.

Drasar, B., Irving, D., 1973. Environmental factors and cancer of the colon and breast. Br. J. Cancer 27 (2), 167–172.

Dukes, C., 1932. The classification of cancer of the rectum. J. Pathol. Bacteriol. 35, 323–332.

Fearon, E., Vogelstein, B., 1990. A genetic model for colorectal tumorigenesis. Cell 61 (5), 759–767.

Fletcher, C., Berman, J., Corless, C., et al., 2002. Diagnosis of gastrointestinal stromal tumors: a consensus approach. Hum. Pathol. 33 (5), 459–465.

Fulcheri, E., Baracchini, P., Pagani, A., et al., 1991. Significance of the smooth muscle cell component in Peutz-Jeghers and juvenile polyps. Hum. Pathol. 22 (11), 1136–1140.

Geboes, K., Ectors, N., Geboes, K., 2005. Pathology of early lower GI cancer. Best Prac. Research Clin. Gastroenterol. 19 (6), 963–978.

Grady, W., 2003. Genetic testing for high-risk colon cancer patients. Gastroenterology 124 (6), 1574–1594.

Haggitt, R., Reid, B., 1986. Hereditary gastrointestinal polyposis syndromes. Am. J. Surg. Pathol. 10 (12), 871–887.

Konishi, F., Morson, B., 1982. Pathology of colorectal adenomas: a colonoscopic survey. J. Clin. Pathol. 35 (8), 830–841.

Kumar, V., Abbas, A., Fausto, N., 2004. Robbins and Cotrans' pathologic basis of disease. seventh ed. Saunders.

Leggett, B., Devereaux, B., Biden, K., et al., 2001. Hyperplastic polyposis: association with colorectal cancer. Am. J. Surg. Pathol. 25 (2), 177–184.

Leslie, A., Carey, F., Pratt, N., et al., 2002. The colorectal adenoma-carcinoma sequence. Br. J. Surg. 89 (7), 845–860.

Longacre, T., Fenoglio-Preiser, C., 1990. Mixed hyperplastic adenomatous polyps/serrated adenomas. A distinct form of colorectal neoplasia. Am. J. Surg. Pathol. 14 (6), 524–537.

Martinez, M., McPherson, R., Annegers, J., et al., 1996. Association of diet and colorectal adenomatous polyps: dietary fiber, calcium, and total fat. Epidemiology 7 (3), 264–268.

Nugent, K., Talbot, I., Hodgson, S., et al., 1993. Solitary juvenile polyps: not a marker for subsequent malignancy. Gastroenterology 105 (3), 698–700.

Perzin, K., Bridge, M., 1981. Adenomas of the small intestine: a clinicopathologic review of 51 cases and a study of their relationship to carcinoma. Cancer 48 (3), 799–819.

Riddell, R., Goldman, H., Ransohoff, D., et al., 1983. Dysplasia in inflammatory bowel disease: standardized classification with provisional clinical applications. Hum. Pathol. 14 (11), 931–968.

Robertson, K., Levison, D., 2006. Pathology of tumours of the small and large intestine. Surgery 24 (4), 126–131.

Rooney, N., Dogan, A., 2004. Gastrointestinal lymphoma. Curr. Diag. Pathol. 10, 69–78.

Rosai, J., 2004. Rosai and Ackerman's surgical pathology. Ninth ed. Mosby.

Rubin, A., Isaacson, P., 1990. Florid reactive lymphoid hyperplasia of the terminal ileum in adults: a condition bearing a close resemblance to low-grade malignant lymphoma. Histopathology 17 (1), 19–26.

Rubin, R., Strayer, D., 2007. Rubin's pathology: clinicopathologic foundations of medicine. fifth ed. Lippincott Williams & Wilkins.

Rudan, N., Nola, P., Popovic, S., 1984. Primary adenocarcinoma of the duodenum. Report of two cases. Cancer 54 (6), 1105–1109.

Sobin, L., 1985. The histopathology of bleeding from polyps and carcinomas of the large intestine. Cancer 55 (3), 577–581.

Stryker, S., Wolff, B., Culp, C., et al., 1987. Natural history of untreated colonic polyps. Gastroenterology 93 (5), 1009–1013.

Syngal, S., Stoffel, E., Chung, D., et al., 2006. Detection of stool DNA mutations before and after treatment of colorectal neoplasia. Cancer 106 (2), 277–283.

Trau, H., Schewach-Millet, M., Fisher, B., et al., 1982. Peutz-Jeghers syndrome and bilateral breast carcinoma. Cancer 50 (4), 788–792.

Vasen, H., Sanders, E., Taal, B., et al., 1996. The risk of brain tumours in hereditary non-polyposis colorectal cancer (HNPCC). Int. J. Cancer 65 (4), 422–425.

Weitz, J., Koch, M., Debus, J., et al., 2005. Colorectal cancer. Lancet 365 (9454), 153–165.

Wickam, R., Lassere, Y., 2007. The ABCs of colorectal cancer. Semin. Oncol. Nurs. 23, 1–8.

Williams, G., Arthur, J., Bussey, H., et al., 1980. Metaplastic polyps and polyposis of the colorectum. Histopathology 4 (2), 155–170.

An introduction to diverticular disease

Robert L. Law

Contents

Introduction

The origin of the word *diverticulum* is suggested to come from the Latin de-verto – to turn aside, at that time implying a by-road (Google, 2008), although perhaps more memorably it has been suggested that it related to a 'wayside house of ill repute' (Tjandra et al., 2008). Nowadays, it is associated with a benign sac-like protuberance that arises from a hollow organ.

Colonic diverticula are more correctly *pseudodiverticula* as it is the mucosa that invaginates through the circular muscle bound by muscularis mucosae and a thin layer of connective tissue. Asymptomatic colonic diverticula identified as an incidental finding are referred to as *diverticulosis*. If diverticula become symptomatic this is known as *diverticular disease*. Inflammation associated with diverticular disease is called *diverticulitis*. During the double contrast barium enema examination, mild uncomplicated diverticula may be noted and ignored except for a short comment in the report.

In this chapter, it is intended to bring to life the humble colonic diverticulum and to provide the reader with an insight into how and why it develops and the complications that can arise.

History

Diverticula of the colon were first described by Littre in 1700. The possibility of diverticula as a site of infection and perforation was first raised in 1849 by

Jean Cruveilhier, an eminent Parisian anatomist (Painter and Burkitt, 1971; Mimura et al., 2002). In 1912, George Haenisch, a roentgenologist, was the first to recognize and describe diverticulitis radiologically.

When considering the etiology of diverticular disease, the most substantiated theory is that of a deficiency in dietary fiber. Following his work as a surgeon in central Africa in the 20th century, Dennis Burkitt appreciated the connection between dietary fiber and the volume and soft nature of feces produced with negligible discomfort by the Africans who lived largely on a vegetarian diet. In 1971, Painter and Burkitt put forward their belief that a *low-residue diet* was the cause of diverticular disease. It was also noted at that time that, in the central parts of Africa, a number of diseases common in the West, including diverticulitis, were rarely observed (Painter and Burkitt, 1971; Story and Kritchersky, 1994; Netter, 2000; Mimura et al., 2002; Stollman and Raskin, 2004).

Anatomy: colon structure as it relates to diverticular disease

To understand the mechanism of how and why diverticula can form, the musculature and blood supply of the colon need to be reviewed. The colon is made up of four layers: mucosa, submucosa, muscularis and serosa. The muscular layer consists of an inner circular muscle and external longitudinal muscle. The circular muscle forms a thin layer over the cecum and colon, forming a thicker layer covering the rectum. The external longitudinal muscle forms a coating of muscle fiber much thinner than that of the circular muscle it covers. On three aspects of the circumference of the colon, the muscle thickens to form three longitudinal bands, the *teniae coli*. Individually, the muscle bands are known as tenia mesocolica, libera and omentalis. The three teniae are shorter than the length of circular muscle causing the colon to concertina and become sacculated. These sacculations are called *haustral folds* between which circular muscle fiber becomes thicker. The three teniae have their origin of attachment at the base of the appendix. In most cases, the bands are spaced equidistant around the circumference of the cecum (Davies, 1969; Netter, 1975) (see also Chapter 4).

In the distal colon, the three teniae fan out at the level of the peritoneal reflection, completely encasing the rectum but forming a thickened portion still recognizable as bands on the anterior and posterior aspects of the rectum (Wolf et al., 2000). Diverticula do not occur distal to the peritoneal reflection, as the anatomical and pathophysiological features are different to that of the colon.

The English physician, Sir David Drummond, described an arterial ring around the colon, the '*marginal artery of Drummond*' (Gunasekera et al., 2003; Floch and Bina, 2004). The *vasa recta* arise at frequent intervals around the marginal artery. Dividing at the tenia mesocolica, the vasa recta branches into nutrient vessels that supply the colon. The nutrient vessels pass deep via a canal either side of mesocolica and on the mesenteric side of teniae libera and omentalis (Bassotti et al., 2003; Floch and Bina, 2004). Along these canals the nutrient artery passes through the circular muscle fiber to its origin. In the right circumstances, these canals constitute the weak points through which the mucosa can protrude creating a diverticulum (Figures 15.1 and 15.2).

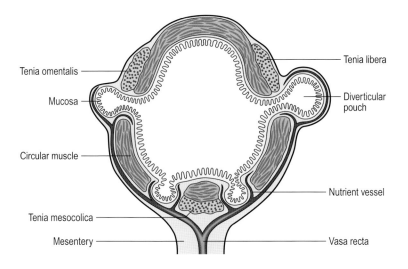

Figure 15.1 Cross-section of the colon with the site of diverticular outpouching.

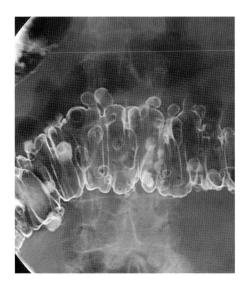

Figure 15.2 **Apparent haphazard formation of diverticula at barium enema.** Sillhouette margin showing diverticula arising from the apex of the haustral folds.

Pathogenesis

Papers by Painter and Burkitt (1971), Smith (1986), Aldoori et al. (1998), Frieri et al. (2006) and Blackwood and Salter (2000) are among the many that support the hypothesis that dietary fiber reduces the risk of diverticular disease and, conversely, the risk being increased by a lack of fiber, particularly the insoluble fiber *hydrocolloid cellulose*.

The dietary fiber hydrocolloid cellulose is a non-digestible carbohydrate found in plant material. Although this cellulose itself has a low water content, it is porous and has a significant capability to retain water within its pores. Hydrocolloid cellulose is also resistant to the effects of enzymes in the small

Table 15.1 Pathogenesis of diverticular disease

Lack of dietary fiber increases the risk of diverticular disease	
High fiber intake	**Low fiber intake**
Cellulose, an insoluble hydrocolloid, is the most relevant dietary fiber	Low bulk, high density stool
Cellulose is indigestible by enzymes in the small bowel	Smaller lumen radius
Cellulose is porous and has a high capacity to retain water	High viscosity and slower stool transit time
Water retained in cellulose forms a bulky stool	Raised intraluminal pressure required to propel stool
Fluid in a bulky stool reduces stool viscosity and therefore transit time	
Lumen radius of colon commensurate to size of stool	

bowel and it can provide support for the growth of microflora in the colon as fermentation takes place. It is the high water-retaining capability of the insoluble element of cellulose that is responsible for the (beneficial) formation of a more bulky stool. This results in the maintenance of colonic lumen diameter commensurate with the stool volume. The fluid retained within the stool as a result of dietary fiber intake reduces fecal viscosity and results in a reduced transit time (Prosky and Dreher, 1999; Bassotti et al., 2003). Painter and Burkitt (1971) reported that, in areas of Africa where the population has a high fiber intake, normal colonic transit time was half that common in the West at that time.

Understanding the widely accepted hypothesis as to what provides and constitutes a good stool enables an understanding of the converse, that a lack of dietary fiber results in a reduction in fecal water content. This leads to the stool being more compact and smaller in diameter and with an increased viscosity. The denser less viscous stool, in conjunction with the reduced diameter of the colon, results in a *higher intraluminal pressure* requirement to pass the fecal column through the bowel. The slower passage of the stool though the colon allows more fluid to be absorbed maintaining the vicious circle that supports the pathogenesis of diverticular disease (Table 15.1).

Pathophysiology

The high intraluminal pressure directed towards the bowel wall identifies the points of least resistance. At the apex of the arc-like haustral folds where the tensile strength is least, the weak points are the canals either side of tenia mesocolica and on the mesenteric side of teniae libera and omentalis through which the nutrient vessels pass.

Pierre-Simon Laplace (1749–1827), a French mathematician, gave his name to a law that provides an explanation as to how the intra- and extraluminal pressure difference, the radius of the colonic lumen and the nature and thickness of the bowel wall can affect the bowel wall tension (Smith, 1986; West, 2006).

BOX 15.1 Pathophysiology of diverticular disease

- Reduction in tensile strength
- High intraluminal pressure
- Law of Laplace explains effect of pressure on colonic wall
- Increased deposits in connective tissue of (e.g.) elastin
- Shortening of the longitudinal muscle
- Thickening of the circular muscle
- Muscular contraction causes segmentation
- Diverticula form through tract of the vasa recta

Basford (2002) considers the *law of Laplace* and its relevance today. One area in which Laplace's law can be demonstrated is *fecal transit* in the colon. The wider diameter of the colonic lumen resulting from a bulky fluid retentive stool provides for a relatively low fecal viscosity and a reduced transit time which together assist in maintaining a low intraluminal pressure requirement for the movement of stool through the large bowel. Normally, the sigmoid region has the narrowest lumen within the colon and thereby lends itself to having the highest intraluminal pressure and thus the greatest propensity towards colonic diverticular disease anywhere where a low fiber diet is usual.

Contractions occur in the colon to help propel fecal material through the lumen and aid its mixing for fluid absorption. These contractions cause *segmentation* in the lumen that are not normally of any clinical relevance when a diet includes a significant proportion of insoluble dietary fiber creating the optimum stool form.

When segmentation becomes occlusive, the likelihood of diverticulosis is increased. *Occlusive segmentation* happens when the structural changes in the connective tissue shortens the longitudinal muscle, thickening the circular muscle layer. Efforts from increased work requirement from the circular muscle results in concertina-like folds narrowing the lumen. In conjunction with these factors, there are associated pathogenetic factors (high intraluminal pressure and high fecal viscosity) which predispose to strong muscular contraction that divides the lumen into segments that can be exaggerated to the point of causing occlusive capsules. Within the occlusive capsule, additional intraluminal pressure is generated that is directed towards the colonic wall.

Arising at the apex of the haustra (where the tensile strength is least), *diverticula* become manifest in a linear array contrary to their apparent irregular distribution demonstrated at barium enema examination (Box 15.1) (Figures 15.2, 15.3A, 15.3B) (Netter, 1975; Whiteway and Morson, 1985; Smith, 1986; Bassotti et al., 2003; Eastwood, 2003; Stollman and Raskin, 2004; Floch and Bina, 2004; West, 2004, 2006; West and Losada, 2004; Ye et al., 2005; Parra-Blanco, 2006).

Epidemiology of right-sided colonic diverticula

The Western tendency towards sigmoid diverticular disease is not reflected in Asian populations where diverticular disease predominantly affects the right colon (Gunasekera et al., 2003). West (2006) reports the suggestion

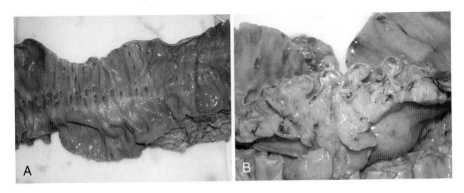

Figure 15.3 (A) Longitudinal dissection of colon demonstrating uniformity of formation; (B) dissection through the bowel wall showing cross-section through diverticula.

that diverticula of the cecum and ascending colon, as commonly found in Asia, differ from the diverticula found in the West, occurring at an earlier age and associated with a *genetic predisposition*. The predisposition of right-sided diverticula in Asians is supported by others (Mimura et al., 2002; Stollman and Raskin, 2004; Kang et al., 2004; Rajendra and Ho, 2005). Etiology of the predominantly right-sided diverticula found in Japan was reported by Nakaji et al. (2002) as similar to left-sided diverticula in the West.

Age

Asymptomatic diverticular disease in the Western world is rare under the age of 40 but is widely recognized as increasing in prevalence with age. A number of papers suggest that diverticulosis might be present in up to 60% of the population, however, there is a variance in the reported age range to which this percentage relates between 60 years and over 80 years of age (Carter and Whelan, 2000; Mimura et al., 2002; Floch and Bina, 2004; West and Losada, 2004).

In a 10-year UK study of diverticular disease hospitalizations, Jeyarajah et al. (2008) reported 1 219 480 patients hospitalized with a diagnosis of diverticular disease with the disease being the primary cause of admission in 567 423 cases and a comorbidity in 652 057 admissions.

With age, structural changes occur in the connective tissue, including increase in submucosal deposits of collagen, elastin and reticular tissue. The association between this and the increased chance of diverticulosis is discussed in the section on pathophysiology in this chapter (Aldoori et al., 1998; Carter and Whelan, 2000; Basford, 2002; Mimura et al., 2002; Eastwood, 2003; Floch and Bina, 2004; West and Losada, 2004; Parra-Blanco, 2006).

Complications

Between 75 and 85% of patients with diverticula will remain asymptomatic (West, 2004; Salzman and Lillie, 2005). The complications that are associated with diverticular disease include bleeding and inflammation, which itself can lead to perforation, abscess formation, obstruction and peritonitis.

Bleeding

The pathogenesis of diverticular bleeding results from the vasa recta becoming stretched over the dome of the forming pseudodiverticular sac, with eccentric intimal thickening with thinning of the walls between the apex of the dome of the sac and the artery. The features predispose to the blood vessel rupturing towards the diverticulum at its apex (Meyers et al., 1976).

Diverticular disease accounts for over 40% of *acute lower gastrointestinal tract bleeding* making it the most common cause of acute bleeding in the lower gastrointestinal tract (Kang et al., 2004; West, 2006). Onset of bleeding is usually abrupt, painless and self-limiting, stopping spontaneously in 70–80% of cases. Bleeding can be significant in 3–5% of cases with a 22–38% chance of a diverticulum re-bleeding. Diverticular bleeding is not considered a feature associated with acute diverticular inflammation (Blackwood et al., 2000; Netter, 2000; Stollman and Raskin, 2004; Frieri et al., 2006; Parra-Blanco, 2006; Kriel and Probert, 2007).

Diverticulitis

Colecchia and Sandri (2003) suggest that diverticulitis will affect 10–25% of patients with diverticular disease. Floch and Bina (2004) advanced further evidence to support the suggestion that fiber deficiency not only leads to the formation of diverticula but is also associated with changes in the colonic microflora. This may be associated with a decrease in the colonic mucosal immune response, supporting referenced evidence that chronic segmental colitis is associated with diverticula. The presented hypothesis was that the *chronic inflammation* occurs in the mucosa associated with the diverticula and is the cause of diverticulitis (Smith, 1986).

Fecal material inspissated within a diverticulum can rasp, irritate and damage the mucosa. While the sac of the diverticulum is bounded by the muscularis, it is provided with extrinsic support. However, once through to the serosa the support is no longer present leading to the potential to perforate, particularly with the increased intraluminal pressure produced with the strain to evacuate. A resultant perforation may only be small, but such a microperforation makes it possible for bacteria to pass into the subserosa and create a local inflammatory reaction within close proximity to the bowel wall, this can result in small contained *pericolic abscess formation* (Figure 15.4).

A local inflammatory process can extend through the full thickness of the bowel wall. The more serious *macroperforation* can lead to abscess and inflammatory mass formation within the peritoneum. Inflammatory mass and *peritoneal abscess development* can result in one or more of a number of complications including: adhesions, scarring, stricturing and free perforation into the peritoneum resulting in *fecal peritonitis*. Where there is inflammatory adhesion to an adjacent hollow organ, such as the bladder or vagina, there is the potential for *fistula formation* (Smith, 1986; Netter, 2000; Colecchia and Sandri, 2003; West and Losada, 2004).

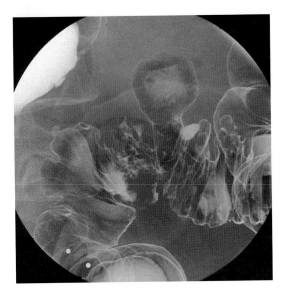

Figure 15.4 Crumpled mucosa of an inflammatory diverticular stricture; large diverticulum, the remains of a pericolic abscess; colocolic fistula.

Fistula

The term fistula originates from the Latin for pipe or tube and denotes a pathologically abnormal passage leading from an abscess cavity or hollow organ to another hollow organ or the skin surface. When a phlegmon or abscess extends from a diverticulum, it has the potential of rupturing into an adjacent hollow organ enabling a fistula to develop (Figure 15.5). *Colovesical fistulae* are the most common variety with a male to female predominance by a factor of 2:1, the female bladder being protected by the uterus. *Colovaginal*

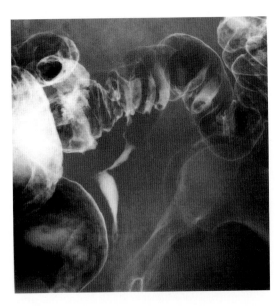

Figure 15.5 Colovaginal fistula seen to arise from a small diverticulum.

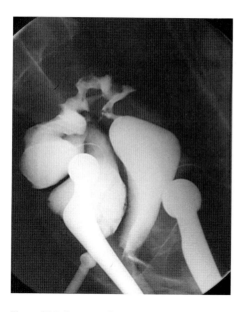

Figure 15.6 Passage of rectal contrast passing directly through a fistulous tract into the vagina.

fistulae constitute 25% of all cases and are the next most common tract formation resulting from diverticulitis (Blackwood et al., 2000; Netter, 2000) (Figures 15.5 and 15.6).

Stricturing and obstruction

Luminal narrowing or obstruction during an acute episode of diverticulitis can occur due to the pericolic inflammation (Figure 15.7) or compression from abscess formation. Diverticular abscess formation is easily diagnosed with CT.

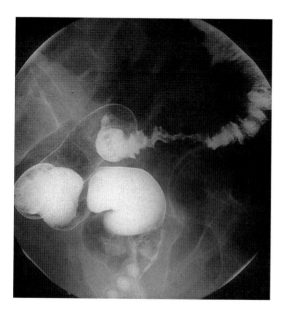

Figure 15.7 Narrow segment associated with an acute diverticulitis.

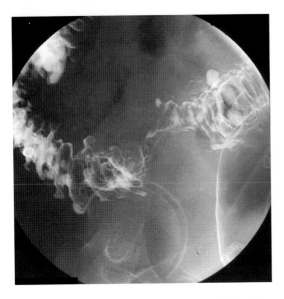

Figure 15.8 Fibrotic stricture: the appearance of the stricture may also suggest a malignancy and will require further imaging to confirm or exclude.

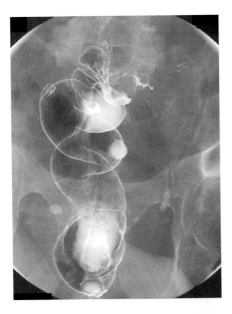

Figure 15.9 Fibrotic stricture: complete obstruction to the retrograde flow of barium, although antegrade passage may still be possible.

Diverticulitis is often self-limiting and responds to drug therapy and with the therapeutic response the associated stricturing can resolve. It is possible for a patient to have recurrent bouts of diverticulitis which appear asymptomatic; these can trigger the development of *fibrotic stricturing* (Figures 15.8 and 15.9) (Box 15.2) (Netter, 2000; Blackwood et al., 2000).

BOX 15.2 Complications of diverticular disease

Bleeding

- The vasa recta may be stretched over the forming diverticula
- 40% of lower GI bleeding is of diverticular origin
- GI bleeding not necessarily related to inflammation

Diverticulitis

- Affects 10–25% of patients with diverticular disease
- Damaged diverticular mucosa can result in micro- or macroperforation
- Microperforation can result in peridiverticular abscess
- Macroperforation can lead to inflammatory mass, peritoneal abscess, free perforation, peritonitis, fistula colonic structuring

---

Additional information

Symptoms associated with diverticular disease and its complications (Chapter 10 – Symptoms of lower gastrointestinal disease).

Diagnosis of diverticular disease and its complications can be found in Chapter 13 – Fluoroscopic investigations of the large bowel; Chapter 17 – Cross-sectional investigations, nuclear medicine and ultrasound of the small and large bowel; Chapter 20 – Endoscopy of the upper and lower gastrointestinal tract.

Surgical management of diverticular disease and its complications (Chapter 21 – Common surgical procedures of the gastrointestinal tract).

References

Aldoori, W.H., Giovannucci, E.L., Rocket, H.R., et al., 1998. A prospective study of dietary fiber types and symptomatic diverticular disease in men. J. Nutr. 128 (4), 714–719.

Basford, J.R., 2002. The law of Laplace and its relevance to contemporary medicine and rehabilitation. Arch. Phys. Med. Rehabil. 83 (8), 1165–1170.

Bassotti, G., Chistolinim, F., Morelli, A., et al., 2003. Pathophysiological aspects of diverticular disease of colon and role of large bowel motility. World J. Gastroenterol. 9 (10), 2140–2142.

Blackwood, A.D., Salter, J., 2000. Dietary fibre, physiochemical properties and their relationship to health. J. Royal Soc. Promo. Health 120 (4), 242–247.

Carter, J.J., Whelan, R.L., 2000. Evaluation and medial management of diverticular disease. Sem. Colon Rectal Surg. 11 (4), 195–205.

Colecchia, A., Sandri, L., 2003. Diverticular disease of the colon: new perspectives in symptom development and treatment. World J. Gastroenterol. 9 (7), 1385–1389.

Davies, D.V., 1969. Gray's anatomy. Longmans, pp. 1488–1508.

Eastwood, M., 2003. Colonic diverticula. Proc. Nutr. Soc. 62 (1), 31–36.

Floch, M.H., Bina, I., 2004. The natural history of diverticulitis: fact and theory. J. Clin. Gastroenterol. 38 (5 Suppl.), S2–S7.

Frieri, G., Pimpo, M.T., Scarpignato, C., et al., 2006. Management of colonic diverticular disease. Digestion 73 (Suppl. 1), 58–66.

Gunasekera, R.T., Akroyd, R., Stoddard, C.J., et al., 2003. Complete rectal obstruction due to ischaemia following elective abdominal aortic aneurysm surgery. Surgeon 1 (2), 114–117.

Jeyarajah, S., Tekkis, P.P., Aylin, P., et al., 2008. British Society of Gastroenterology (BSG) Abstracts. Diverticular disease hospitalisations have a rapidly increasing impact on the health service and affect younger people and deprived socioeconomic groups. Gut 57 (Suppl.1), A17.

Kang, J.Y., Melville, D., Maxwell, J.D., et al., 2004. Epidemiology and management of diverticular disease of the colon. Drugs Aging 21 (4), 211–228.

Kriel, H., Probert, C.S., 2007. Diverticular disease. Medicine (Abingdon) 35 (6), 317–319.

Meyers, M.A., Alonso, D.R., Morson, B.C., et al., 1976. Pathogenesis of bleeding colonic diverticulosis. Gastroenterology 76 (4), 577–583.

Mimura, T., Emanuel, A., Kamm, M.A., et al., 2002. Pathophysiology of diverticular disease. Best Pract. Res. Clin. Gastroenterol. 16 (4), 563–576.

Nakaji, S., Danjo, K., Munakata, A., et al., 2002. Comparison of etiology of right-sided diverticula in Japan with that of left sided diverticula in the West. Int. J. Colorectal Dis. 17 (6), 365–373.

Netter, F.H., 2000. Atlas of human anatomy, 2nd ed. Novartis.

Netter, F.H., 1975. The Ciba collection of medical illustrations, Vol. 3. Digestive system, Part 2: Lower digestive tract.

Painter, N.S., Burkitt, D.P., 1971. Diverticular disease of the colon: a deficiency disease of western civilization. Br. Med. J. 2, 450–454.

Parra-Blanco, A., 2006. Colonic diverticular disease: pathophysiology and clinical picture. Digestion 73 (Suppl.), 47–57.

Prosky, L., Dreher, M.L., 1999. Complex carbohydrates in food, CRC Press.

Rajendra, S., Ho, J.J., 2005. Colonic diverticular disease in a multiracial Asian patient population has an ethnic predilection. Eur. J. Gastroenterol. Hepatol. 17 (8), 871–875.

Salzman, H., Lillie, D., 2005. Diverticular disease: diagnosis and treatment. Am. Fam. Physician 72 (7), 1229–1234.

Smith, A.N., 1986. Colonic muscle in diverticular disease. Clin. Gastroenterol. 15 (4), 917–935.

Stollman, N., Raskin, J.B., 2004. Diverticular disease of the colon. Lancet 363, 631–639.

Story, J.A., Kritchersky, D., 1994. Denis Parsons Burkitt (1911–1993) (Biographical article). J. Nutr. 124, 1551–1554.

Tjandra, J.J., Clunnie, G.J.A., Kaye, A.H., et al., 2008. Textbook of Surgery, 3rd ed. Blackwell Publishing, p. 211.

West, A.B., Losada, M., 2004. The pathology of diverticulosis coli. J. Clin. Gastroenterol. 38 (Suppl. 1), S11–S16.

West, B., 2004. The pathology of diverticulosis coli. J. Clin. Gastroenterol. 38 (Suppl. 1), s11–s16.

West, B., 2006. The pathology of diverticulosis: classical concepts and mucosal changes in diverticula. J. Gastroenterol. 40 (3), S126–S131.

Whiteway, J., Morson, B.C., 1985. Elastosis in diverticular disease of the sigmoid colon. Gut 26 (3), 258–266.

Wolf, B., Nichols, D.M., Munro, A., et al., 2000. Acute small bowel ischaemia complicating emergency colectomy. J. R. Coll. Surg. Edinb. 45, 64–65.

Ye, H., Losada, M., West, A.B., 2005. Diverticulosis coli: update on a 'Western' disease. Adv. Anat. Pathol. 12 (2), 74–80.

Further reading

Chaplin, M., 2007. Dietary fiber and health. http://www.lsbu.ac.uk/water/hyhealth.html

Kruis, W., Forbes, A., Jauch, K.W., et al., 2006. Diverticular disease: emerging evidence in a common condition. Falk Symposium 148, Springer.

Mimura, T., Emanuel A Kamm, M.A., 2002. Pathophysiology of diverticular disease. Best Pract. Res. Clin. Gastroenterol. 16 (4), 563–576.

Netter, F.H., 1975. The Ciba collection of medical illustrations, Vol 3. Digestive system, Part 2: Lower digestive tract.

Painter, N.S., Burkitt, D.P., 1971. Diverticular disease of the colon: a deficiency disease of western civilization. Br. Med. J. 2, 450–454.

Prosky, l., Dreher, M.L., 1999. Complex carbohydrates in foods. CRC Press.

Stollman, N., Raskin, J.B., 2004. Diverticular disease of the colon. Lancet 363, 631–639.

Additional information

CHAPTER 15

Introduction to inflammatory conditions of the small and large bowel

Ian S. Shaw
Images courtesy of Robert L. Law

Contents

Introduction

Inflammatory disorders account for a significant proportion of bowel related disease. The two main inflammatory conditions – ulcerative colitis and Crohn's disease, which are collectively referred to as *inflammatory bowel disease (IBD)* – affect up to 1 in 200 of the European and North American population between them (Kappelman et al., 2007). There are also a number of other inflammatory conditions that can affect the bowel, usually as part of wider systemic disease involving other organs, but these occur much less commonly (Table 16.1). This chapter will therefore largely focus on inflammatory bowel disease, although brief reference will be given to some of these other conditions.

Inflammatory bowel disease

The term inflammatory bowel disease (IBD) is the umbrella term for ulcerative colitis and Crohn's disease, which are discrete inflammatory conditions of the gut that share many common features.

Table 16.1 Inflammatory conditions affecting the bowel

Inflammatory bowel disease	Connective tissue disease with gut involvement
Ulcerative colitis	Behçet's
Crohn's disease	Systemic lupus erythematosus
Microscopic colitis	Rheumatoid arthritis
	Systemic sclerosis
	Polyarteritis nodosum
	Wegener's granulomatosis
	Henoch-Schönlein
	Sarcoid

Ulcerative colitis, the slightly more common of the two conditions, causes inflammation of the colon, whereas *Crohn's disease* can affect any part of the gastrointestinal tract from the mouth through to the anus. Both conditions tend to follow a chronic relapsing and remitting course and can lead to disabling symptoms and complications.

Studies have shown similar rates of IBD in Europe and North America where the *estimated incidence* of ulcerative colitis ranges from 8.8 to 13.4 new cases per 100 000 population per year, with slightly lower rates for Crohn's disease of 5.6 to 8.6/100000/year. The incidence of Crohn's disease appears to be increasing, while that of ulcerative colitis is stable (Loftus et al., 2007). Rates of IBD in Africa and Asia are thought to be much lower, although limitations in case definition may have led to some underestimation. All *age groups* can be affected, although the condition is unusual in infancy, with the peak age of diagnosis occurring between the ages of 15 and 30 years, with a second peak between the ages of 50 and 80. Women and men are affected equally (Gunesh et al., 2008).

Etiology

The exact cause of IBD remains unknown, but a number of recent developments, particularly in the field of genetics, have led to better understanding in this area. It is now widely accepted that causation involves interplay between genetic, environmental and microbial factors that lead to alterations within the gut immune system.

Genetic factors

It has been known for a long time that *first degree relatives* of patients with IBD are between 3 and 20 times more likely to develop IBD themselves and that the risk for twins with IBD was much higher (Thompson et al., 1996). A number of genes have now been identified to explain this observation and a complex picture is emerging with at least 30 different genes involved (Barrett et al., 2008). It seems likely that certain genes confer susceptibility to specific patterns of IBD, which becomes activated if other trigger factors arise. The best example and the gene about which most is known is the *IBD1* or *NOD2 gene*, present on chromosome 16. Mutations of this gene have been shown to be associated with increased rates of Crohn's disease involving the ileum. The gene itself codes for a protein that is involved in the interaction between the gut's immune system and gut bacteria and it seems likely that Crohn's disease can be triggered in an IBD1 individual who comes into contact with certain bacteria that they are unable to deal with effectively. Unfortunately, at the moment, the bacteria or group of bacteria involved have not been identified (Hisamatsu et al., 2003).

Environmental factors

Many environmental agents have been suggested as factors in the development of IBD, although the evidence for most of these has been limited. Many of the earlier studies were looking for a direct causal role, whereas our current understanding of genetics makes it likely that environmental factors could contribute to disease in genetically susceptible individuals.

The strongest evidence for an environmental trigger relates to *cigarette smoking*, which has intriguingly been shown to confer a risk of developing Crohn's disease, while protecting individuals from ulcerative colitis. The mechanism of this effect has not been identified, but it is also recognized that Crohn's disease can be more aggressive in smokers compared with non-smokers, whereas the converse is true in ulcerative colitis (Mahid et al., 2006).

Other environmental factors that have been suggested include the *oral contraceptive pill* and various *dietary factors* such as food additives, processed fats and refined sugars, although the evidence for most of these is limited (Reif et al., 1997).

Microbial factors

As with environmental factors, most of the early work in this field focused on trying to identify 'the' infective cause of IBD. Potential candidates included *Mycobacterium paratuberculosis*, which is known to cause a Crohn's-like illness in cattle called Johne's disease. However, this has always been controversial and, to date, no clear cause has been identified, despite large amounts of research, although it remains possible that *M. paratuberculosis* may play some part in the IBD story (Freeman and Noble, 2005). Other equally controversial studies have focused on the *measles virus* and the potential link between measles vaccine and Crohn's disease (Thompson et al., 1995) but, once again, this association has not been confirmed. Consequently, recent research has tended to move away from looking at specific organisms and has focused on the interaction between the gut and the microflora of bacteria it contains. This shows potential as an area for research, although, like the field of genetics, the area is hugely complex; for example, it has now been shown that IBD patients are more likely to have received antibiotics in childhood (Hildebrand et al., 2008), which is just one of the many factors that could have an impact on gut flora.

Signs and symptoms

The signs and symptoms of inflammatory bowel disease largely depend on the site affected and the nature of bowel involvement at the site. Consequently, the symptoms of ulcerative colitis, which only involves the colon, are more predictable than those of Crohn's disease, which can occur anywhere within

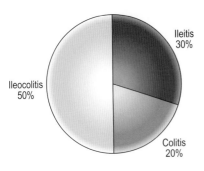

Figure 16.1 **Distribution of Crohn's disease.**

Table 16.2 Extra-intestinal features of IBD (frequency in IBD cases in brackets)

Eye	Skin	Joints	Liver
Episcleritis (5%)	Erythema nodosum (15%)	Seronegative arthritis – spine (25%)*	Primary sclerosing cholangitis (5%)*
Uveitis (0.5%)*	Pyoderma gangrenosum (5%)*	Rheumatoid-like acute (10%)	Gall stones (25%)*
		Rheumatoid-like chronic (3%)*	

*Indicates conditions that can persist despite control of bowel disease

the gastrointestinal (GI) tract (Figure 16.1). However, a number of patterns can be recognized. In addition, both ulcerative colitis and Crohn's disease can be associated with a number of symptoms that occur outside of the GI tract (Table 16.2), particularly when the disease involves the colon (Orchard, 2003).

Ulcerative colitis

Ulcerative colitis (UC) causes *superficial inflammation* of the colon, so the major symptoms are those of bowel upset in the form of diarrhea, urgency to pass stool and the passage of blood-stained stools. Unlike Crohn's disease, fistula formation and bowel strictures are relatively uncommon and the lack of deep inflammation means that pain is not usually a significant symptom.

The *relapsing and remitting nature* of UC means patients experience symptoms at times when the disease is active, commonly referred to as a *flare*, interspersed by periods without symptoms. Symptoms tend to build up gradually and often last for several weeks at a time. The severity of symptoms is at least in part explained by the extent of colon affected. The rectum is inflamed in all patients, but the extent of proximal colonic inflammation varies, with approximately 30% of sufferers having disease confined to the rectum, 40% with disease of the left colon and 30% developing total colonic inflammation (Jess et al., 2006). Individuals tend to follow the same pattern with each flare leading to inflammation in the same part of the colon, with only around 15% of patients experiencing extent progression over time.

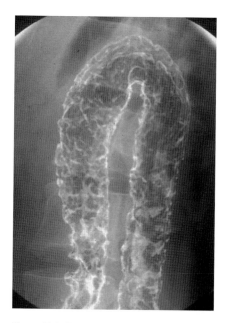

Figure 16.2 Focal image of the splenic flexure demonstrating a florid ulcerative colitis.

Most patients with *proctitis and left-sided colitis* present with relatively mild or moderate symptoms with little or no systemic upset and are managed as outpatients, whereas patients with *pan colonic involvement* (Figure 16.2) often have a more aggressive presentation with malaise, anemia, fever, tachycardia and abdominal pain. A proportion of patients presenting with severe disease will fail to settle despite treatment and, in the past, this type of presentation was associated with significant mortality. However, this is now largely avoided by ensuring that patients who fail to settle have surgery to remove the inflamed colon (colectomy) before complications such as bowel perforation develop. Factors that help predict patients at risk of not settling have been developed and most centers find that about 20–30% of patients presenting acutely with severe symptoms will require colectomy (Travis et al., 1996).

Crohn's disease

Like ulcerative colitis, the symptoms of Crohn's disease tend to reflect the site of affected bowel and, as Crohn's disease can occur anywhere within the GI tract, there is a wider variety of presentations than in UC. The inflammation in Crohn's disease involves the *full thickness* of the bowel wall (Figures 16.3 and 16.4) and, consequently, healing with fibrosis leading to scar tissue and narrowing of the bowel or '*stricturing*' is common (Figure 16.5). Holes in the bowel wall can also develop and these often lead to communication between the bowel and skin or other abdominal structures, known as *fistulae* (Figure 16.6). Over time, it is estimated that between 30 and 50% of Crohn's patients will develop fistula, with the majority involving communication between the bowel and the peri-anal skin (Schwartz et al., 2002). General *systemic features*, such as lethargy and abdominal pain, are also more common in Crohn's disease.

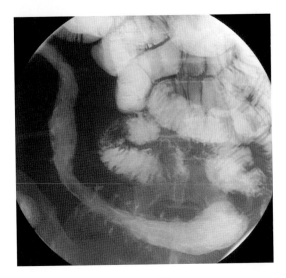

Figure 16.3 Deep ulcers: terminal ileum.

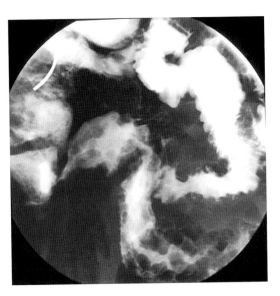

Figure 16.4 Cobblestone ulceration: terminal ileum.

Colonic Crohn's disease

Approximately 20% of Crohn's patients have disease that is limited to the colon (Figure 16.7). Symptoms tend to be similar to those in ulcerative colitis, although, unlike in UC, the rectum is not always involved – so bleeding is less common.

Ileo-colonic Crohn's disease

This is the commonest pattern of Crohn's disease occurring in around 50% of patients. Inflammation involves both the colon and the small bowel, most commonly in the region of the terminal ileum. Symptoms reflect a mixture of

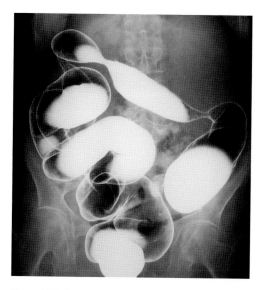

Figure 16.5 Prone abdomen: inflammation in stricture at splenic flexure, with two fibrotic strictures in transverse colon.

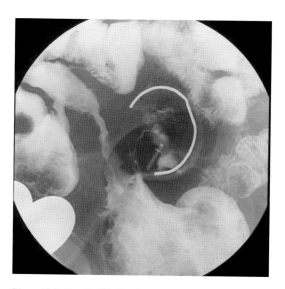

Figure 16.6 Terminal ileal stricturing with pre-stenotic dilatation, entero-enteric fistulae and deep 'rose thorn' ulcers.

colonic related bowel upset combined with symptoms from the small bowel involvement such as abdominal pain and excessively noisy bowel activity (borborygmi). *Small bowel strictures* commonly occur (Figure 16.8), leading to intermittent episodes of bowel obstruction, characterized by severe colicky abdominal pain, bloating and borborygmi, which classically come on within an hour of eating. Patients with more extensive small bowel involvement will often experience *marked weight loss* due to a combination of disease activity and reduced absorption of nutrients.

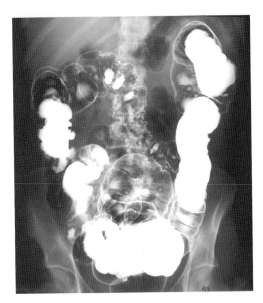

Figure 16.7 Colonic Crohn's disease: aphthous ulcers in the transverse and sigmoid colon, identified by barium pooling in ulcer craters with a surrounding (dark) edematous ring.

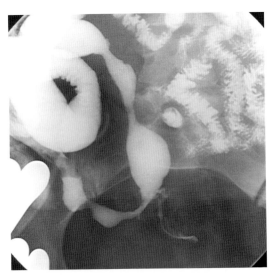

Figure 16.8 Fibrotic strictures with associated prestenotic stricturing in the distal ileum. Demonstrates a fistulous tract communicating with sigmoid colon.

Isolated ileitis or small bowel involvement

This pattern accounts for about 30% of Crohn's disease. Symptoms can be similar to those experienced by patients with ileo-colonic disease, although diarrhea may be less marked and even absent in some cases. Weight loss and systemic features may predominate.

Peri-anal disease

This can occur in isolation, or in association with any of the other patterns of disease distribution described, although it is more common in patients with colonic involvement. Potential presentations include anal fissure, peri-anal fistula, peri-anal abscess and inflammatory skin tags. *Anal fissure* involves a small break or inflamed area within the anal margin, which results in extreme pain on defecation. Rectal examination is usually impossible due to pain and resultant spasm of the anal sphincter muscles. *Peri-anal fistulae* are very common and lead to discharge of bowel content through tracts onto the peri-anal skin. These frequently become infected and lead to *peri-anal abscess formation*, involving the build up of infected material under the peri-anal skin leading to painful subcutaneous swelling and systemic symptoms of infection.

Upper gastrointestinal Crohn's disease

Crohn's disease involving the esophagus, stomach or duodenum is relatively uncommon and collectively occurs in only 5% or so of patients (Figure 16.9). Symptoms that raise the possibility of upper GI involvement include dysphagia or painful swallowing (odynophagia), ulcer-like epigastric pain and pain occurring immediately or very soon after eating. This form of disease can be difficult to treat and warrants aggressive therapy.

Oral Crohn's disease

Mouth ulcers commonly occur in patients with Crohn's disease affecting other sites within the GI tract. However, oral Crohn's disease can also present in isolation and may sometimes require systemic treatment.

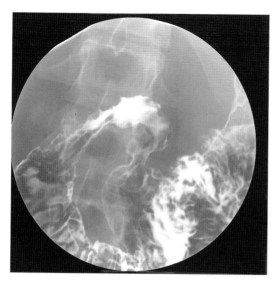

Figure 16.9 Post bulbar duodenal Crohn's stricture, aphthous ulceration in distal aspect of stricture.

Pathophysiology

Both forms of inflammatory bowel disease are characterized by chronic inflammation of the bowel and, while the exact etiology of the conditions remains unknown (see above), the pathological consequences of the disease are well documented.

The pathological hallmark of *Crohn's disease* is full thickness inflammation of the intestine, with associated granuloma formation. Involvement is often patchy with normal areas of intestine interspersed between areas of inflammation. This contrasts with *ulcerative colitis* where the inflammation is more superficial and always continuous, starting at the rectum and extending proximally to the limit of the disease. Macroscopically, both conditions manifest themselves through ulceration of the bowel mucosa with related mucosal swelling (edema) and loss of the normal appearance of bowel features. The ulcers in Crohn's disease are typically deeper and more defined than those seen in ulcerative colitis, although there is considerable overlap and, where Crohn's disease does present as confluent inflammation in the colon, the two conditions can be difficult to distinguish (Williams et al., 2003).

Diagnosis and management

Diagnosis

The diagnosis of inflammatory bowel disease relies on a high index of *clinical suspicion* based on the symptoms, coupled with appropriate investigation to confirm the presence of the characteristic pathological features (Carter et al., 2004). Despite our increased understanding about inflammatory bowel disease, patients still often experience a delay before being diagnosed; for example, a study from the USA found that the average time from symptom onset to diagnosis was over 7 years for Crohn's patients and just over a year for ulcerative colitis (Pimentel et al., 2000). This most likely reflects the rather non-specific nature and gradual onset of symptoms in some patients with Crohn's disease and serves as a reminder that clinical vigilance is necessary to make the diagnosis.

When a patient presents with symptoms suggestive of inflammatory bowel disease, the initial step is usually to look for confirmatory features such as raised markers of inflammation in *blood tests*. If there remains concern about the diagnosis following this, then further investigation is targeted according to the suspected site of disease involvement. For ulcerative colitis patients, the disease can be diagnosed relatively easily by *endoscopic assessment* of the rectal and lower colonic mucosa. This can be achieved in the outpatient setting using a rigid sigmoidoscope to examine the rectal mucosa, but is more reliably done using a fiberoptic flexible sigmoidoscope or colonoscope. Here, detailed assessment of the mucosa can be obtained and biopsies taken for histological assessment. Ileo-colonic Crohn's disease can be diagnosed in a similar way, although full *colonoscopy* after preparation of the patient's bowel with laxative is necessary to ensure views of the proximal colon and terminal ileum are obtained.

Crohn's disease involving the more proximal small bowel is less accessible to endoscopic diagnosis and diagnosis has tended to rely on demonstration of typical features of small bowel Crohn's using *radiological techniques*. This has the limitation of not obtaining tissue for histological analysis, but a combination of typical features in a patient with symptoms suggestive of the diagnosis is usually reliable. The imaging of the small bowel is considered in more detail in earlier chapters and it seems likely that there will be an increasing trend towards using *magnetic resonance imaging* in this setting (Masselli et al., 2008), although emerging endoscopic tests such as *wireless capsule endoscopy* and *balloon assisted enteroscopy* may play a complementary role (Chong et al., 2005).

Management

The treatment of inflammatory bowel disease is complex and, for many patients, involves a combination of medical therapy to control the inflammatory process, emotional support to assist with the impact for the patient from their chronic disease, nutritional support and surgical treatment for resistant disease or where complications such as strictures or abscess develop. Treatment decisions depend on clear identification of the nature and extent of the bowel that is affected (Carter et al., 2004).

Ulcerative colitis

Active disease that is limited to the rectum or left colon can often be treated with *topically acting drugs* that are inserted into the bowel through the rectum, either in the form of suppositories or enema. More extensive disease usually requires *systemic therapy*, which is sometimes given in combination with topical therapy. For mild disease flares, *mesalazine* based drugs are usually used. These have a good safety record and come in a range of oral and rectal preparations with delivery mechanisms that allow them to be targeted at the area of active disease. For more severe attacks, *steroids* are often introduced. Very severe colitis with systemic upset is usually managed in hospital to facilitate close observation and treatment with intravenous steroids in the first instance. Patients who do not settle are at risk of complications, such as toxic dilation of the colon with subsequent perforation, and second line treatment with powerful *immunosuppressive drugs*, such as ciclosporin, may be required. Up to 30% of patients will still fail to settle even with aggressive therapy and require colectomy.

Once patients have recovered from an acute episode of colitis, *maintenance therapy* is usually instigated to reduce the risk of further problems. Mesalazine is the most commonly used agent, but azathioprine or other immunosuppressive drugs are being used more frequently for patients with troublesome disease.

Crohn's disease

Like ulcerative colitis, treatment of Crohn's disease is dictated by the disease severity and site of bowel involved. Colonic Crohn's disease is treated similarly to ulcerative colitis, although mesalazine treatment

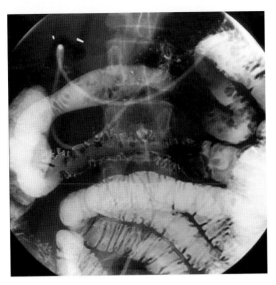

Figure 16.10 Loop of quiescent jejunal Crohn's disease with post-inflammatory filiform polyps.

tends to be less effective and, consequently, more patients will end up on immunosuppressive therapy. Small bowel disease usually requires *immunosuppressive therapy* to control inflammation. *Steroids* are commonly used in the short term, but have limited efficacy in the long term due to side effects. Conventional immunosuppressive drugs, such as *azathioprine* and *methotrexate*, can be highly effective but, like steroids, can be limited by side effects. They also have a delayed onset of action, meaning that other drugs are often needed to bridge the time period until they become effective. *Infliximab* and *Adalumimab* are two relatively new drugs that were developed specifically to block tumor necrosis factor (TNF), which is one of the many chemicals (cytokines) involved in triggering and sustaining the inflammatory process in Crohn's disease. Results have been encouraging with response in up to 70% of patients treated (Figure 16.10) and the use of these drugs is steadily increasing, despite treatment costs averaging around £10000 per year. However, some concern remains about their long-term effectiveness and safety profile (Peyrin-Biroulet et al., 2008).

Despite the advances in medical therapy for Crohn's disease, *surgery* is still required by up to 50% of Crohn's patients within the first 10 years after diagnosis and, for many patients, close liaison between surgeon and physician is required to enable optimal management (Fichera and Michelassi, 2007). Common surgical procedures in Crohn's disease include drainage of abscesses with correction of fistula and resection of segments of strictured bowel (Figure 16.11). Carefully planned and expertly performed surgery is essential to minimize loss of bowel, as patients frequently require several operations over their lifetime and the impact of cumulative bowel loss remains a concern for some patients.

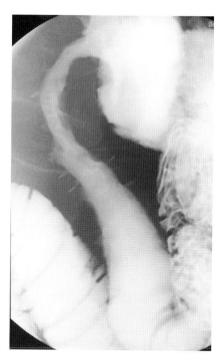

Figure 16.11 Right hemi-colectomy: neo-terminal ileal Crohn's disease demonstrating deep fissure ulcers.

Differential diagnoses

The conditions that need to be considered in the differential diagnosis of inflammatory bowel disease are largely dictated by the type of symptoms involved and can usually be distinguished based on the clinical history and results of initial investigation. Table 16.3 provides a reference to some of the common conditions that can mimic certain presentations of inflammatory bowel disease.

Table 16.3 Differential diagnosis of IBD

IBD symptoms	Common conditions included in differential diagnosis
Acute bloody diarrhea (UC or Crohn's)	Infective enteritis, e.g. *Campylobacter* Diverticular disease Ischemic colitis Colon cancer NSAID-induced colitis
Chronic diarrhea (Crohn's or UC)	*Giardia* Celiac disease Bile salt malabsorption Bacterial overgrowth Microscopic colitis Lactose intolerance Irritable bowel syndrome

(Continued)

Table 16.3 Differential diagnosis of IBD—cont'd

IBD symptoms	Common conditions included in differential diagnosis
Severe abdominal pain (Crohn's)	Any cause of an acute abdomen, e.g. appendicitis
Chronic abdominal pain (Crohn's)	Diverticular disease Irritable bowel syndrome Abdominal malignancy Pelvic inflammatory disease Endometriosis Chronic pancreatitis Biliary pathology Peptic ulceration Connective tissue disease of gut Adhesions
Malabsorption/weight loss	Celiac disease Jejunal diverticula Pancreatic insufficiency Anorexia Addison's disease Abdominal tuberculosis

NSAID, non-steroidal anti-inflammatory drugs

Prognosis

Ulcerative colitis

Ulcerative colitis tends to follow a relapsing and remitting course over time, with about 50% of patients in full remission at any time. Once a patient achieves *remission* following an attack they have about a 70% chance of having a further flare during the next year. This risk can be reduced but not avoided by use of maintenance therapy. For all patients, the risk of having a colectomy within the first 10 years of diagnosis is in the region of 25%, although this is likely to be lower for patients with limited or left-sided disease (Langholz et al., 1994). The prognosis following a severe attack of colitis has been discussed previously but, with modern treatment, the risk of death should not exceed 1%. Overall life expectancy is thought not to be reduced, but there is a clearly documented increased risk of developing *bowel cancer* among UC patients, with a likelihood of developing bowel cancer in the region of 5–10% after 20 years. This risk seems to be focused on patients with extensive disease of the colon and it is conventional to offer such patients regular surveillance.

Crohn's disease

Like ulcerative colitis, Crohn's disease also follows a relapsing and remitting course over time but, unlike UC, the natural history tends to involve the *gradual development of complications* such as strictures and fistulae. These in turn lead to the need for surgical correction, with around 50% of patients requiring surgery within 10 years from diagnosis (Solberg et al., 2007). In contrast to UC, surgery is not curative and the disease frequently recurs with about 50% of patients requiring a further operation within 10 years of their first procedure. A proportion of patients have disease that appears to follow an aggressive course, characterized by frequent relapse and rapid development of complications. In the past, these patients were at risk of developing intestinal failure over time but, fortunately, aggressive modern management of Crohn's disease appears to be reducing this rate. However, most studies still show that average life expectancy is slightly reduced among patients with Crohn's disease.

References

Barrett, J.C., Hansoul, S., Nicolae, D.L., et al., 2008. Genome-wide association defines more than 30 distinct susceptibility loci for Crohn's disease. Nat. Genet. 40 (8), 955–962.

Carter, M.J., Lobo, A.J., Travis, S.P.L., 2004. British Society of Gastroenterology Guidelines for the management of inflammatory bowel disease in adults. Gut 53 (Suppl. V), v1–v16.

Chong, A.K., Taylor, A., Miller, A., et al., 2005. Capsule endoscopy vs. push enteroscopy and enteroclysis in suspected small-bowel Crohn's disease. Gastrointest. Endosc. 61 (2), 255–261.

Fichera, A., Michelassi, F., 2007. Surgical treatment of Crohn's disease. J. Gastrointest. Surg. 11 (6), 791–803.

Freeman, H., Noble, M., 2005. Lack of evidence for Mycobacterium avium subspecies paratuberculosis in Crohn's disease regulation of immunity. Inflamm. Bowel Dis. 11 (8), 782.

Gunesh, S., Thomas, G.A.O., Williams, G.T., et al., 2008. The incidence of Crohn's disease in Cardiff over the last 75 years: an update for 1996–2005. Aliment. Pharmacol. Ther. 27 (3), 211–219.

Hildebrand, H., Malmborg, P., Askling, J., et al., 2008. Early-life exposures associated with antibiotic use and risk of subsequent Crohn's disease. Scand. J. Gastroenterol. 43 (8), 961–966.

Hisamatsu, T., Suzuki, M., Reinecker, H.C., et al,, 2003. CARD15/NOD2 functions as an antibacterial factor in human intestinal epithelial cells. Gastroenterology 124 (4), 993–1000.

Jess, T., Riis, L., Vind, A., et al., 2006. Changes in clinical characteristics, course and prognosis of inflammatory bowel disease during the last 5 decades: a population based study from Copenhagen, Denmark. Inflamm. Bowel Dis. 13, 481–489.

Kappelman, M.D., Rifas- Shiman, S.L., Kleinman, K., et al., 2007. The prevalence and geographic distribution of Crohn's disease and ulcerative colitis in the United States. Clin. Gastroenterol. Hepatol. 5, 1424.

Langholz, E., Munkholm, P., Davidsen, M., et al., 1994. Course of ulcerative colitis: analysis of changes in disease activity over years. Gastroenterology 107 (1), 3–11.

Loftus, C.G., Loftus EV Jr, Harmsen, W.S., et al., 2007. Update on the incidence and prevalence of Crohn's disease and ulcerative colitis in Olmstead County, Minnesota, 1940–2000. Inflamm. Bowel Dis. 13 (3), 254–261.

Mahid, S.S., Minor, K.S., Soto, R.E., et al., 2006. Smoking and inflammatory bowel disease: a meta-analysis. Mayo Clin. Proc. 81, 1462–1471.

Masselli, G., Casciani, E., Polettini, E., et al., 2008. Comparison of MR enteroclysis with MR enterography and conventional enteroclysis in patients with Crohn's disease. Eur. Radiol. 18 (3), 438–447.

Orchard, T., 2003. Extraintestinal complications of inflammatory bowel disease. Curr. Gastroenterol. Rep. 5 (6), 512–517.

Peyrin-Biroulet, L., Deltenre, P., De Suray, N., et al., 2008. Efficacy and safety of tumor necrosis factor antagonists in Crohn's disease: meta-analysis of placebo-controlled trials. Clin. Gastroenterol. Hepatol. 6, 644–653.

Pimentel, M., Chang, M., Chow, E.J., et al., 2000. Identification of a prodromal period in Crohn's disease but not ulcerative colitis. Am. J. Gastroenterol. 95 (12), 3458–3462.

Reif, S., Klein, I., Lubin, F., et al., 1997. Pre-illness dietary factors in inflammatory bowel disease. Gut 40 (6), 754–760.

Schwartz, D.A., Loftus, E.V. Jr., Tremaine, W.J., et al., 2002. The natural history of fistulizing Crohn's disease in Olmsted County, Minnesota. Gastroenterology 122 (4), 875–880.

Solberg, I.C., Vatn, M.H., Hoie, O., et al., 2007. Clinical course in Crohn's disease: results of a Norwegian population-based ten-year follow-up study. Clin. Gastroenterol. Hepatol. 5 (12), 1430–1438.

Thompson, N.P., Driscoll, R., Pounder, R.E., et al., 1996. Genetics versus environment in inflammatory bowel disease: results of a British twin study. Br. Med. J. 312, 95–96.

Thompson, N.P., Montgomery, S.M., Pounder, R.E., Wakefield, A.J., 1995. Is measles vaccination a risk factor for inflammatory bowel disease? Lancet 345 (8957), 1071–1074.

Travis, S.P.L., Farrant, J.M., Ricketts, C., 1996. Predicting outcome in severe ulcerative colitis. Gut 38, 905–910.

Williams, G., Sloan, J., Warren, B., et al., 2003. Morson and Dawson's gastrointestinal pathology, fourth ed. Blackwell, Oxford.

Cross-sectional investigations, nuclear medicine and ultrasound of the small and large bowel

Jessie Aw, S. Gandhi

Contents ||||||||||||||||||||||||||||||||||||||||||||||||||||||||||||||||||||||||||||||||||||||

Introduction

The role of cross-sectional imaging is an integral part of the hospital service and an essential part of the multidisciplinary team approach to the care of the patient both in hospital and in the community. Imaging can clarify clinical assessment, provide presurgical roadmaps, postsurgical complications and aid management decisions. Cross-sectional imaging is also a prerequisite for preassessment planning and performance of an interventional procedure. It is critical in the multidisciplinary meetings and fundamental in the patient care pathway.

Most abdominal imaging is performed to investigate general abdominal symptoms, such as pain, weight loss, bloating or abdominal distension. Abdominal imaging involves a multitude of complex investigations to the uninitiated. Ultrasound, computed tomography (CT), magnetic resonance imaging (MRI) and radionuclide scanning are all important adjuncts to first line imaging: *the abdominal radiograph*. They are complementary to each other and the majority of clinical questions can be answered by cross-sectional imaging. Occasionally specialist investigations will be required e.g. indium-111 labelled white cell nuclear scintigraphy when the other imaging modalities have been negative and there are ongoing clinical symptoms or concern. Each investigative method is appropriate for certain clinical questions, when used appropriately it will help make an accurate diagnosis, preventing any treatment delays. To understand the role of each imaging modality you must understand the principle technique, including its value and limitations.

Evidence-based medicine can be defined as the integration of best available research with clinical expertise and patient values (Erturk et al., 2006). You can apply evidence-based practice to any clinical discipline using five basic principles:

1 Formulate an answerable question
2 Analyze the best current available evidence
3 Appraise critically
4 Apply findings to practice
5 Evaluate performance.

Evidence-based radiology (EBR) is an effective tool for radiologists, radiographers, advanced practitioners and clinicians skilled in a particular radiological skill to regularly update their knowledge, deepen their understanding of research methods and (if applicable to clinical setting EBR) can allow effective clinical practice. More importantly for patients this can translate to providing the most up to date clinical practice and care.

Ultrasound

Ultrasound (US) imaging uses high-frequency (greater than 20 kHz) sound waves, which are emitted and received by the ultrasound probe and are inaudible to humans. The frequency of the sound humans hear determines the pitch. *Frequency* is defined as the number of oscillations per second and Hertz is the unit measurement of frequency. Medical imaging normally uses higher frequencies, in the range of 2.5–10 mHz, with specialist imaging such as intravascular studies requiring frequencies of 20 mHz or more mHz.

The basic essential component of an *ultrasound probe* is the *piezoelectric (PZE) crystal* in a shape of a rectangle or disk. When an alternating (AC) current is applied to the crystal, it expands and contracts with the same frequency: this is the *'piezoelectric effect'*. This produces sound waves or echoes. The echoes are transmitted undergoing 'reflection', returning at different velocities depending on the media the echoes have encountered within the body. Different tissues will have different *acoustic impedance*. The proportion of energy (or sound) reflected and transmitted depends on the acoustic impedances of the two materials. In physics terms, the acoustic impedance of a material is defined as the product of the density of the material and the velocity of the sound within it. The greater the acoustic impedance mismatches between two materials the greater the fraction of sound which is reflected and thus imaging is limited. The reflected/returning sound waves act on the PZE crystal in the ultrasound probe to produce an electric signal. The probe is connected to a powerful computer processor that converts the electrical signal into a cross-sectional image. The images are captured in real

BOX 17.1 Advantages of ultrasound

- Safe (no radiation)
- Low cost
- Portable
- Quick
- Non-invasive
- Real-time imaging
- Real-time ultrasound guided interventional procedures
- Excellent local detail using endoluminal ultrasound (applications: endoanal, endoluminal local staging for esophageal carcinoma)

BOX 17.2 Limitations of ultrasound

- Operator dependent
- High body mass index can attenuate the sound waves and deep penetration cannot be achieved
- Limited spatial resolution
- Attenuated by bone and large amount of air/gas

time and it can show the solid organs and the movement and flow through blood vessels using a special technique of *Doppler ultrasound*. The image is then displayed on a monitor and may be stored or printed.

The properties of ultrasound are unique. Unlike x-rays or light waves, which can travel through a vacuum, sound waves require a material medium to travel through and thus cannot penetrate air gaps. Ultrasound cannot image through bone or large collections of air. There is also a high acoustic impedance mismatch between the patient's skin and the probe. This is overcome by the use of *ultrasound scanning gel*. The advantages and limitations of ultrasound as an imaging modality are outlined in Boxes 17.1 and 17.2.

Doppler ultrasound

The Doppler effect occurs when there is a relative movement between a sound source and a sound receiver. This occurs in everyday life, when you hear a police siren. As the siren is travelling towards you (the receiver), the sound waves are compressed producing a higher frequency, then as it passes and moves further away the sound waves are further apart producing a lower frequency. This principle is used in *Doppler imaging*: the change in sound wave frequency is used to detect movement and the change in frequency can be calculated in order to quantify the blood flow. Doppler is used clinically for detection and assessment of peripheral arterial disease, deep venous thrombosis, portal vein thrombosis, assessing arterial and venous flow. This is very useful in native and transplanted kidneys and livers to assess any evidence of rejection.

Colour Doppler is an augmentation of the Doppler principle. The colours are superimposed on the cross-sectional imaging to allow instant assessment of the direction of flow. Blood flowing towards the transducer is colored red and away from the transducer is colored blue. In venous imaging, any poor infilling of color with associated turbulence of color is suggestive of a vascular stenosis or narrowing secondary to a mural thrombus.

The combination of two-dimensional ultrasound imaging with Doppler ultrasound is known as *duplex ultrasound*. Duplex is an important technique for the examination of arteries and veins.

Applied terminology

The tissues within the human body produce various degrees of sound wave reflection; this is termed *echogenicity*. The echoes are the ultrasound waves.

Hyperechoic: on the gray scale a hyperechoic lesion is bright, white or light gray, e.g. muscularis mucosae of the bowel wall. Hyperechoic lesions reflect more sound than a tissue of low echogenicity.

Hypoechoic: dark gray, nearly black, e.g. fat, muscularis propria of the bowel wall.

Isoechoic: gray lesion, e.g. liver substance or gut wall.

Anechoic: a very dark lesion, black, e.g. pure fluid; it does not reflect any sound waves back, i.e. all the sound passes through.

Acoustic enhancement: occurs when sound passes through an anechoic structure. The echoes all pass through the anechoic lesion and more sound is available.

Acoustic shadowing: this is produced when a sound wave encounters a very echo dense structure and nearly all the sound is reflected back, resulting in an acoustic shadow.

Clinical indications for ultrasound assessment

- Abdominal pain – ascites
- Query intussusception
- Esophageal local staging – endoluminal ultrasound
- Anal pain – endoanal ultrasound
- Weight loss – liver query metastases
- Enlarged abdominal organs – hepatomegaly in cirrhosis, splenomegaly in hematological disorders
- Pancreas – pseudocyst post pancreatitis, pancreas mass
- Gallbladder – stones and their complications
- Assess intrahepatic and extrahepatic ducts
- Appendicitis – appendix is identified and has thickened wall; however, if the appendix is not identified this does not exclude the diagnosis.

Clinical contraindication

- There is no absolute contraindication for an ultrasound examination, as ionizing radiation is not involved. However, you must be aware of the limitations of an ultrasound examination (see Box 17.2).

Patient preparation

Ultrasound of abdomen

Nil by mouth for 8–12 hours pre-test and a fat-free meal the evening before the test. This is to keep the gallbladder distended. Smoking should also be avoided as this can contract the gallbladder.

Ultrasound of the kidneys

To evaluate the bladder, it must be distended fully. This is achieved by drinking one litre of water or more, an hour before the examination. If the patient is catheterized it should be clamped off, again to fill the bladder. If the bladder is only partially filled, then only comment can be made on any gross/large abnormalities. Small lesions cannot be confidently detected.

Ultrasound of the bowel

Normal sonographic bowel wall anatomy

The sonographic appearance of the normal bowel wall consists of five concentric layers of alternating hypoechoic and echogenic interfaces. We will describe from inside out (Figure 17.1).

Layer 1 This represents the superficial mucosal interface – a thin echogenic layer

Layer 2 The deep mucosa including the muscularis mucosa – hyperechoic layer

Layer 3 This represents the submucosa and muscularis propria interface – hyperechoic layer

Layer 4 This represents the muscularis propria – hypoechoic layer

Layer 5 The marginal interface to the serosa – a thin hypoechoic layer.

Normal gut wall thickness is 2–4 mm on average (Ledermann et al., 2000).

Ultrasound of small and large bowel

Ultrasound of the bowel is a sub-specialist technique only performed in specialist centers worldwide. The technique, however, has been found to be of value in the diagnosis of the acute abdomen, in particular diagnosis of *acute appendicitis*. It is one of the commonest causes for an acute abdomen for the surgical on-call team.

Acute appendicitis in experienced hands is usually diagnosed on history, physical examination and laboratory investigations. The aim of imaging is either to confirm or refute the diagnosis; however, if the appendix is not visualized then appendicitis cannot be excluded. In a female, diagnoses which mimic appendicitis include enlarged ovarian cysts or torsion of the ovaries. Thickening of the wall of a normal appendix wall to 6 mm (3 mm or less is normal) is suggestive of appendicitis (Guillerman and Ng, 2005). Other features include non-compressibility and round in cross-section rather than oval.

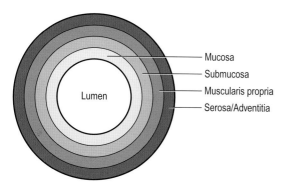

Figure 17.1 Normal bowel wall anatomical layers.

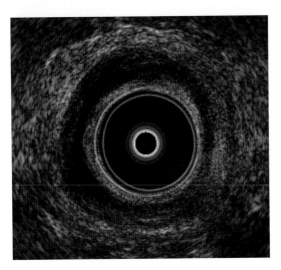

Figure 17.2 Endoanal ultrasound depicting the different sonographic layers of the mid rectum.

Ultrasound of the bowel can be used for bowel obstruction and in Crohn's disease. *Bowel obstruction* is considered present at sonography when the lumen of the fluid-filled small bowel loops were dilated more than 3 cm and the length of a segment of the dilated small bowel was over 10 cm; peristalsis of the dilated segment was increased. This is shown by rapid progression or whirling movement of bowel content (Ko et al., 1993).

Ultrasound can be used for the diagnosis of *Crohn's disease* (an inflammatory bowel disease that may involve various segments of the GIT, although ileal and/or colonic involvement is most frequent); however, the specificity and sensitivity of any test depends on the prevalence of the disease in the population (i.e. the pre-test probability) (Fraquelli et al., 2005).

Endoluminal ultrasound is performed using an axial endoscopic type probe with a 7.5–10 MHz transducer. It is a mechanically rotated probe that produces a 360 degrees cross-sectional image.

Endoluminal ultrasound is excellent for local staging of *esophageal cancer*. It can define tumor infiltration, as well as local nodal staging. This has major prognostic and management implications, and associated morbidity of open surgery if lesions are detected early. Puncture endosonographic scopes have also been developed to enable fine needle aspiration of lymph nodes and more accurately stage nodal burden (Binmoeller, 1999).

Endoanal ultrasound (Figure 17.2) essentially follows the same principle and has several specific indications. It is used to assess the anal–rectal region, in particular the sphincters. The main indication for endoanal ultrasound is in the investigation of fecal incontinence as well as anal pain (Rottenberg and Wiiliams, 2002).

These are specialized techniques requiring specific training and are preformed in tertiary referral centers.

Computed tomography (CT)

CT uses x-rays to produce the cross-sectional images. The x-ray tube is mounted on a *gantry*, which is a set of circular rotating metal rings. Directly opposite the x-ray tube is a set of *detectors*, which collect the information that is analyzed by a powerful computer and displayed on high resolution monitors. The gantry is positioned at the level of interest and the x-ray tube rotates 360 degrees on the gantry. The patient passes through the gantry and the image is acquired in a spiral fashion (or by multislice techniques); previously only one slice was acquired at a time. CT previously was long and cumbersome with respiratory and motion artefact causing limitation in the information acquired. When we discuss spiral or multislice imaging, imagine that the x-ray tube is mounted on an imaginary large Slinky around the patient. These data are transformed into a cross-sectional image using a mathematical technique called *Fourier's transformation*. The cross-sectional data are called a data set, just like a stack of coins. The computers give an illusion of one continuous image, when in fact you are scrolling through the data set.

The x-ray beam passes through the patient and is detected on the corresponding side. The x-rays are attenuated to varying degree according to the different tissue densities of the body. High density components (e.g. bone, calcium, metal or contrast material) are attenuated to a greater degree than lower density tissues (fat or soft tissues) and appear white. Fat, soft tissues and lung/air allow more x-rays to pass through and appear black. The image can be manipulated using the computer by altering the 'window' settings. Thus you can concentrate on looking at just the lung, bone or soft tissue settings. Figures 17.3, 17.4, 17.5 and 17.6 are examples of abdominal CT anatomy.

Advances in modern computers, software platforms, medical physics and detector technology have all allowed greater imaging capability with improved detail and image manipulations. The data set can be reconstructed into *multiplanar reconstruction* (MPR) images (all three orthogonal planes; sagittal, coronal and axial) or *maximum image projection* (MIP) images. The advantages and limitations of CT are outlined in Boxes 17.3 and 17.4.

Applied terminology

Attenuation: the energy loss of the x-ray beam as it passes through a material. High attenuation – white; low attenuation – dark, gray/black; isoattenuation – gray/light gray.

Density can be used as an alternative to attenuation.

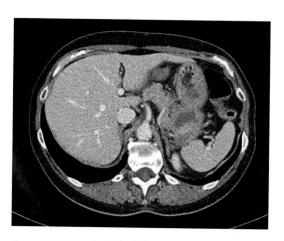

Figure 17.3 Abdominal CT with intravenous contrast (portal venous phase) at the level of the origin of the celiac axis.

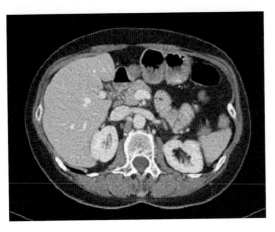

Figure 17.4 Abdominal CT with intravenous contrast at the level of the kidneys.

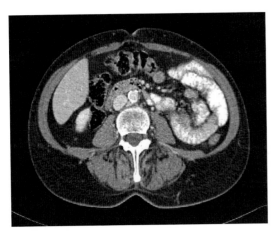

Figure 17.5 Abdominal CT with intravenous contrast at the level of the distal aorta.

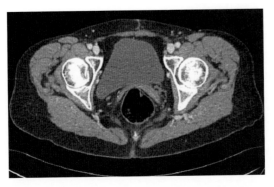

Figure 17.6 Abdominal CT with intravenous contrast at the level of the bladder.

BOX 17.3 Advantages of CT

- Modern scanners are very fast and whole abdomen can be scanned within a minute
- Excellent for bone detail
- Excellent for trauma cases. CT provides a global view of the abdomen and is quick. Most life support systems are compatible with CT, whereas specialist equipment is needed for MR imaging
- Minimum preparation for the colon

BOX 17.4 Limitations of CT

- Use of ionizing radiation
- Contrast allergy
- Lack of portability
- Certain areas of the body are poorly imaged (e.g. the pituitary fossa)
- Contrast detail in certain areas is inferior to MRI, e.g. liver, rectal MRI

Hounsfield unit: a unit of measurement for CT densities, named after Geoffrey Hounsfield, the inventor of CT.

Windowing: manipulation of the CT image to display differences in the gray scale.

Clinical indications for CT assessment

- Abdominal trauma
- Staging of local and distant metastatic disease (Figure 17.7)
- Cancer follow-up for disease recurrence
- Cause for bowel obstruction
- Diagnosis of postoperative complication for an unwell patient
- Presurgical planning with minimal preparation for the colon

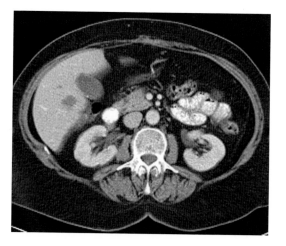

Figure 17.7 Axial CT of the abdomen shows ill-defined low density lesions (proved to be liver metastases) in the liver.

Clinical contraindication for CT assessment

- Absolute: allergy to iodine-based contrast medium.

Future developments

CT examination was initially obtained as single slice images, it was prolonged, cumbersome and only 2D views were possible. The advent of *multislice CT* with improved high performance software and powerful computers has added a new dimension to all radiological specialities. Examinations are obtained as spiral acquisitions with thin slices. This equates to faster scanning and thus fewer motion artefacts, especially useful for severely sick patients, patients with respiratory compromise (shorter breath hold) and the pediatric population. Overlapping data are obtained which can be mathematically remodeled to produce *3D multiplanar reconstructed images*. The narrow slices obtained with multislice CT result in improved spatial resolution. Currently, there are 4, 16, 32 and 64 slice multidetector CT (MDCT) readily available on the market. Future developments include 256 MDCTs which will allow greater temporal and spatial resolution with a non-significant increase in radiation doses. Temporal resolution is essential for cardiac imaging when capturing small coronary vessels at a rapid heart rate.

Appropriate windowing with review on work stations with the original data set is crucial. This is a potential pitfall if only thick axial slices are used to interpret from. Also altering the window levels is useful, as certain pathologies will be made more apparent to the human eye by changing the relative contrast. Reconstructing the original thin axial dataset with the 3D reconstruction function in the three orthogonal planes is invaluable both for reporting and demonstrating the abnormalities to the clinicians.

Magnetic resonance imaging (MRI)

MRI physics is highly complex; further details can be found in the recommended text. We will cover the basics only.

MRI uses the properties of a *hydrogen atom* which is highly abundant in the human body. The hydrogen nucleus has a single proton and a single electron. Water is the biggest source of protons in the body, followed next by fat.

The proton has a positive electric charge and spin. Imagine the proton represents the Earth; it has a North and a South pole and a spin along an axis which is slightly tilted off the centre (Figure 17.8). This is occurring in the human body; the protons are spinning along their axis but spinning randomly. However, once placed inside the *magnetic bore*, the protons will align in one of two stable states. They will either align parallel (spin-up) or antiparallel (spin-down) to the strong external magnetic field. A greater proportion will align in the parallel direction and so the *net vector* (the net direction) will be in the direction of the magnetic field (known as B zero).

Then a second phenomenon on the spinning protons occurs due to the influence of the magnetic field. The B zero causes a secondary spin known as *precession*. The frequency of the precession is an inherent property of the hydrogen atom in a specific magnetic field strength and is known as the

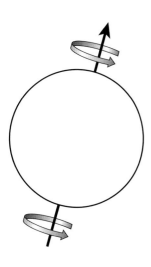

Figure 17.8 Illustration of a proton spinning on its axis.

Larmor frequency. Larmor frequency will change depending on the magnetic field strength.

Then, with a second magnetic coil; the *radiofrequency (RF) coil*, we will apply a strong magnetic field, the RF pulse. The RF pulse causes the net vector to turn 90 degrees towards the transverse plane and to precess in phase (synchronously). This has given energy to the proton called *excitation*. When RF is removed, the protons want to return to the stable lowest energy state. The extra energy is dissipated to the surroundings in a process known as T1 relaxation. The process of dephasing is known as T2 relaxation.

The net vector in the transverse plane induces a current in magnetic coils known as *radiofrequency* and the RF receiver coils pick up the signal, to be converted to an image. The advantages and limitations of MRI are given in Boxes 17.5 and 17.6.

BOX 17.5 Advantages of magnetic resonance imaging

- Excellent soft tissue characterization
- Safe (no ionizing radiation)
- Multiplanar capabilities
- Lack of artefacts from adjacent bony structures

BOX 17.6 Limitations of magnetic resonance imaging

- Claustrophobia
- Bowel peristalsis artefact
- Respiratory movement artefact
- Costly
- Poor sensitivity for calcification detection as compared with CT
- MRI compatible anesthetic and resuscitation equipment required
- Timely preparation required for anesthetized patients; this is an issue for unstable patients on ITU
- Many absolute contraindications

Applied terminology

The accepted MRI terminology is *signal characteristics*.

- High signal – this shows as white
- Low signal – this shows as black
- Iso-signal – this shows as light or dark gray.

The MR signal characteristics in physics terms are dependent on the T1 and T2 properties of a given tissue. Every tissue in the human body has its own T1 and T2 value.

T1 weighting: This is the spin/lattice interaction, where energy is given off to surrounding tissue. It is used to indicate an image where most of the contrast between tissues is due to differences in the T1 value. A T1-weighted magnetic resonance image (Figure 17.9) is created typically by using short TE (time to echo) and TR (time to relaxation) times.

Lesions with short T1 are (bright in T1-weighted sequences):

- fat (lipoma)
- paramagnetic agent (gadolinium)
- protein-containing fluid (colloid cyst)
- metastatic melanoma (melanotic).

T2 weighting: This is spin/spin interaction which is the dephasing of magnetic moment. It is created typically by using longer TE and TR times.

Lesions with short T2 are (dark in T2-weighted sequences) (Figure 17.10):

- physiologic iron (iron in liver of patients with iron overload)
- mucinous lesions (mucinous carcinoma of the pancreas).

Lesions with long T2 are bright.

- Bile
- Oedema
- CSF

MR physics is beyond the scope of this chapter and further excellent text is available. Please see recommended reading list.

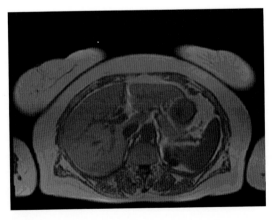

Figure 17.9 MR axial T1-weighted image of the liver.

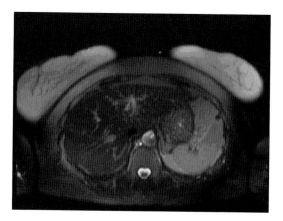

Figure 17.10 MR axial T2-weighted image of the liver.

Clinical indications for magnetic resonance imaging

- Indeterminate liver lesions on a background of cirrhotic liver disease or past medical history of carcinoma
- Rectal carcinoma local tumor MR staging: coronal T1-weighted (Figure 17.11) and sagittal T2-weighted (Figure 17.12) images demonstrate a large tumor in the mid to upper rectum (arrowed). The tumor is annular and there is extramural spread involving the peritoneal reflection. There are a few enlarged mesorectal lymph nodes with a large annular tumor in mid-upper rectum. It is radiologically staged as T4 N1 M0 (Strassburg, 2004).
- Magnetic resonance cholangiopancreaticography
- Indeterminate adrenal masses.

Clinical contraindication for magnetic resonance imaging

- *Absolute:* allergy to gadolinium contrast medium/cardiac pacemaker
- *Relative:* metal fragments or MRI-incompatible surgical prostheses or intracerebral aneurysm clips, severe renal dysfunction (see the 2007 guidelines on the Royal College of Radiologists website)

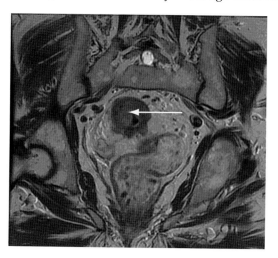

Figure 17.11 Rectal MR: coronal T1W image. (Courtesy of Dr E. Loveday.)

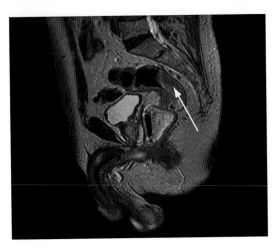

Figure 17.12 Rectal MR: sagittal T2W image. (Courtesy of Dr E. Loveday.)

Magnetic resonance cholangiopancreaticography

The image is heavily T2-weighted so the signal from solid parenchyma is suppressed and fluid-filled structures are highlighted (Figure 17.13).

CT, MR colonography and enteroclysis

Each year in the UK, around 16 000 people die from colorectal cancer. At disease presentation, around 55% of people have advanced cancer that has spread to lymph nodes, metastasized to other organs or is so locally advanced that surgery is unlikely to be curative (Dukes' stage C or D) (Drug Therapy Bulletin, 2006). Overall 5-year survival for colorectal cancer in the UK is around 47–51% (compared to 64% in the USA), but only 7% at most in those presenting with metastatic disease (Drug Therapy Bulletin, 2006). It is now

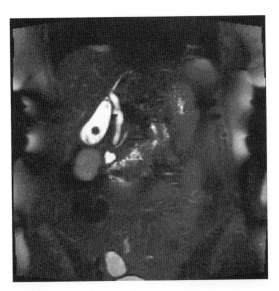

Figure 17.13 Magnetic resonance cholangiopancreaticography. (Courtesy of Dr E. Loveday.)

known that colorectal carcinoma can start as an adenomatous (precancerous) polyp then develop to carcinoma in-situ and finally to frankly invasive. The risk of malignant progression increases with the increasing size of the polyp: generally adenomatous polyps 5 mm and below have 0.5% risk, greater than 10 mm have 3–10% risk and greater than 20 mm have 10–50% risk (Dahnert, 2003). Thus there is a significant advantage in detecting adenomatous polyps. Direct colonoscopy is the reference standard as simultaneous biopsy and polyp removal can be achieved. However, it is painful, requires analgesia ± sedatives, may not reach the right side of the colon and has a risk of perforation (Lee et al., 1994). (Please refer to Chapter 20 for a more detailed discussion.)

Developments such as *MR and CT colonography* (CTC) allow examination of the colon and rectum with the possibilities of detecting polyps and/or carcinomas (Pickhardt et al., 2003). It can be used in both symptomatic and asymptomatic patients who have a high risk of developing cancer or even those of average risks.

CTC (Figures 17.14, 17.15, see color insert and 17.16) is less invasive with no clinically significant complications (Yee et al., 2001; Pickhardt et al., 2003) unlike direct colonoscopy; though full bowel preparation is required so fecal residue is not misinterpreted. Antispasmodic prior to the scan is given and a distended colon to patient's toleration, with full distention being the optimum situation. Distention is achieved by insufflation with air or carbon dioxide and spiral acquisition with breath hold in both supine and prone positions (National Institute for Clinical Excellence). The data obtained are used to produce a 2- and 3-dimensional image of the entire colon and rectum, the software enabling the operator to manipulate the data set in order to define lesions. CTC has high average sensitivity and specificity for large and medium polyps in the symptomatic population, but the findings in the asymptomatic population have not been established due to heterogeneity and small numbers in the cohort groups for the various studies (Halligan et al., 2005). CTC techniques are explored further in Chapter 18.

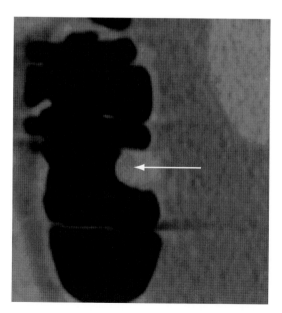

Figure 17.14 Original dataset of CT colonography showing an intraluminal colonic polyp arrowed.

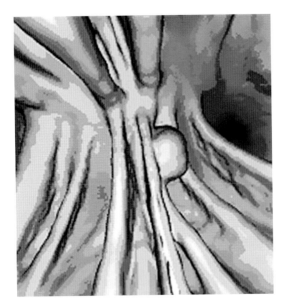

Figure 17.16 Reconstructed CT colonographic image of the colonic polyp as seen in the original dataset of Figure 17.14.

MR colonography on the other hand has no radiation exposure but still requires antispasmodics to minimize bowel peristalsis and spasm. The colon is distended with several litres of tap water with the patient in the prone position. Once complete filling is achieved with adequate colonic distention, intravenous gadolinium is given. The examination is only performed in the prone position and generally it is well tolerated (Lauenstein et al., 2002).

MR enteroclysis imaging is a technique for evaluation of the small bowel, in particular patients with Crohn's disease. The technique involves administration of 1.5–2 litres of isosmotic water solution through a nasojejunal catheter, which ensures distention of the bowel and facilitates identification of wall abnormalities. This is similar to the traditional enteroclysis technique, but an antiperistaltic agent is essential to acquire images free of motion artefacts. The patient is then imaged with special MRI sequences: FISP (fast imaging with steady state precession) and HASTE (half Fourier acquisition single shot turbo spin echo) (Prassopoulos et al., 2001). The major advantage is the lack of ionizing radiation especially in patients who are diagnosed at a young age with inflammatory bowel disease and will have to have repeated examinations for follow up, disease status or its complications. It provides excellent soft tissue contrast with 3-dimensional images and is able to provide extramural information. However, the spatial resolution is not yet sufficient to delineate superficial abnormalities. It is emerging, but it is not the initial investigation of choice as its clinical utility has not been fully established.

Nuclear medicine

Nuclear medicine uses *radioactive labeled pharmaceuticals*, which are injected into the patient, and the image is captured by a *gamma camera*. The radionuclide emits gamma rays (majority of cases); the most commonly used radionuclide is *technetium*. The radionuclide compound used depends on the area

BOX 17.7 Advantages of scintigraphy

- High sensitivity
- Functional information
- Patient acceptability

BOX 17.8 Limitations of scintigraphy

- Non-specific, i.e. an isolated 'hot spot' on an isotopic bone scan can be due to infection, tumor or trauma. Clinical correlation is necessary
- Cost and an extra license is required to handle the radioactive material and its disposal
- Separate area is needed in order to separate the patients, in order to minimize radiation exposure
- Breast feeding – certain radiotracers can be excreted in the breast milk

to be examined. The gamma camera detects the gamma rays and converts the absorbed energy into an electrical signal; this is analysed by a computer and then displayed as an image.

Nuclear scintigraphic examinations are highly sensitive to pathology and can detect abnormalities early before changes are apparent on any other cross-sectional imaging. Anatomically detail is not specific but broad anatomical regions can be read. Its other strength is that it provides *functional imaging*, i.e. how an organ is working or not. The advantages and limitations of scintigraphy are given in Boxes 17.7 and 17. 8.

Applied terminology

Hot: an area of increased radionuclide activity.

Photopenic/cold: an area of decreased radionuclide activity.

Nuclear medicine in abdominal imaging

The role of nuclear medicine in relation to the detection of GI bleeding has specific indications. *GI bleeding* is typically intermittent and requires active bleeding to be localized. When other investigations have been unable to detect the exact site, it is imperative to 'stop the tap' in patients where the bleeding is massive or recurrent. This will determine who may benefit from aggressive treatment and who would be appropriate for medical management. The full scintigraphy protocol has been set by the Society of Nuclear Medicine, which can be downloaded from the website (www.snm.org). It must be emphasized that only hemodynamically stable patients should undergo nuclear scintigraphic scan and the unstable patients should immediately undergo angiography (Hastings, 2000). A high level of certainty in localizing the site of bleeding is possible when located in the stomach or the colon. Localizing the bleeding site is less sensitive in the small bowel, especially from the jejunum and ileum (Holder, 2000).

Table 17.1 Clinical application for scintigraphic assessment in abdominal imaging

Organ	Radionuclide	Clinical application
Liver/spleen	99 mTc	Liver/splenic masses
Bile ducts/gallbladder	99 mTc-IDA	Acute cholecystitis, biliary obstruction, biliary atresia, post liver transplant
Adrenal medulla	131I-MIBG	Localization of pheochromocytoma, staging of neuroblastoma (pediatric population in particular)
Gastrointestinal bleeding	99 mTc-labeled red blood cells	Acute gastrointestinal bleeding
Occult infections	67gallium, 111 indium	Patients with abdominal abscess or pyrexia of unknown origin

There are several scintigraphic factors which affect the differences in detecting bleeding sites: they include dynamic imaging, delayed imaging and the extra large field of view needed to visualize the upper and lower gastrointestinal tract simultaneously.

Physiological factors affecting detection are: the bleeding flow rate (rapid, moderate, slow, intermittent, minimal, antegrade and retrograde bleeding); the specific bleeding site; and any previous bowel surgery. An indication of the clinical application for scintigraphic assessment in abdominal imaging is given in Table 17.1.

Positron emission tomography CT (PET-CT)

PET-CT is a relatively new imaging technique. PET requires radionuclides that decay by *positron emission*. A cyclotron produces positron-emitting isotopes. The radionuclide is attached to a biological compound to form a radiopharmaceutical. This is injected into the patient and a PET camera detects the emission. PET is similar to the other scintigraphic examinations: it provides functional information, but similar to other nuclear medicine investigations, it is not specific anatomically (Figures 17.17, 17.18, see color insert).

Then, after the acquisition of the PET examination, a CT examination is performed for anatomical localization. The images from the examinations are fused. There are now specific single *PET-CT machines* where the patient is on a long gantry, the PET is acquired then the CT in a single session. The alternative is two separate machines, whereby the examinations are acquired separately. The disadvantage of this is that the fusion of the examinations is less than ideal.

The fusion of modalities provides functional and specific anatomical information. Its main role is in *oncology imaging*, whereby primary, secondary sites and recurrences can be identified. Identification can occur prior to the development of a significant mass by which time the carcinoma may be only amenable for palliative therapy.

Acknowledgment

I would like to acknowledge Emma Hornsby and Dinesh Ranatunga for their help in proof reading.

References

Binmoeller, K.F., 1999. Endoluminal ultrasound for oesophageal cancer. Dig. Endosc. 11 (1), 3–6.

Dahnert, W., 2003. Radiology review manual, fifth ed. Lippincott Williams & Wilkins, ISBN 0–7817–4822–4.

Drug Therapy, Bulletin, 2006. Population screening for colorectal cancer. Drug Ther. Bull. 44 (9), 65–68.

Erturk, S.M., Ondategui-Parra, S., Otero, H., Ros, P.R., 2006. Evidence-based radiology. J. Am. Coll. Radiol. 3 (7), 513–519.

Fraquelli, M., Colli, A., Paggi, S., et al., 2005. Role of ultrasound in detection of Crohn's disease: Meta-analysis. Radiology 236: 95–101.

Guillerman, R.P., Ng, C.S., 2005. Ultrasound of appendicitis. Ultrasound 13 (2): 78–85.

Halligan, S., Altman, D.G., Taylor, S.A., et al., 2005. Evidence-based practice. CT colonography in the detection of colorectal polyps and cancer: systematic review, meta-analysis, and proposed minimum data set for study level reporting. Radiology 237, 893–904.

Hastings, G.S., 2000. Angiographic localization and transcatheter treatment of gastrointestinal bleeding. Radiographics 20, 1160–1168.

Holder, L.E., 2000. Radionuclide imaging in the evaluation of acute gastrointestinal bleeding. Radiographics 20 (4), 1153–1159.

Ko, Y.T., Lim, J.H., Lee, D.H., Lee, H.W., Lim, J.W., 1993. Small bowel obstruction: sonographic evaluation. Radiology 188, 649–653.

Lauenstein, T.C., Goehde, S.C., Ruehm, S.G., Holtmann, G., Debatin, J.F., 2002. MR colonography with barium-based faecal tagging: initial clinical experience. Radiology 223, 248.

Ledermann, H.P., Borner, N., Strunk, H., Bongartz, G., Zollikofer, C., Struckmann, G., 2000. Review: bowel wall thickening on transabdominal sonography. Am. J. Radiol. 174, 107–117.

Lee, P.Y., Fletcher, W.S., Sullivan, E.S., Vetto, J.T., 1994. Colorectal cancer in young patients: characteristics and outcome. Am. Surg. 60, 607–612.

National Institute for Clinical Excellence, Interventional procedures programme. Interventional procedures overview of computed tomography colonography (virtual colonoscopy). www.nice.com

Pickhardt, P.J., Choi, J.R., Hwang, I., et al., 2003. Computed tomographic virtual colonoscopy to screen for colorectal neoplasia in asymptomatic adults. N. Eng. J. Med. 349, 2191–2199.

Prassopoulos, P., Papanikolaou, N., et al., 2001. MR enteroclysis imaging of Crohn disease. Radiographics 21, S161–S172.

Rottenberg, G.T., Williams, A.B., 2002. Pictorial review: Endoanal ultrasound. Br. J. Radiol. 75, 482–488.

Society of Nuclear Medicine procedure guidelines for gastrointestinal bleeding and Meckel's diverticulum scintigraphy, 1999. Version 1.0. www.snm.org

Strassburg, J., 2004. The MERCURY experience of MRI. Tech. Coloproctology 8, S16–S18.

Yee, J., Akerkar, G.A., Hung, R.K., et al., 2001. Colorectal neoplasia: performance characteristics of CT colonography for detection in 300 patients. Gastrointest. Imag. 219, 685–692.

Further reading

Farr, R.F., Allisy-Roberts, P.J., 2002. Physics for medical imaging. W.B. Saunders.

McRobbie, D.W., Moore, E.A., Graves, M.J., Prince, M.R., 2002. MRI from picture to proton. Cambridge University Press.

Wheater, P.R., Burkitt, H.G., Daniels, V.G., 1996. Functional histology. A text and colour atlas, second ed. Churchill Livingstone, 201–224.

CT colonography

Christine Bloor

Contents

Introduction

Colon cancer is the third most common malignancy in men and the second most common malignancy in women with 35 599 new cases reported in the UK in 2005 (Cancer Research UK, 2008). Most colon cancers arise from *pre-existing adenomatous polyps* where the incidence of malignancy increases with size. There are well known risk factors to developing colon cancer, such as hereditary polyposis syndromes and chronic inflammatory bowel disease, but most cancers occur in patients with no predisposing risk factors other than advancing age (Tolan et al., 2007).

Computed tomography colonography (CTC) was first described in 1994 as dual position, helical computed tomography (CT) of a cleansed, gas distended colon (Vining et al., 1994). Since that time, the examination has steadily evolved to the point where it is not only advocated for the investigation of patients with symptoms of colon cancer but also as a screening test for asymptomatic patients (Levin et al., 2008).

Meta-analysis of published data demonstrates that CTC has high sensitivity and specificity rates (using conventional colonoscopy as the reference standard) for large and medium size polyps and a high reported diagnostic accuracy for symptomatic cancer (Pickhardt et al., 2003; National Institute for Health and Clinical Excellence, 2005). However, diagnostic accuracy falls with polyp size and, as with conventional colonoscopy, there may be low sensitivity in detecting flat colonic lesions (Hoon et al., 2003). Studies have also shown that CTC is significantly more sensitive than barium enema at polyp detection and has the additional advantage of being able to demonstrate significant *extracolonic pathology* in approximately 9% of patients (Yee et al., 2005; Spreng et al., 2005; Taylor et al., 2006; Tolan et al., 2007).

Research shows that the diagnostic accuracy of CTC is highly dependent on the quality of the examination and that meticulous attention must be given to both examination and interpretation techniques in order to achieve acceptable diagnostic performance (Ho Park et al., 2007; Rockey et al., 2007).

CTC technique

Patient information

Patient compliance is vital to achieve an optimal CTC examination, therefore, it is most important that high quality, *accurate written information* should be available so that patients are aware of the bowel preparation, the dietary restrictions and their effect on the diagnostic outcome. A description of what the procedure involves must be included so patients are forewarned about what they will undergo, especially the need to distend the colon with gas and the administration of spasmolytic drugs and contrast media. The information leaflet should clearly explain the risks, benefits and alternatives to the procedure, including the risk of perforation, contrast reaction, side effects of the spasmolytic drugs and the radiation dose. The information should also include advice for patients with diabetes on where and how to obtain specific information on glycemic control and specialist information for those taking Metformin (Tolan et al., 2007).

Bowel preparation and fecal tagging

Reliable detection of small polyps at CTC is heavily dependent on optimum bowel preparation. The presence of fecal residue and retained fluid can cover colonic mucosa, hide pathology and reduce the sensitivity and specificity of the examination (Mang et al., 2007).

There is currently no consensus as to the *optimum bowel preparation regime* for CTC, although it is generally recognized that a clean, dry colon is required. Picolax (sodium picosulphate and magnesium citrate) is widely used in the UK for barium enema and colonoscopy bowel preparation (Box 18.1) and there is evidence to support its efficacy for CTC (Taylor et al., 2003a). Patient safety and tolerance should also be considered in the choice and administration of bowel preparation as *vulnerable groups*, such as the elderly and those with renal impairment, may be at risk of dehydration and electrolyte

BOX 18.1 Standard bowel preparation

The day before the procedure

0800	Take one sachet of Picolax Then drink as much clear fluid as you can, including clear soups, Oxo, Bovril, jelly and sweet, fizzy drinks
1600	Take the second sachet of Picolax Continue to drink as much clear fluid as you can, including clear soups, Oxo, Bovril, jelly and sweet, fizzy drinks until your examination

BOX 18.2 Full purgation with stool/fluid tagging: University of Wisconsin (standard regimen)

24h before	Clear liquids only
18h before	Fleet phosphosoda (45 ml) undiluted followed by 1–2 l of clear fluids
15h before	Barium 2.1% (250 ml) (plus 296 ml of magnesium citrate if bowel cleansing not commenced). Further 1–2 l of clear fluid
12h before	60 ml gastrograffin (Bracco Diagnostics) with clear fluids
8h before	Nil by mouth until examination

(Tolan et al., 2007)

disturbance. Patients with diabetes should be advised to contact departments so they can be scheduled first on the list and to contact a diabetic nurse specialist to obtain advice regarding glycemic control for the period of dietary restriction (Tolan et al., 2007).

It is recognized that full bowel preparation does not always result in a completely clean colon. Techniques have been developed that allow residue and fluid to be labeled or tagged using oral contrast agents in order to avoid them being confused with pathology. There are a number of *tagging protocols* in use which include barium compounds, iodinated contrast media or a combination of the two (Box 18.2). It is suggested that barium is superior at tagging solid residue and iodinated contrast media is better at tagging fluid, although there is undoubtedly some overlap (Figure 18.1). The diagnostic accuracy of CTC can be further increased by using specialized computer software to perform '*electronic cleansing*'. This allows the opacified colonic fluid and barium tagged stool to be digitally removed at the post processing stage so that it does not obscure the visualization of polyps or significant pathology (Rockey et al., 2007; Mang et al., 2007).

CHAPTER 18

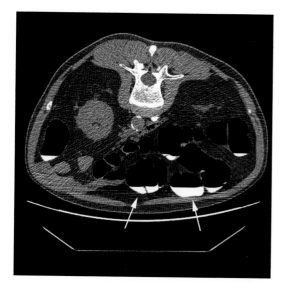

Figure 18.1 Prone view showing tagging with iodinated contrast media (arrows).

The development of fecal tagging protocols and 'electronic cleansing' has resulted in some centers reducing the laxative regime given to patients. This undoubtedly increases *patient acceptability* as the bowel preparation is often considered the most intolerable part of the examination. It also allows CTC to be performed with reduced or no laxation in those patients where it may be harmful, e.g. the elderly and those with significant comorbidity (O'Hare and Fenlon, 2006; Laudi et al., 2008).

Colonic insufflation

Good colonic distension is fundamental to obtaining a high quality examination and optimal mucosal visualization. Imaging under-distended or collapsed segments of bowel can render the examination non-diagnostic, necessitating a repeat examination or referral for colonoscopy. It may also result in pathologies being missed or lead to a false positive diagnosis. There are several strategies currently used to achieve good *colonic distension* which include the use of different catheters and insufflation devices, administering spasmolytics and obtaining images in the prone and supine position (Burling et al., 2006a; Mang et al., 2007).

Insufflation techniques vary between centers and a number of methods are currently used to distend the colon. These include *manual insufflation* of room air or carbon dioxide or the use of a commercially available *automated carbon dioxide colon inflator*. Inflating carbon dioxide is preferable to room air as it is more readily absorbed, resulting in less post-procedural discomfort and bloating (Burling et al., 2006a).

A small caliber (20F), *soft flexible catheter* is adequate to obtain optimal colonic distension and is well tolerated by the patient. Large, rigid rectal catheters of the type used for barium enema examinations have not been found to improve colonic distension and, in some cases, have led to rectal perforation and their use should be actively discouraged (Sosna et al., 2006).

The practice of using a *retention balloon* varies and, although the occurrence of perforation during barium enema examination is estimated to increase by a factor of 2.5 when a retention balloon is used, there are no published data to suggest this is the case during CTC. If an inflated rectal catheter balloon is used, it should be deflated during the prone series, which best visualizes the lower rectum. This, together with performing a per rectal (PR) examination, will minimize the risk of missing a low rectal tumor (Burling et al., 2006a; Tolan et al., 2007).

Manually inflating room air or carbon dioxide has the advantage of being relatively cheap and readily available. The automated colon inflator (PROTOCO2L E-Z-Em) has the advantage of using carbon dioxide as well as maintaining constant pressure and adequate insufflation of the colon throughout the study by regulating the pressure and volume of gas administered. It has also been found significantly to improve colonic distension when compared to manual insufflation. The disadvantages of the automated colon inflator are the high capital cost of the machine and the ongoing costs of the consumables (rectal catheter and tubing) (Burling et al., 2006a).

Whichever method of gas insufflation is used, there is always a risk of *colonic perforation* and care must be taken throughout the procedure. If gas insufflation proves difficult or the patient complains of undue discomfort,

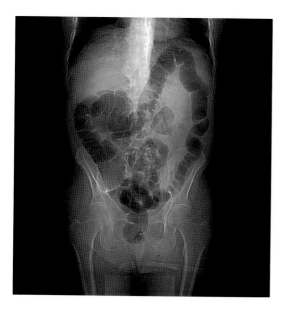

Figure 18.2 Scout view showing good colonic distension.

careful consideration of the causes must be made. Symptoms of bloating and mild cramping are usually good indicators that reasonable distension has been achieved. If there is any doubt a *scout view* should be obtained to assess the level of distension (Figure 18.2) or identify any abrupt cut off in the colonic gas pattern which may represent the presence of an *obstructing stricture or mass* (Tolan et al., 2007).

Patient positioning and technique

It is widely accepted that patients must be imaged in two positions in order to maximize distension of all dependent parts of the colon. Changing position also allows better recognition of fecal and fluid contamination as it tends to move to the dependent wall of the colon. The *prone and supine positions* have been found to maximize colonic distension and there is no consensus as to the order in which the views should be obtained. If the patient cannot lie in either position, then imaging in the *decubitus or recovery position* may be helpful. The supine images are often the most valuable and this position is often better tolerated by the patient. If IV contrast is to be administered, it is easier to do so with the patient in the supine position.

CTC insufflations/technique protocols will vary between centers and a typical technique protocol is outlined in Box 18.3. In order to reduce the duration of patient discomfort and to ensure an optimum examination is obtained, it is important the CTC is performed by well-trained, motivated staff with a special interest. Ideally, the primary read of the axial images should take place while the patient is in the examination room so that full staging can be performed if a colon cancer or extra colonic pathology is demonstrated (Tolan et al., 2007).

BOX 18.3 CTC technique using automated or manual insufflation

- Obtain consent and cannulate patient (out of examination room)
- Introduce patient to the staff conducting the examination
- Position the patient in the left lateral position on the examination table
- Perform a digital rectal examination
- Insert rectal catheter
- Inject spasmolytic
- For automated insufflation, zero the volume reading and set pressure to 25 mmHg or start manual insufflation
- Insufflate about 1.5–2 l of CO_2 or about 20 bulb puffs for manual distension
- Turn the patient prone with their arms in front of them
- Advance patient into gantry to start position for scout
- Wait until 2.5–4 l of CO_2 and pressure has risen to 20 mmHg or a further 20 bulb puffs have been performed
- Perform scout view
- Review scout view for adequacy of distension. If inadequate continue distension and repeat scout view
- Acquire prone series
- Stop automatic insufflator or reduce pressure to 15 mmHg
- Review unreconstructed images at the work station to assess distension and identify pathology
- Remove patient from gantry
- Turn patient supine
- Connect IV contrast to patient if required
- Insert patient into gantry
- Restart CO_2 insufflator and add an additional 500 ml–1 l of CO_2 or another few manual bulb puffs
- Scout immediately
- Review scout for adequacy of distension (if inadequate, continue insufflation and re-scout)
- Acquire supine series 65–70 seconds after IV contrast administration (300 mg/ml)
- Pause automated insufflation
- Review unreconstructed images to assess for distension and obvious tumor
- Consider undertaking chest series if tumor present
- Remove patient from gantry, disconnect IV injector pump and remove rectal catheter

Antispasmodics

Antispasmodics are used routinely in gastrointestinal imaging to improve colonic distension and reduce patient discomfort. There are currently two anti-spasmodics in general use in the UK – hyoscine-N-butylbromide (Buscopan) and glucagon (Glucagen).

Hyoscine-N-butylbromide (Buscopan) is widely used in barium enema practice and has also been shown significantly to improve colonic disten-sion during CTC. It is only effective for about 15 minutes after injection so should be administered just before insufflation begins to allow enough time to acquire the prone and supine data sets with optimum distension. Due to the drug's anticholinergic effect, caution must be used when giving it to patients with a cardiac history or a history of glaucoma (Taylor et al., 2003a).

Glucagon is often used in barium enema practice when Buscopan is contraindicated. However, it has been shown that during CTC, distension of the colon is not significantly improved after glucagon and that patients often experience nausea and vomiting (Rogalla et al., 2005).

Intravenous contrast

Image enhancement with IV contrast can be helpful in differentiating polyps from fecal residue and improving the detection of polyps in a poorly prepared colon. Currently, the use of IV contrast in the *screening population* is not advocated due to the increased risk involved and the uncertain cost effectiveness. However, IV contrast enhancement has been shown to be of benefit in *symptomatic patients* where the examination of extracolonic organs and detection of extracolonic abnormalities is of clinical benefit. The symptoms of colon cancer can be very non-specific and it has been demonstrated that significant extracolonic findings are relatively frequent in older symptomatic patients (Rockey et al., 2007; Soo Lee et al., 2007).

If IV contrast is administered, it is easier for both the patient and operator if this is done during the supine acquisition. Acquisition of images during the *arterial phase* (45s) may be more appropriate for the purposes of polyp detection since bowel wall enhancement is maximized and polyps are better visualized in this phase. However, in reality, acquisition of images in the *portal phase* (65–70s) is more appropriate to maximize extracolonic evaluation and optimize tumor staging (Spreng et al., 2005; Tolan et al., 2007).

CT acquisition technique

The ability of CT colonography to detect colorectal polyps is dependent on the CT acquisition parameters including slice thickness. The *slice thickness* should be at least half of the target polyp size to minimize partial volume averaging with adjacent air. Therefore, in practice, slice thickness should be no more than 2.5 mm, however, in reality much thinner slices are obtained with modern 16 and 64 slice scanners. Faster tube rotation times and increased detectors permit *faster table speeds* so that patients can be scanned quicker, reducing the chance of movement artefact and allowing scans to be acquired during one breath hold. It is generally accepted that the thin sections and faster scanning times provided by multidetector CT scanners are required for optimum results. The American College of Radiology practice guidelines (2006) recommend a KVp of 120 KV and a *tube current* of <100 mA for routine colonography examinations in adult patients; if IV contrast is given then normal dose settings should be employed. Typical protocols using a 16 and 64 detector CT are given in Box 18.4 (Taylor et al., 2003b; Tolan et al., 2007).

Supine with contrast

	16 section	64 section
Voltage	120 KV	120 KV
Effective current	100 mA (current modulation to minimum dose)	
Acquisition	16 × 0.75 mm	64 × 0.6 mm
Collimation	0.75 mm	0.6 mm
Feed/rotation	12 mm	26.9 mm
Increment	1 mm	0.7 mm
Reconstructed section thickness		1 mm

Prone without contrast

As above but reduce tube current to 30–50 mA (with tube current modulation)
Consider increasing mA in obese patients

Post CTC patient care

Patients who have undergone CTC require specific after care due to the combined effects of the bowel preparation, abdominal distension and intravenous injection of IV contrast and a spasmolytic. Once the rectal catheter is removed, the patient should be assisted to sit up slowly and advised to sit on the examination couch for a few minutes. The patient should be warned and reassured about abdominal pain. They should be escorted to a toilet which must be immediately available and near by; ideally, a shower should also be available. The patient should be offered refreshments, e.g. a cup of tea or coffee and a light snack which should be taken in a comfortable quiet environment. They should be advised to remain in the department for 15–30 minutes, especially if IV contrast has been administered (the cannula should be removed before they leave). *Verbal and written information* must be given with advice about the side effects of the spasmolytic drugs, the possible complications that can occur and symptoms to look out for as well as reassuring advice about abdominal pain caused by the gas (Tolan et al., 2007; Burling et al., 2006b).

Interpretation and reporting

CTC images can be reviewed as two-dimensional (2D) or three-dimensional (3D) images. *2D image review* refers to the sagittal images of the colon from the rectum to the cecum viewed by scrolling through the serial images in a stack mode. *3D image review* refers to an optical colonoscopy-like *endoluminal fly-through* of a 3D reconstructed colon (Figure 18.3) and relies on specialized computer software to manipulate the data set (Figure 18.4, see color insert).

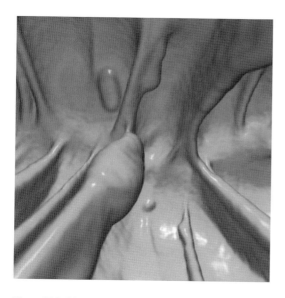

Figure 18.3 3D endoluminal view demonstrating a polyp (Courtesy of Viatronix, Inc).

The *primary 2D read* should ideally occur in the CT control room while the patient is still in the examination room. This allows any significant colonic or extracolonic pathology to be identified and means that any additional imaging such as chest images or images with IV contrast may be acquired (Figure 18.5).

Formal CTC interpretation must take place at a *dedicated workstation using specialist software*. Optimized interpretation of CTC requires specialist reader training and robust audit practices. The method of image interpretation is the personal choice of the reporter and may consist of a primary 2D read, where the axial images are interrogated first, or a primary 3D read, where the colon

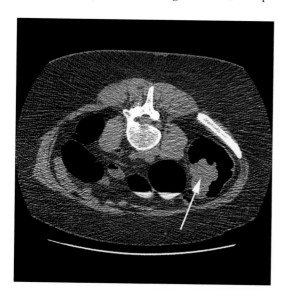

Figure 18.5 Large cecal tumor (arrow) demonstrated on a prone image – this patient could proceed immediately to tumor staging protocols.

is examined principally using the 3D endoluminal images. However, standard practice appears to consist of a simultaneous review of the prone and supine 2D images viewed side by side. This allows tracing of the colonic outline on each image to find small contour abnormalities which can be compared in the supine and prone view (Figures 18.6 and 18.7). 3D endoluminal fly through images can be obtained as antegrade and retrograde in both the supine and prone positions (see Figure 18.4). Taking advantage of this plethora of data can make CTC interpretation extremely time consuming and, in reality, the 3D endoluminal views are often used to problem solve in a segment of abnormal colon, to confirm the presence of a polyp (Figure 18.8) or to help distinguish between fecal residue and polyp (Rockey et al., 2007).

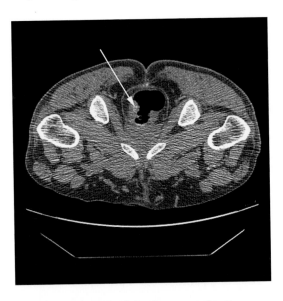

Figure 18.6 Rectal tumor (arrow) on a prone image.

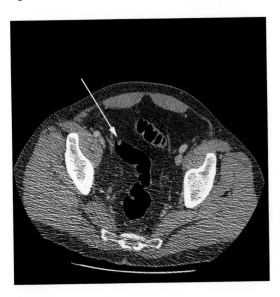

Figure 18.7 Small sigmoid polyp visible on the supine view (arrow).

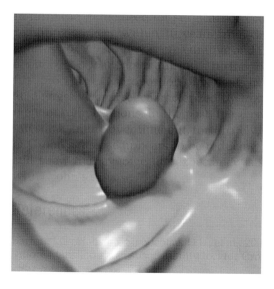

Figure 18.8 Endoluminal view clearly demonstrates a sessile polyp (Courtesy of Viatronix, Inc.).

A recent development in CTC interpretation has been the availability of *computer-aided detection* (CAD). This is currently an area of active research and will undoubtedly have an impact on the future of CTC interpretation. CAD has the potential to improve the sensitivity for polyp detection and has already been incorporated into several commercial CTC reporting software systems. Although it has many advantages, CAD has the potential, when incorporated into established reading strategies, to increase reporting time and reduce specificity. Most established readers currently use CAD as a 'second reader', reading the data set first without using the CAD prompts, then repeating the analysis using CAD (Yoshida and Nappi, 2007).

References

American College of Radiology, 2006. ACR Practice guideline for the performance of computed tomography (CT) colonography in adults.

Burling, D., Taylor, S.A., Halligan, S., et al., 2006a. Automated insufflation of carbon dioxide for MDCT colonography: distension and patient experience compared with manual insufflation. Am. J. Roentgenol. 186, 96–103.

Burling, D., Halligan, S., Slater, A., et al., 2006b. Potentially serious adverse events at CT colonography in symptomatic patients: national survey of the United Kingdom. Radiology 239, 464–471.

Cancer Research UK. UK Bowel Cancer Incidence Statistics. <http://www.info.cancerresearchuk.org/cancerstats/tyoes/bowel/incidence/> Accessed 28/09/2008.

Ho Park, S., Yee, J., Hyung Kim, S., et al., 2007. Fundamental elements for successful performance of CT colonography. Korean J. Radiol. 8 (4), 264–275.

Hoon, J., Rolnick, J.A., Haker, S., et al., 2003. Multislice CT colonography: current status and limitations. Eur. J. Radiol. 47 (2), 123–134.

Laudi, C., Campanella, G., Galatola, G., et al., 2008. PA.246 virtual colonoscopy (VC) using same day faecal tagging and limited bowel preparation. Dig. Liver Dis. 40 (1), S165.

CTC technique

CHAPTER 18

Levin, B., Lieberman, D.A., McFarland, B., et al., and for the American Cancer Society Colorectal Cancer Advisory Group, the US Multi-Society Task Force and the American College of Radiology Colon Cancer Committee, 2008. Screening and surveillance for the early detection of colorectal cancer and adenomatous polyps. A joint guideline from the American Cancer Society, the US Multi-Society Task Force on Colorectal Cancer and the American College of Radiology. Cancer J. Clin. 58, 130–60.

Mang, T., Graser, A., Schima, W., et al., 2007. CT colonography: techniques, indications, findings. Eur. J. Radiol. 61 (3), 388–399.

National Institute for Health and Clinical Excellence, 2005. Computed tomographic colonography. (virtual colonoscopy). Interventional procedure guidance 129. <http://www.nice.org.uk/Guidance/IPG129> Accessed 29/09/08.

O Hare, A., Fenlon, H., 2006. Virtual colonoscopy in the detection of colonic polyps and neoplasms. Best Pract. Res. Clin. Gastroenterol. 20 (1), 79–92.

Pickhardt, P.J., Choi, R.J., Hwang, I., et al., 2003. Computed tomographic virtual colonoscopy to screen for colorectal neoplasia in asymptomatic adults. N. Engl. J. Med. 349 (23), 2191–2200.

Rockey, D., Barish, M., Brill, J.V., et al., 2007. CT colonography standards. Standards for gastroenterologists for performing and interpreting diagnostic computed tomographic colonography. Gastroenterology 133, 1005–1024.

Rogalla, P., Lemboke, A., Ruckert, J.C., et al., 2005. Spasmolysis at CT colonography: butyl scopolamine versus glucagon. Radiology 236, 184–188.

Soo Lee, S., Ho Park, S., Choi, E.K., et al., 2007. Colorectal polyps on portal phase contrast-enhanced CT colonography: lesion attenuation and distinction from tagged feces. Am. J. Roentgenol. 189, 35–40.

Sosna, J., Blachar, A., Amitai, M., et al., 2006. Colonic perforation at CT colonography: assessment of risk in a multicenter large cohort. Radiology 239, 457–463.

Spreng, A., Netzer, P., Mattich, J., et al., 2005. Importance of extracolonic findings at IV contrast medium-enhanced CT colonography versus those at non enhanced CT colonography. Eur. Radiol. 15, 2088–2095.

Taylor, S.A., Halligan, S., Goh, V., et al., 2003a. Optimizing colonic distension for multi-detector row CT colonography: effect of hyocine butylbromide and rectal balloon catheter. Radiology 229, 99–108.

Taylor, S.A., Halligan, S., Bartram, C.I., et al., 2003b. Multi-detector row CT colonography: effect of collimation, pitch, and orientation on polyp detection in a human colectomy specimen. Radiology 229, 109–118.

Taylor, S.A., Halligan, S., Slater, A., et al., 2006. Comparison of radiologists' confidence in excluding significant colorectal neoplasia with multidetector-row CT colonography compared with double contrast barium enema. Br. J. Radiol. 79, 208–214.

Tolan, D.J.M., Armstrong, E.M., Burling, D., et al., 2007. Optimization of CT colonography technique: a practical guide. Clin. Radiol. 62 (9), 819–827.

Vining, D.J., Gelfand, R.E., Bechtold, R.E., et al., 1994. Technical feasibility of colon imaging with helical CT and virtual reality. Am. J. Roentgenol. 162 (Suppl.), 104.

Yee, J., Kumar, N.N., Godara, S., et al., 2005. Extracolonic abnormalities discovered incidentally at CT colonography in a male population. Radiology 236, 519–526.

Yoshida, H., Näppi, J., 2007. CAD in CT colonography without and with oral contrast agents: progress and challenges. Comput. Med. Imag. Graph. 31 (4–5), 267–284.

Introduction to the reporting of gastrointestinal (GI) radiological procedures

David Gary Culpan

Contents

Introduction

Reporting standards

Practical skills

- Observation and interpretation
- Reporting style and structure

- Communication
- Terminology

Audit of reporting practice

Conclusion

References

Introduction

The reporting of radiological (medical imaging) procedures has traditionally been performed by radiologists (specialist medical doctors). However, initially in medical ultrasound (US), due to increasing workload and a shortage of radiologists beginning in the 1970s, there has been a gradual shift within the UK to reporting duties being undertaken by allied healthcare practitioners, predominantly radiographers (Fernando, 1999).

The precedent from US imaging was expanded into Accident and Emergency (A&E) radiographic imaging, initially with an *abnormality flagging system*, often called the 'red dot' system (Berman et al., 1985; Nuttall, 1995). This subsequently developed into reporting of a wider range of plain radiographs by radiographers (Quick, 1993; Robinson, 1996a; Robinson et al., 1999a) and from there expanded into most other subspecialties of medical imaging (Culpan, 2006).

Although there is no specific requirement that the *delegation of medical image reporting* be to a specific professional group (General Medical Council, 2001), the delegation process should be robust and take into account the skills base of those to whom the task is delegated.

This concept is well developed for the radiography profession in the UK and has involved liaison and co-operation between the relevant professional bodies. These include:

- The College of Radiographers (CoR), the professional body for radiographers
- The Society of Radiographers (SoR), the trade union for radiographers

- Health Professions Council (HPC), the regulatory and registration body for allied health professionals
- Royal College of Radiologists (RCR), the professional body for clinical radiologists
- General Medical Council (GMC), the regulatory body for doctors.

In the field of GI imaging, the first area of delegated practice to be undertaken (and subsequently reported) by radiographers was the double contrast barium enema (DCBE) (Mannion et al., 1995). *Radiographer reporting of DCBE was shown to be of similar accuracy to radiologist reporting* (Law et al., 1999; Culpan et al., 2002, 2003; Booth and Mannion, 2005).

Reporting standards

Standards of reporting are important, not least because cases may be tested in a Court of Law. As such, the standards achieved by the healthcare professional undertaking the delegated reporting role must at least match the standards of the professional group which had previously performed the role, namely the clinical radiologists (Dimond, 2002, 366-7). The RCR produced *standards for reporting for radiologists* (The Royal College of Radiologists, 2006) which consequently must also apply to all others undertaking the reporting role.

Ensuring that the reporting skills of the allied health practitioner match those of the radiologist(s) who previously undertook the task can be achieved by appropriate training, education and subsequent audit of performance.

In the UK, several universities run post registration courses, predominantly delivered by radiography lecturers, which cover the basic skills required for the generation of a medical imaging report and also covers the range of anatomy, normal variants and pathology which may be demonstrated on medical images. Most such courses require course delegates/students to have a fundamental understanding of the imaging process at the outset.

Practical skills

Observation and interpretation

To understand and interpret medical images, an individual needs an understanding of the process by which the images were created. Almost all medical imaging in the UK is now in *digital format*, be that the output from the image intensifier in fluoroscopy, static images in fluorography, computed radiography (CR) images, direct digital radiography (DR), computed tomography (CT), magnetic resonance (MR) imaging, radionuclide imaging (RNI) and ultrasound (US).

Digital format has several advantages (e.g. the potential for manipulation of the image after it has been captured); however, the uninitiated may simulate or mask/obscure pathology by incorrect manipulation of images. *Transfer of images* in digital format is also simplified; no longer does the reporting professional have to wait for 'hard copy' images or carry around stacks of photographic film. Electronic digital image files can now be transferred to image reporting stations within (and outside) the healthcare facility in which they are acquired.

It is important to acknowledge that *image reporting workstations* have specific requirements for monitor quality. Three megapixel monitors are used for reporting in medical imaging departments, but satellite facilities on hospital wards or outpatient clinics may not have such high resolution monitors (often standard computer displays are utilized) and it must be recognized that abnormalities may go undetected if healthcare professionals use these to try to interpret and diagnose from medical images.

Building on the basic understanding of medical images, the next skill required is to understand how pathological/disease processes affect imaging appearances. Although much of this can be learned in the classroom on a theoretical basis, there is no substitute for actual/real clinical experience and all taught courses in the UK have embedded such clinical perspective within them.

Many healthcare professionals learning the skills of medical image reporting start off using a technique known as '*pattern recognition*'. This involves subconsciously matching the viewed image against a preconceived pattern or '*template*', such that matches and mismatches are recognized immediately by the viewer. This process is integral to *human perception* (a full discussion of how this works is beyond the scope of this chapter) due to the way image information is built up within separate areas of the brain and finally brought together into a recognizable form.

Patterns can be built up over a period of time so that specific pathological findings are immediately recognized without conscious thought because they had been experienced in the past. The radiological community has adopted the term 'Aunt Minnie' type pattern recognition for this and there is a commercial website named after the phenomenon (auntminnie.com) which also promotes educational activities.

Although pattern recognition has its uses, there are potential downfalls to relying on the process. For instance, if a pattern demonstrated is not one that the viewer has seen before, or is not one they are completely familiar with, it may not be recognized. In such cases, even quite obvious abnormalities may be ignored as the individual is only looking for 'what they know'. To overcome this limitation, the trainee reporting practitioner is taught to review medical images systematically, interrogating the whole image sequentially, looking at all parts of an image and all images within each particular examination or study. This may be quite challenging since with multidetector CT examinations (MDCT) and multisequence MR studies, there may be 300–500 individual images in a single study (Fishman, no date). When, therefore, it is not possible to scrutinize each image in detail, pattern recognition remains the primary method of review. This process may be facilitated by *computer-assisted detection* (CAD) software, application specific programs being commonplace for virtual colonoscopy (VC) for instance, to highlight potential pathology.

It is also important that personnel involved in image interpretation and reporting understand the *clinical information* provided by the referring clinician (The Royal College of Radiologists, 2006). In the UK, there is a legal requirement that this is sufficient to enable the radiologist or radiographer to 'justify' the examination with respect to the ionizing radiations (medical imaging) regulations (IR(ME)R 2000) (Department of Health, 2000). Clinical information in the referral should convey any relevant signs and symptoms elicited from the patient's medical history, physical examination and laboratory tests and should give a provisional diagnosis or suggest differentials. The referral is often expressed in terms of a *'clinical question'*, for instance, a patient with unexplained iron deficiency anemia may be referred for a range of diagnostic tests such as initial esophago-gastroduodenoscopy (OGD) and subsequent DCBE or colonoscopy to confirm or refute the presence of a colonic source of bleeding such as a cecal tumor.

Reporting style and structure

Report styles vary across institutions, the range including simple 'normal/abnormal' flag systems (such as red dot), informal commenting systems and definitive free text reporting.

The *definitive report* is the permanent legal record of the medical imaging examination. This is now typically stored electronically within a *radiology information system* (RIS) with a paper or electronic copy in the individual patient record (clinical or medical notes).

Most medical imaging reporters use a free text type report, although alternatives include a pre-defined proforma style, where specific questions are answered or pre-coded standard phrases selected (Naik et al., 2001). Each style has its own strengths but the recommended structure expected of medical imaging reports is defined by the The Royal College of Radiologists (2006). Initially, a report should contain *patient identifying information* to ensure that a specific report can be related to a specific patient on a specific occasion, as mis-identification can have significant, potentially serious adverse consequences.

Next, *procedural information* should be included. Often this is part of the electronic patient record, but it is important to check that the planned examination did actually happen; for instance, if a request for a DCBE was made but the patient was not fit enough to participate in the full/complete examination, a less demanding, but less diagnostically sensitive test such as a single contrast barium enema may have been performed. The significance of altering/modifying the requested examination must be made clear to the referrer in the report. Similarly, it is important to acknowledge limitations within the report when the findings are based upon sub-optimal images.

Since medical imaging examinations are usually performed to answer a specific clinical question, the *clinical question* is also usually included within the main body of the report.

Next should follow a *description of the imaging findings* (The Royal College of Radiologists, 2006) in terms of size, shape, outline contour, position and radiographic characteristics. The overall radiological findings must then be related to the presence or absence of pathology. Comments can be made on normal findings where this refutes the clinical question or where there is a variance of normal anatomy, e.g. malrotation of the colon or situs inversus.

Communication

Communication of the report to the referrer is of paramount importance as the report is the end result of the imaging examination (The Royal College of Radiologists, 2007). It is important that the referrer can understand the report and that it is written in plain language, devoid of jargon and obscure terminology.

The distinction between a *'descriptive report'* offered by an allied healthcare professional and a *'medical report'* offered by a clinical radiologist is one that should be made on the grounds of authorship (Robinson, 1996b). Only a medical practitioner can provide a 'medical report', anything else is considered a 'descriptive report' regardless of content, thus the authorship and professional status of the reporter should be stated in the report somewhere (Dimond, 2002).

Where there are *urgent or unexpected abnormal findings*, e.g. obstructing tumor, these should be communicated rapidly to the referring clinician and this procedure documented (The Royal College of Radiologists, 2006). To ensure that the referrer is aware of the situation, direct communication, such as face-to-face or telephone conversation is always best, as a written note, memo, letter, fax, e-mail or voice mail may be ignored, lost, erased in error, or its urgency or significance may not be appreciated if it is received by an inappropriate member of the healthcare team.

In recognition of this issue, the National Patient Safety Agency (NPSA, 2007) reported a number of incidents which had led to patient fatalities and significant long-term harm when there had been failures to follow up on medical imaging reports.

It is unusual for patients to be told the results of a medical imaging investigation at the time of the investigation. This is because the referrer will be the person with all the relevant information pertaining to the range of clinical, laboratory and imaging investigations and how the results of these all fit together to inform the care or treatment plan for the individual patient. It is often frustrating for patients to be told that they must see the referring clinician again for the results, but allied healthcare professionals (AHPs) must be trained to deal with such delicate situations. There are some situations where AHPs do give results (e.g. in obstetric ultrasound) but this is only after specific training has been undertaken and is within the remit of an agreed protocol which outlines their responsibility and scope of practice (Simpson, 2001).

Terminology

The terminology used in imaging reports (and of course in the clinical history provided by the referrer) is important; all parties involved need to understand the terms and phrases used. It is very easy to use abbreviations, acronyms and technical or professional jargon, which are perfectly reasonable in context, but are open to misinterpretation. Some examples of terms with multiple meanings are shown in the Table 19.1.

In the same way, use of ambiguous reporting terminology is to be discouraged when describing medical imaging findings. Although conventions are important, key stakeholders need to know what the conventions are. For instance, diverticulosis, seen on a DCBE, may be described as mild, moderate or severe, but it is important to ensure that there is consistency between individual reporting personnel so that the referrer knows just what degree of disease is implied when each term is used. If one observer states that disease is moderate while another calls it severe and a third observer calls it moderately severe, the clinician will find it unhelpful. To avoid this, a local agreement/consensus should be reached, for example, *mild* diverticulosis might be defined as 'some scattered diverticula', *moderate* disease as more concentrated in a particular segment and includes circular muscle thickening, and

Table 19.1 Standard abbreviations and their multiple clinical meanings

Abbreviation	Possible meanings
Ca	Calcium Carcinoma Cardiac arrest Contrast agent Chronological age Citric acid
MS	Multiple sclerosis Mitral stenosis Musculoskeletal Medical student Medical surgical Metabolic syndrome Munchausen's syndrome Morphine sulfate
IHD	Ischemic heart disease Intermittent hemodialysis Intrahepatic duct(s) Implantable hearing device
DM	Diabetes mellitus Doctor of medicine Dopamine Dextromethorphan Dermatomyositis Dystrophia myotonica Diastolic murmur
NAD	No abnormality detected No active disease No acute distress No apparent distress Nicotinamide adenine dinucleotide Nitric acid dihydrate
PMH	Past medical history Psychiatric/mental health Profoundly mentally handicapped Postmenopausal hormone
CF	Cystic fibrosis Cardiac failure Cerebrospinal fluid Cervical fracture Contributing factor Childfree Caucasian female Confer (Latin: Compare)

Table 19.1 Standard abbreviations and their multiple clinical meanings—cont'd

Abbreviation	Possible meanings
PID	Prolapsed intervertebral disk
	Protruded intervertebral disk
	Pelvic inflammatory disease
	Pain intensity difference
	Phosphotyrosine interaction domain
	Photoionization detector
	Picture image directory
	Plasma iron disappearance
	Plus integral plus derivative
	Poisons information database
	Postinertia dyskinesia
	Postinfection day
	Postinoculation day
	Preimplantation diagnosis
	Primary immunodeficiencies
	Primary immunodeficiency diseases
	Principal immunodominant domain
	Proliferative intraocular disorders
	Proportional-integral-derivative
OGD	Esophago-gastroduodenoscopy
	Osteoglophonic dysplasia
	Osteoglophonic dwarfism
	Old granulomatous disease

Adapted from GlobalRPh.com 2007.

the term *severe* reserved for cases where the disease interferes with confidence of diagnosis or exclusion within a particular segment. Such agreement must involve all interested parties, i.e. referrers and reporters.

Inconsistency may also exist in the way that the reporter states that the imaging investigation shows no evidence of active disease. Phrases in common use include: NAD (no abnormality detected), normal, completely normal, within normal limits, no significant abnormality, no definite abnormality. All these statements indicate lack of pathology to a greater or lesser degree, although the intent of the reporter and the understanding of the report recipient may be discrepant. The reporter thus needs to be aware of the connotations of the language used in their reports and choose words and phrases carefully.

As in any specialty, specialized language is often used in relation to specific imaging techniques such as 'signal intensity', 'enhancement pattern' or 'echogenicity' but, wherever possible, 'jargon' terms should be kept to a minimum unless the reporter is sure that the intended recipient (referrer) will understand the terms used. Where there is evidence of a pathological process, this should be commented upon and interpreted as either *significant findings* (related to the current signs and symptoms) and thus requiring some intervention, or be categorized/classified as *insignificant findings* where incidental findings such as degenerative disease, inactive colitis or diverticulosis are not considered to be responsible for the patient's current presentation. Significant findings must be analyzed to suggest a diagnosis or list of differentials. Occasionally, specific findings cannot be attributed to a single pathological process. For example, extrinsic compression of the colon noted at DCBE can have a range of causes which produce the same imaging appearances (Blakeborough et al., 2001). In such cases, the *differential list* should start with the most likely possibility. Wherever possible, the report should contain a *recommendation as to any further investigations* that might be suitable for clarifying such a diagnostic dilemma; in the aforementioned example, this might include abdominal and pelvic CT to characterize the nature of an extrinsic mass.

Some indication of the *diagnostic certainty* should be included in the report. This can be expressed in terms of the language used such as 'there is' rather than 'there may be' or 'this represents' rather than 'appearances are compatible with'.

Where findings are *equivocal*, 'don't know' might be an appropriate answer to the clinical question. In such cases, it is important to include a recommendation for further investigation. For instance, it may not be possible to tell during a DCBE whether a particular filling defect is due to residual feces, a mucosal fold or if it represents a true polyp, in such a case it is appropriate to suggest that endoscopy would be a useful adjunct.

Clinical coding systems, such as READ or SNOMED CT are used in administration systems to ensure compatibility and standardization across institutions/ electronic recording systems (NHS, 2007), but are not used in the generation of medical imaging reports at the time of writing. Hypothetically, this might be a future development with computerized reporting systems in medical imaging departments linking electronic/voice recognition reporting with the applications codes to keep the report as an integral part of the image file.

When static images are available for a particular examination, a *'double reporting'* process is recommended in some areas of medical imaging. Such practice is routine in mammographic breast screening, as it is more cost effective in terms of reducing the number of 'false positive' recalls for further assessment than single reading and it increases the cancer detection rate (Brown et al., 1996). Double reporting has been recommended for use in DCBE as it increases the sensitivity but inevitably decreases specificity of the examination (Markus et al., 1990; Anderson et al., 1991). However, where the examination images are dynamic, such as in ultrasound or videofluoroscopy, double reporting is problematic unless the entire study is stored and available for review on a separate workstation. This was not realistically feasible before the advent of PACS (picture archiving and communication system) due to the large data storage requirements and the time constraints of second real-time review of a dynamic study, i.e. at least the same length of time as taken to perform the original study. However, the benefits of being able to review *dynamic studies* digitally and frame by frame or in slow motion should not be underestimated.

Audit of reporting practice

In keeping with the clinical focus of reporting training at UK universities, these courses have some form of clinical assessment of report writing skills. For many this involves an audit of the student's reports and these are compared to the reports which were issued – to check for concurrence. Typically, 95% *concurrence* (Table 19.2) is required in plain film reporting and this may be

Table 19.2 Definitions of key terms associated with measurement of reporting accuracy

Radiological term	Definition
Reference (gold) standard	Standard against which accuracy is measured. May be another observer (e.g. experienced radiologist) or against another test
True positive (TP)	A correct decision which identifies abnormality when it is present
True negative (TN)	A correct decision which identifies normality when no pathology is present
False positive (FP)	An incorrect decision which identifies abnormality when none is present
False negative (FN)	An incorrect decision which identifies normality when a pathology is present. Also known as a perception error
Sensitivity	The ability to identify pathology within a population. The true positive percentage $TP/(TP+FN) \times 100$
Specificity	The ability to identify normality within a population. The true negative percentage $TN/(TN+FP) \times 100$
Accuracy	How often we make the *correct* decision. A combination of sensitivity and specificity values $TP + TN/\text{total number of cases} \times 100$
Concurrence	Complete inter-observer agreement
Partial concurrence	General inter-observer agreement, but: minor pathology missed extent of disease incorrectly identified
Non-concurrence	Disagreement between observers – a false positive or false negative in which patient management would have been affected
Reproducibility	How often we get the same result (not necessarily the correct result!)
Error	Those interpretations which differ from the consensus view of a panel of 'experts'. Types of error = technical; perceptual; interpretational; communication
Observer variation	Where experts fail to achieve consensus

(Continued)

Table 19.2 Definitions of key terms associated with measurement of reporting accuracy—cont'd

Radiological term	Definition
Discrepancy	Reporting errors which come to light at a later date with the benefit of additional information
Critical incident	A critical incident occurs when an error results in mismanagement of the patient with resultant morbidity or mortality, requiring mandatory further investigation

RCR, 2001; Robinson (1997)

carried over to more complex examinations, although it must be recognized that variation between observers is likely to be higher (Robinson, 1997) as no-one is perfect and disagreements are likely on the more difficult cases. One hundred percent *accuracy* is not the norm expected of radiologists reporting medical imaging studies and there has historically been research to assess the *level of errors and variation* for various types of medical imaging examinations (Robinson, 1997); a 5% error rate is deemed acceptable of competent individuals (Dimond, 2002).

Since the Accident and Emergency department was one of the first places where reporting was delegated by radiologists to other healthcare professionals, most often radiographers, this is one area where discussion of potential error rates has been widest (Robinson et al., 1999b). These discussions involve comparing radiologists with casualty doctors, radiologists with radiographers, casualty doctors with nurses and there has been a wide range of published papers covering these issues, each showing that, while different healthcare professionals can be compared to each other, there is no agreed standard across the professional boundaries. Clinical radiologists are deemed competent by passing the FRCR examinations, radiographers will have to prove themselves during a post graduate M-level course at one of the universities, casualty doctors have little or no specific reporting training and nurses generally match themselves to this latter group.

If the reporting practitioner has proven during the training phase to be able to produce reports with a less than 5% error rate, then during the practice of reporting this standard must be maintained and this is checked by regular *audits of performance and accuracy*. This varies between hospitals and departments from monthly random samples of reports to annual audits where the reporter is required to repeat an audit of reports. Departments undertaking DCBE will undertake an annual *audit of colorectal cancer detection* as laid down by the RCR and inherent in this is a check of report quality since it is the accuracy of reporting of cancer by which the test is judged (Tawn et al., 2005).

Whichever audit process is utilized, this should be applied to all staff producing medical imaging reports to ensure that, in the absence of National standards, the highest possible standard is maintained.

Conclusion

Traditionally, the reporting of medical images has been undertaken by clinical radiologists but, over a period of time, it has become accepted that non-radiologists can undertake this task, either other doctors or allied healthcare professionals.

The position of the Royal College of Radiologists has changed to reflect this progress; they state that:

> Reporting of GI examinations may be undertaken by clinical radiologists, but increasingly this task is being delegated to allied healthcare professionals who are trained to undertake and report either specific examinations or a range of examinations of a particular body system or organ (The Royal College of Radiologists, 2006).

Specifically with DCBE in the UK, it is often common practice for the examination to be performed and double reported by radiographers with no input from radiologists except for the inevitable 'difficult' cases where their medical experience is required. Having proven themselves in this area, radiographers have also been able to show that they can provide a similar service for a wider range of GI and fluoroscopy examinations and there are pockets of such practice scattered across the UK.

The *Gastrointestinal Radiographers Special Interest Group (GIRSIG)* was set up in 1998 to support such practice, whether it was established or in development and there is a wide support network of local groups feeding into a national group which has an active website (www.girsig.co.uk), biannual magazine and biennial conference to continue this support.

References

Anderson, N., Cook, H.B., Coates, R., 1991. Colonoscopically detected colorectal cancer missed on barium enema. Gastrointest. Radiol. 16 (2), 123–127.

Berman, L., de Lacey, G., Twomey, E., Twomey, B., Welch, T., Eban, R., 1985. Reducing errors in the accident department: a simple method using radiographers. Br. Med. J. 290 (6466), 421–422.

Blakeborough, A., Chapman, A.H., Swift, S., Culpan, G., Wilson, D., Sheridan, M.B., 2001. Strictures of the sigmoid colon: barium enema evaluation. Radiology 220, 343–348.

Booth, A.M., Mannion, R.A.J., 2005. Radiographer and radiologist perception error in reporting double contrast barium enemas: a pilot study. Radiography 11, 249–254.

Brown, J., Bryan, S., Warren, R., 1996. Mammography screening: an incremental cost effectiveness analysis of double versus single reading of mammograms. Br. Med. J. 312 (7034), 809–812.

Culpan, D.G., 2006. Development of radiographer reporting into the 21st century. Imag. Oncol. 38–45.

Culpan, D.G., Mitchell, A.J., Hughes, S., Nutman, M., Chapman, A.H., 2002. Double contrast barium enema sensitivity: a comparison of studies by radiographers and radiologists. Clin. Radiol. 57, 604–607.

Culpan, G., Mitchell, A., Rock, C., Ackerley, C., 2003. Radiographer reporting accuracy of double contrast barium enema (DCBE) examinations. UKRC 2003.

Department of Health, 2000. The Ionising Radiation (Medical Exposure) Regulations 2000. Department of Health. <http://www.opsi.gov.uk/si/si2000/20001059.htm> Accessed 08 May 2008.

Dimond, B.C., 2002. Legal aspects of radiography and radiology. Blackwell Science Ltd, Oxford.

Fernando, R., 1999. The radiographer reporting debate – the relationship between radiographer reporting, diagnostic ultrasound and other areas of role extension. Radiography 5, 177–179.

Fishman E.K., 2008. General, multidetector CT scanning (MDCT): a primer of practical decision making. Ctisus. <http://www.ctisus.org/multidetector/syllabus/multidetector_article1.html> Accessed 08 May 2008.

General Medical Council, 2001. Good medical practice. General Medical Council.

GlobalRPh.com. 2007. Common medical abbreviations. <http://www.globalrph.com/abbrev.htm> Accessed 08 May 2007.

Law, R.L., Longstaff, A.J., Slack, N., 1999. A retrospective 5-year study performed on the accuracy of barium enema examination performed by radiographers. Clin. Radiol. 54, 80–84.

Mannion, R.A.J., Bewell, J., Langan, C., Robertson, M., Chapman, A.H., 1995. Barium enema training programme for radiographers: a pilot study. Clin. Radiol. 50, 715–719.

Markus, J.B., Somers, S., O'Malley, B.P., Stevenson, G.W., 1990. Double-contrast barium enema studies: effect of multiple reading on perception error. Radiology 175, 155–156.

Naik, S.S., Hanbidge, A., Wilson, S.R., 2001. Radiology reports: examining radiologist and clinician preferences regarding style and content. Am. J. Roentgenol. 176, 591–598.

National Patient Safety Association, 2007. Safer practice notice. Early identification of failure to act on radiological imaging reports. February 2007. <http://www.npsa.nhs.uk/nrls/alerts-and-directives/notices/radiological/> Accessed 20/10/08.

NHS, 2007. Connecting for health. SNOMED CT – the language of the NHS care records service: a guide for NHS staff in England. HMSO, London.

Nuttall, L., 1995. Changing practice in radiography. In: Patterson, A., Price, R. (Eds.), Current topics in radiography 1. WB Saunders, London.

Quick, J., 1993. Radiographers to interpret films. Radiogr. Today 59, 1.

Robinson, P.J., 1996a. Short communication: plain film reporting by radiographers – a feasibility study. Br. J. Radiol. 69 (828), 1171–1174.

Robinson, P.J.A., 1996b. The nature of image reporting. In: Patterson, A., Price, R. (Eds.), Current topics in radiography 2. WB Saunders, London.

Robinson, P.J.A., 1997. Radiology's Achilles heel: error and variation in the interpretation of the Roentgen image. Br. J. Radiol. 70, 1085–1098.

Robinson, P.J.A., Culpan, G., Wiggins, M., 1999a. Interpretation of selected accident and emergency radiographic examination by radiographers: a review of 11000 cases. Br. J. Radiol. 72, 546–551.

Robinson, P.J.A., Wilson, D., Coral, A., Murphy, A., Verow, P., 1999b. Variation between experienced observers in the interpretation of accident and emergency radiographs. Br. J. Radiol. 72, 323–330.

Simpson, R., 2001. 'I'm not picking up a heart-beat': experiences of sonographers giving bad news to women during ultrasound scans. Br. J. Med. Psychol. 74, 255–272.

Tawn, D.J., Squire, C.J., Mohammed, M.A., Adam, E.J., 2005. National audit of the sensitivity of double-contrast barium enema for colorectal carcinoma, using control charts. Clin. Radiol. 60, 558–564.

The Royal College of Radiologists, 2001. To err is human. The case for review of reporting discrepancies. Royal College of Radiologists, London.

The Royal College of Radiologists Board of the Faculty of Clinical Radiology, 2006. Standards for the reporting and interpretation of imaging investigations. Royal College of Radiologists, London.

The Royal College of Radiologists Board of the Faculty of Clinical Radiology, 2007. Making the best use of clinical radiology services, sixth ed. Royal College of Radiologists, London.

Conclusion

CHAPTER 19

Endoscopy of the upper and lower gastrointestinal tract

Anne M. Pullyblank, Christopher Wong

Contents ||||||||||||||||||||||||||||||||||||||||||||||||||||||||||||||||||||||

Introduction

'Endoscopy' simply refers to examining the inside of the body with a scope. Nowadays, we generally consider 'endoscopy' to be an examination of the gastrointestinal tract. Since the introduction of the flexible fiberoptic endoscopes in the 1960s, endoscopy has come a long way from the days of rigid sigmoidoscopy or rigid esophagoscopy. Modern endoscopes are used to carry out day-to-day diagnostic and therapeutic procedures of the gastrointestinal tract. For the purpose of this chapter, we will concentrate on flexible endoscopy.

Indications

Upper gastrointestinal tract (GI) endoscopy and lower gastrointestinal tract endoscopy means direct inspection of the esophagus, stomach, duodenum, small intestines and the colon using a flexible fiberoptic endoscope. A *gastroscopy* (aka esophago-gastroduodenoscopy or OGD) refers to the examination of the esophagus, stomach and duodenum, whereas *enteroscopy* refers to examination of the small intestines. Full examination of the colon to the cecum is known as *colonoscopy*, examination of just the left colon to the splenic flexure is known as *flexible sigmoidoscopy*.

Endoscopy and fluoroscopy can be used to investigate the GI tract, but there are advantages to endoscopy which may be taken into account when a clinician decides which test to request:

1   Endoscopy is preferable when direct inspection of the mucosa is desirable or where subtle mucosal changes may not be demonstrated on fluoroscopy, e.g. mild esophagitis, gastritis, inflammatory bowel disease, proctitis or angiodysplasia. Endoscopy also allows tissue biopsy

2   Therapeutic intervention can be performed, e.g. esophageal stricture balloon dilatation (Figure 20.1, see color insert), polypectomy or banding of hemorrhoids

3   The functional aspects of the upper GI tract (i.e. esophageal motility and gastric emptying) are better investigated by fluoroscopic studies than direct inspection

4   Endoscopy is useful where pathologies coexist and where fluoroscopy may be less accurate, e.g. if there is a suggestion of a polyp in a segment of severe diverticular disease (Thomas et al., 1995)

5   For a tissue diagnosis of a fluoroscopy detected lesion, e.g. stricture (Figure 20.2, see color insert).

Both endoscopy and fluoroscopy complement each other in the assessment of the GI tract. Gastroscopy is the investigation of choice for upper GI investigation and colonoscopy often follows radiological investigation. It could be argued that endoscopy would be preferable in every case as the patient could have both diagnosis and treatment in a single test. However, in many hospitals, endoscopy services are overstretched and a barium enema is often a good first line test in selected patients. Endoscopy also carries a risk of morbidity and even mortality as discussed below.

Types of endoscopy

Upper gastrointestinal endoscopy

Most upper GI endoscopy is carried out by a forward looking *gastroscope*. This investigation will allow examination to and in some cases into the proximal jejunum. To examine the small bowel, an *enteroscope* (essentially a very long gastroscope) or *capsule endoscopy* is used. In practice, patients would usually have undergone prior fluoroscopic investigation by means of barium follow-through or enteroclysis.

To prepare for upper gastrointestinal endoscopy patients are asked not to eat or drink for 4–6 hours prior to the procedure. The procedure can be done under local anesthetic to the throat or under sedation. The gastroscope is passed via the mouth, through the cricopharyngeal sphincter and into the esophagus. Once intubation is achieved the examination of the esophagus, stomach and duodenum is relatively straightforward (Figures 20.3, 20.4 and 20.5, see color insert). There are several *blind spots* that merit special attention. The view of the esophageal mucosa is often lost at the point of passage through the sphincter and lesions can be missed. If this is suspected, the patient should undergo a barium swallow or a rigid esophagoscopy. Another potential blind spot is the superior part of the gastric antrum and angulus. It is important to retroflex the gastroscope in the antrum to gain a good view of this area.

Small bowel endoscopy

Enteroscopy is used to examine mainly the proximal small bowel. This is a much more involved procedure than gastroscopy. *Enteroscopy* is indicated for diagnosis of small bowel diseases including obscure gastrointestinal bleeding, malabsorption, obtaining tissue biopsies following abnormal fluoroscopic studies as well as therapeutic procedures for treating small bowel bleeding or polyps.

Colorectal endoscopy

Visualization of the lower bowel can be performed using a rigid or flexible endoscope. Rigid sigmoidoscopy and proctoscopy usually occur in the outpatient clinic. The Association of Coloproctology of Great Britain and Ireland recommends that a patient referred for barium enema should have had at least a rigid sigmoidoscopy prior to referral (Guidelines for Management of Colorectal Cancer, 2007). The reason for this is that lesions very low down in the rectum may be missed on barium enema but seen on proctoscopy or rigid sigmoidoscopy. A rigid examination is especially important in patients presenting with bright red rectal bleeding as common pathologies such as distal proctitis or hemorrhoids may not be demonstrated on barium enema.

Proctoscopy involves inserting a rigid instrument approximately 10 cm long into the distal rectum. No air insufflation is used but there is a light source attached giving good visualization of piles/mucosal prolapse but only limited views of the lower rectum. For full visualization of the rectum a *rigid sigmoidoscope* is used. This is a 25 cm long rigid tube connected to a light source with air insufflation to give a good luminal view. The word 'sigmoidoscopy' is actually a misnomer as it is difficult to negotiate the various mucosal folds required to enter the sigmoid with a rigid instrument. However, it is useful diagnostic tool and may influence the investigation subsequently chosen. For example, if a polyp is seen at rigid sigmoidoscopy, it is preferable to go straight to colonoscopy where a therapeutic procedure can be performed at the same time. Likewise, if distal colitis is seen, colonoscopy may be more appropriate than barium enema to determine extent and get a tissue diagnosis.

Flexible endoscopic examinations of the lower GI tract fall into two tests – flexible sigmoidoscopy and colonoscopy. Previously, there were separate endoscopes for each test but, in practice, a *colonoscope* is used for both. A colonoscope is a 160 cm long fiberoptic telescope that is inserted via the anus.

For a *flexible sigmoidoscopy*, the left colon is examined to the splenic flexure. This is usually performed for rectal bleeding as red blood passed per rectum is usually coming from the left colon. If the origin of the bleeding is more proximal, it manifests as altered blood by the time it is passed per rectum (PR). The majority of cancers in patients presenting with rectal bleeding and/or change in bowel habit (CIBH) without any other significant diagnostic factors occur within 60 cm of the anal verge and can be diagnosed by flexible sigmoidoscopy (Guidelines for Management of Colorectal Cancer, 2007). Flexible sigmoidoscopy is also useful for indeterminate lesions detected on barium enema, e.g. strictures. It is mandatory for suspected rectal cancers where a tissue diagnosis is needed before starting neoadjuvant therapy (Guidelines for Management of Colorectal Cancer, 2007).

Colonoscopy requires the telescope to be inserted to the cecum. With a straight colonoscope, the cecum is approximately 80 cm from the anal verge. However, *distance from the anal verge* is notoriously unreliable in terms of judging position in the colon. This is because there may be redundant loops of colon causing the colonoscope to loop within the patient. Rather than using centimeters as a measure, the endoscopist uses the *visual landmarks* of the colon to judge position, for example the triangular appearance of the mature transverse colon (Figure 20.6, see color insert).

Identification of the cecum requires identification of the ileocecal valve, appendix orifice and tri-radiate fold (Figure 20.7, see color insert).

Trans-illumination is unreliable since the experienced fluoroscopist will know that the cecum can lie in a variety of positions. The gold standard for proof of a complete colonoscopy is intubation of the ileocecal valve with a terminal ileal biopsy but, in practice, this can be difficult. This may be clinically necessary where terminal ileal Crohn's disease is suspected but the Guidelines for Management of Colorectal Cancer (2007) suggest that a printed picture of the ileocecal valve may be adequate for patients who are undergoing colonoscopy for colorectal cancer.

Although colonoscopy might be considered the gold standard for visualizing the colon, it is operator dependent. There are data from a UK study of 9223 colonoscopies demonstrating cecal intubation rates as low as 56% (Bowles et al., 2004) and one-third of 55 endoscopists failed to achieve a cecal intubation rate of 90% in 5905 colonoscopies (Taylor et al., 2004). It has been demonstrated that continuous quality assessment and training can increase standards (Ball et al., 2004) and there are now improved standards for training (Joint Advisory Group on Gastrointestinal Endoscopy, 2004). National quality standards for endoscopy have been set by the Department of Health using a global rating scale (GRS) (www.grs.nhs.uk) and by the British Society of Gastroenterology (www.BSG.org.uk).

There are differences between flexible sigmoidoscopy and colonoscopy in terms of bowel preparation. For flexible sigmoidoscopy, a phosphate enema is adequate and can give good views to the transverse colon. The patient lies in the left lateral position with a pulse oximeter attached and the procedure is usually performed without sedation. For colonoscopy, full bowel preparation is needed similar to the barium enema, although with colonoscopy fluid residue is not an issue. Again, the patient starts in the left lateral position with monitoring but sedation and analgesia are given. The patient may need to be moved during the procedure to enable intubation to the cecum. Altering the position of the patient can open up difficult bends. Unlike barium enema where the table can be tilted, movement is limited to right and left lateral positions or prone and supine. The sedation is usually a benzodiazepine with amnesic effects such as midazolam. Most endoscopists would aim to use a dose of 2–3 mg with a maximum of 5 mg. The analgesic used varies but is usually pethidine or fentanyl. The aim is for 'conscious sedation' meaning that the patient is able to maintain verbal communication throughout the test. In practice, most patients do not remember the test due to the amnesic effects of midazolam.

Therapeutic endoscopic procedures

The simplest procedure is a *biopsy* where small fragments of tissue are sampled using forceps that are passed down the endoscope. This type of biopsy is used for benign or malignant lesions or to sample mucosal abnormalities such as colitis (Figure 20.8, see color insert).

A *hot biopsy* utilizes the same tissue forceps but with the application of diathermy. This is mainly used to biopsy small sessile polyps less than 5 mm across. The advantage of diathermy is that it coagulates potentially friable tissue but also the heat destroys tissue. This has the effect of both biopsying and destroying the polyp at the same time.

Snare polypectomy is used for pedunculated polyps. This involves lassoing the polyp with an extendable wire loop. The wire loop is passed around the polyp stalk, pulled snug and diathermy is used to coagulate as the wire cuts through the tissue (Figure 20.9, see color insert). The polyp can then be retrieved with a variety of devices such as a basket. *Argon beam (plasma) coagulation* combines a jet (beam) of ionized argon gas and electrocoagulation to create rapid vaporization of tissue and coagulation with eschar formation. This can be used to destroy large carpeting rectal lesions in unfit patients or to ablate angiodysplasia, Barrett's esophagus and gastric antral vascular ectasia (GAVE).

Endoscopic mucosal resection (EMR) is a technique proliferated in Japan for large mucosal as well as submucosal lesions. In its simplest form, a lesion can be raised by infiltration of adrenaline solution to create a pseudopolyp before the lesion is excised by snare polypectomy technique. Other variations involve using specialist attachments to the endoscope to remove lesions in a technique not too dissimilar to variceal banding (Soetikno et al., 2003).

Variceal banding, sclerotherapy and endoscopic clips are used to treat bleeding problems including esophageal varices, bleeding ulcers and angiodysplasia. *Variceal banding* involves fitting a cap pre-loaded with rubber bands to the end of the gastroscope that is connected to a firing mechanism. The varix is sucked into the cap before the rubber band is fired, resulting in ligation. *Injection sclerotherapy* involves injection of sclerosant or fibrin glue into the ulcer base/varices/lesion to stop bleeding or induce shrinkage of the lesion. Mechanical *endoscopic clips* can be applied to bleeding points to stop bleeding.

Dilatation and stent insertion can be carried out endoscopically for treating achalasia and strictures. Traditionally, *dilatations* have been done with Savoury-Gillard or Mallory bougies under semi-blinded or radiology control. Modern *hydrostatic pneumatic balloons* have allowed dilatation under direct vision and better control of the rate and extent of the dilatation (Figure 20.1). There is a risk of perforation associated with dilatations and the results have favored balloon dilatations over the other methods (Hernandez et al., 2000).

Percutaneous insertion of gastrostomy tube into the stomach is also widely used. This utilizes the gastroscope to distend the stomach with air and, using the transilluminated light as a target, a guide wire is inserted into the stomach and retrieved by the gastroscope. A gastrostomy tube can then be placed and positioned in the stomach via the mouth. This procedure is done under local anesthetic with or without sedation which obviates the need for a general anesthetic and formal surgery.

Complications of GI endoscopy

Endoscopy is a very safe procedure but, nonetheless, it is associated with its attendant risk and complications. Several large studies, including the National Confidential Enquiry into Patient Outcome and Death (2004), have highlighted cardiopulmonary and sedation-related complications as the major complications, together with a number of procedure-related complications.

The general complications include over-sedation that may induce respiratory depression with hypoxia, bleeding, perforation, hyper- or hypotension, aspiration, cardiac events including angina and myocardial infarction and strokes (Green, 2006). *Cardiopulmonary complications* account for 50% of serious morbidity and approximately 50% of all gastrointestinal endoscopy related deaths (Daneshmend et al., 1991). Respiratory depression from *over-sedation* from midazolam and opiates have an antidote in the form of flumazenil or naloxone, respectively, allowing the sedation to be reversed if an adverse event occurs (Bell and Quine, 2006).

The *perforation* risk in diagnostic gastroscopy is estimated to be 0.03%. Perforation can occur anywhere from the pharynx to the duodenum. This may be caused by pushing the gastroscope blindly, taking biopsy and esophageal tears from eosinophilic esophagitis. There is an increased perforation risk with all therapeutic procedures, e.g. dilatations, stent insertion, EMR and sclerotherapy. Mild bleeding following taking biopsy and polypectomy in the upper GI tract is not uncommon but major hemorrhage is rare. *Bleeding* (17%) is common after EMR, but the majority stop spontaneously without requiring further intervention. It is estimated that hemorrhage following EMR is approximately 2% (Riley and Alderson, 2006).

Perforation from colonoscopy is associated with greater risks than fluoroscopy. Full colonoscopy carries more risk than flexible sigmoidoscopy and therapeutic procedures produce more complications than diagnostic scopes. The main risks are perforation and bleeding (Epstein, 2006).

Perforation is rare following flexible sigmoidoscopy, but the risk increases with colonoscopy and/or therapeutic procedures. Perforation is more likely if transmural inflammation or ulceration is present and the risks are greater in the right colon where the bowel wall of the colon is thinner and subject to higher pressures (Epstein, 2006). Perforation rates have been quoted as 1.96 per 1000 procedures for colonoscopy and 0.88 per 1000 procedures for flexible sigmoidoscopy (Gatto et al., 2003) with similar figures of 1.9/1000 for 10 486 colonoscopy and 0.4/1000 out of 49 501 sigmoidoscopies (Anderson et al., 2000). However, the flexible sigmoidoscopy screening trial in the UK demonstrated a perforation rate of only one per 40 674 for flexible sigmoidoscopies and four out of 2131 colonoscopies (UK flexible screening trial investigators, 2002).

The perforation can be due either to direct trauma from the colonoscope or a thermal injury from diathermy and the diagnosis is often delayed (Hall et al., 2005; Epstein, 2006). If the bowel is perforated, free air may be seen on erect chest x-ray but a CT or contrast enema may be necessary to confirm the diagnosis. Some patients can be managed non-operatively as they have had full bowel preparation and hence have a clean colon limiting contamination, but others will require surgery. The surgery carried out depends on the extent of the injury and the bowel pathology. A resection ± stoma may be necessary or just oversewing of the perforation.

Barium enema, on the other hand, carries a risk of only one serious complication per 9000, perforation of the rectum in one in 25 000 and one death attributable to barium enema in one in 60 000 (Blakeborough et al., 1997).

Mild bleeding can occur after any biopsy or polypectomy with an incidence of 0.001–0.24% (Guidelines for Management of Colorectal Cancer, 2007). This is not usually severe and is usually self-limiting. More *severe bleeding* can occur after snare polypectomy, especially if the polyp has a thick stalk with a large vessel within it. Again, this is usually self-limiting but, if it persists or is severe, this can be treated endoscopically. Primary bleeding can be dealt with by coagulation, adrenaline injection or by applying a small metal clip to the bleeding vessel (endoclip).

As discussed above, colonoscopy is only complete if the cecum, or preferably the terminal ileum, is reached. Patients are usually warned during the consent process that an *incomplete examination* may occur. If it is recognized that the cecum has not been reached, a completion barium enema may be requested to examine the residual colon not inspected at colonoscopy.

References

Anderson, M.L., Pasha, T.M., Leighton, J.A., 2000. Endoscopic perforation of the colon: lessons from a 10 year study. Am. J. Gastroenterol 95, 3418–3422.

Ball, J.E., Osborne, J., Jowett, S., et al., 2004. Quality improvement programme to achieve acceptable colonoscopy completion rates: prospective before and after study. Br. Med. J. 239 (7467), 665–667.

Bell, G.D., Quine, A., 2006. Cardiopulmonary and sedation related complications. BSG guidelines in Gastroenterology. <http://www.bsg.org.uk/bsgdisp1.php?id = 48c1b0bcae9daa89d36a&m = 00023>

Blakeborough, A., Sheridan, M.B., Chapman, A.H., 1997. Complications of barium enema examinations: a survey of UK consultant radiologists 1992–1994. Clin. Radiol. 52, 142–148.

Bowles, C.J., Leicester, R., Romaya, C., et al., 2004. A prospective study of colonoscopy practice in the UK today: are we adequately prepared for national colorectal cancer screening tomorrow? Gut 53 (2), 277–283.

Daneshmend, T.K., Bell, G.D., Logan, R.F.A., 1991. Sedation for upper gastrointestinal endoscopy: results of a nationwide survey. Gut 32, 12–15.

Epstein, O., 2006. Complications of colonoscopy. BSG guidelines in Gastroenterology. <http://www.bsg.org.uk/bsgdisp1.php?id = 48c1b0bcae9daa89d36a&m = 00023> Accessed 10.11.08.

Gatto, N.M., Frucht, H., Sundararajan, V., et al., 2003. Risk of perforation after colonoscopy and sigmoidoscopy: a population based study. J. Natl. Cancer. Inst. 95, 230–236.

Green, J., 2006. Complications of gastrointestinal endoscopy. BSG guidelines in Gastroenterology. <http://www.bsg.org.uk/bsgdisp1.php?id = 48c1b0bcae9daa89d36a&m = 00023> Accessed 10.1.08.

Guidelines for Management of Colorectal Cancer, 2007. Association of Coloproctology of Great Britain and Ireland, third ed.

Hall, C., Dorricott, N.J., Donovan, I.A., et al., 2005. Colon perforation during colonoscopy: surgical versus conservative management. Br. J. Surg. 78 (5), 542–544.

Hernandez, L.V., Jacobson, J.W., Harris, M.S., 2000. Comparison among the perforation rates of Maloney, balloon, and savary dilation of esophageal strictures. Gastrointest. Endosc. 51 (4 Pt 1), 460–462.

Joint Advisory Group on Gastrointestinal Endoscopy, 2004. Guidelines for training, appraisal and assessment of trainees in gastrointestinal endoscopy and for the assessment of units for registration and re-registration.

National Confidential Enquiry into Patient Outcome and Death, 2004. Scoping our practice. <http://www.ncepod.org.uk/reports2.htm> Accessed 10.11.08.

Riley, S., Alderson, D., 2006. Complications of upper gastrointestinal endoscopy. British Society of Gastroenterology guidelines in Gastroenterology. <http://www.bsg.org.uk/bsgdisp1.php?id = 48c1b0bcae9daa89d36a&m = 00023> Accessed 10.1.08.

Soetikno, R.M., Gotoda, T., Nakanishi, Y., et al., 2003. Endoscopic mucosal resection. Gastrointest. Endosc. 57, 567–579.

Taylor, K.M., Arajs, K., Rouse, T., et al., 2004. A prospective audit of colonoscopy quality in Kent and Medway, UK. Endoscopy 40 (4), 291–295.

Thomas, R.D., Fairhurst, J.J., Frost, R.A., 1995. Wessex regional radiology audit: barium enema in colorectal carcinoma. Clin. Radiol. 50, 647–650.

UK flexible screening trial investigators, 2002. Single flexible sigmoidoscopy screening to prevent colorectal cancer: baseline findings of a UK multicentre randomised trial. Lancet 359, 1291–1300.

Common surgical procedures of the gastrointestinal tract

Anne M. Pullyblank, Christopher Wong

Contents |||||||||||||||||||||||||||||||||||||||||||||||||||||||||||||||||||||||||||||||||

Introduction

Gastrointestinal (GI) surgery is a vast topic encompassing many different techniques. These procedures can be performed by the traditional open surgery or more and more commonly laparoscopically (keyhole). Whether surgery is open or laparoscopic, the procedures should remain the same.

The range of operations in upper GI surgery can be conveniently divided into benign and cancer surgery. This is in contrast to lower GI surgery where the same operations are performed for both benign and neoplastic conditions. The aim for this chapter is to give the reader a broad idea of what is involved in each procedure.

Upper gastrointestinal procedures

Cancer surgery

The principle of cancer surgery is to remove the tumor completely with histologically proven margins and the lymph nodes that drain the tumor. Histologically, completeness of tumor clearance from the resection margins is classified R0, R1 and R2. An R0 resection is defined as one where all margins are histologically free of tumor. An R1 resection is defined as one in which microscopic residual disease has been left behind. An R2 resection is defined as incomplete resection with macroscopic residual disease.

Esophagectomy

Indication: esophageal cancers and occasionally benign esophageal strictures.

Area resected: lower third to entire esophagus and lesser curve of stomach. The surrounding lymph nodes are also removed enbloc with the specimen.

Main blood vessels divided: left gastric artery and esophageal arterial branches.

Reconstruction: the continuity of the GI tract is reconstructed commonly by using the stomach. Occasionally the jejunum or transverse colon may be used to reconstruct continuity.

Postoperative barium appearance: barium will run from esophageal remnant or pharynx directly into the stomach (or other conduit), which is now situated in the mediastinum.

Subtotal gastrectomy

Indication: gastric cancer situated in the distal part of stomach, complicated gastric ulcer disease.

Area resected: the distal half to two thirds of stomach with the surrounding lymph nodes.

Main blood vessels divided: left and right gastric arteries, right gastroepiploic artery.

Reconstruction: historically, the continuity was usually reconstructed by carrying out a simple gastrojejunostomy. This can result in significant biliary reflux which can cause anastomotic ulcerations. A *roux-en-Y reconstruction* negates biliary reflux and is generally the preferred option of reconstruction (Figures 21.1A, 21.1B).

Postoperative barium appearance: barium passes from the stomach into the drainage roux loop. Reflux of barium may occur at the jejunoje-junostomy.

Total gastrectomy

Indication: gastric cancer located in the proximal part or body of the stomach.

Area resected: whole stomach and surrounding lymph nodes.

Main blood vessels divided: left and right gastric arteries, right and left gastroepiploic arteries and short gastric arteries.

Reconstruction: A roux-en-Y reconstruction with or without a neogastric pouch. This is akin to a J-shaped ileoanal pouch (see ileoanal pouch) (Figures 21.2A, 21.2B and 21.3A, 21.3B).

Postoperative barium appearance: barium will flow from esophagus into a small gastric pouch and down the roux limb.

Benign surgery

Antireflux procedures

Indication: Gastro-esophageal reflux disease including repair of hiatus hernia.

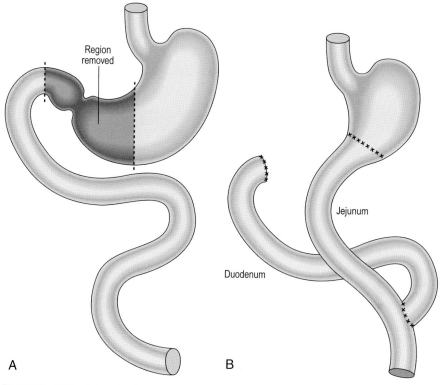

Figure 21.1 (A) Partial gastrectomy, resection margins; (B) partial gastrectomy, reconstruction.

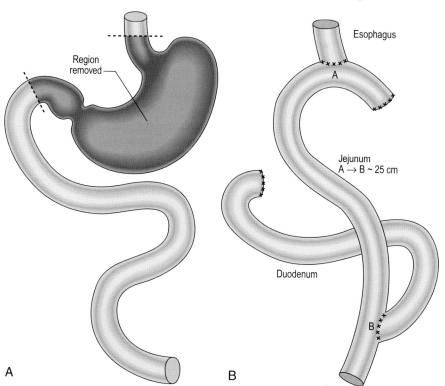

Figure 21.2 (A) Total gastrectomy, resection margins; (B) total gastrectomy, roux-en-Y reconstruction.

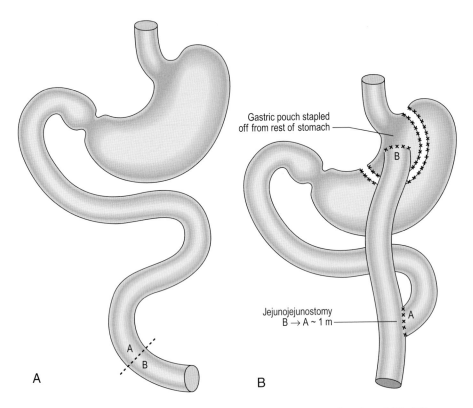

Gastric pouch stapled
off from rest of stomach

B

Jejunojejunostomy
B → A ~ 1 m

A

A

B

Figure 21.3 (A) Roux-en-Y, gastric bypass (note resection margins A and B); (B) roux-en-Y reconstruction. Resection margin 'A' forming a jejunojejunostomy; resection margin 'B' anastomosed to gastric pouch.

Procedure: Performed laparoscopically, this procedure essentially consists of two parts:

1   to reduce the hiatus hernia (if present) and repair the diaphragmatic hiatal defect
2   to create an antireflux mechanism using the fundus of the stomach.

Antireflux surgery has a number of variations; however, the two gold standard procedures were described by the German surgeon Rudolph Nissen (1896–1981) and the French surgeon Andre Toupet born in 1915. *Nissen's fundoplication* is a complete (360 degrees) wrap with the fundus round the lower esophagus and *Toupet's fundoplication* is one where the fundus wraps the posterior aspect of the lower esophagus, variations suggest between 180 and 270 degrees (Figures 21.4 A–F).

Main blood vessel divided: the short gastric vessels may be divided.

Postoperative barium appearance: the lower esophagus is slightly narrowed by the wrap and the esophagus may have a *bird's beak appearance*. Barium often has a slight delay before passing into the stomach.

Heller's myotomy

Indication: achalasia. This is caused by dysmotility of the smooth muscle layer of the esophagus in lower esophageal or cardiac sphincter. This results in a functional stenosis.

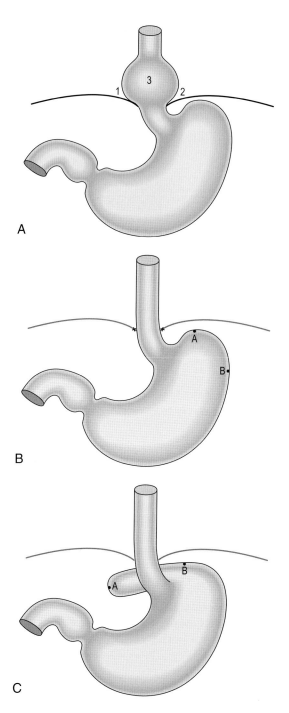

Figure 21.4 (A) Wide diaphragmatic hiatus (1–2), gastric herniation (3); (B) gastric herniation reduced and the hiatus repaired. A retro-esophageal tunnel is created to allow for fundoplication; (C) gastric fundus pulled through to the right of the esophagus;

(*Continued*)

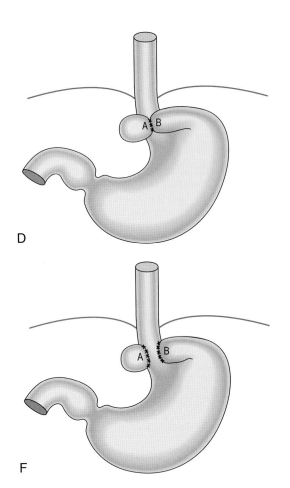
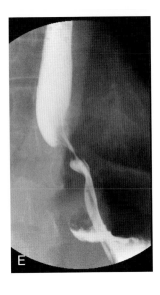

D

E

F

Figure 21.4—cont'd (D) the Nissen 360 degrees wrap created by suturing points 'A' and 'B'; (E) Nissen wrap at barium swallow; (F) the alternative Toupet 270 degrees wrap can be created by suturing points 'A' and 'B' to the sides of the esophagus.

Procedure: this procedure is carried out laparoscopically. A longitudinal incision down to but not beyond the mucosa is made in the lower esophagus extending into the gastric cardia. The smooth muscle is parted preventing it from forming a ring when contracted. Many patients will suffer from gastro-esophageal reflux following this and a partial fundoplication is often performed to reduce this.

Main blood vessels divided: none.

Postoperative barium appearance: the lower esophagus is widened and barium should pass easily into the stomach.

Ulcer surgery

Indication: perforated duodenal or gastric ulcer. With the introduction of H$_2$ antagonist (e.g. ranitidine) and proton pump inhibitors (e.g. omeprazole), ulcer surgery, like highly selective vagotomy, has been consigned to history books. Modern day ulcer surgery is refined to emergency surgery for perforated or bleeding ulcers.

Procedure: this procedure is carried out laparoscopically. Gastric and duodenal ulcers may bleed or perforate. A *gastrectomy* should be considered if there is suspicion that the gastric ulcer may be malignant. Otherwise a *wedge excision* of the ulcer can be performed with the stomach wall simply repaired.

Torrential bleeding from duodenal ulcers are almost always sited posteriorly with the gastroduodenal artery involved. The duodenum is opened and the bleeding ulcer is under-run with sutures to ligate the bleeding vessel. With perforation, the perforation may be closed primarily or plugged by using the greater omentum.

Main blood vessels divided: none.

Postoperative barium appearance: often back to normal or may well show some residual scarring.

Surgery to the small bowel

The most common small bowel procedure is the *small bowel resection*. However, where small bowel conservation is paramount, such as when the patient is at risk of developing short gut syndrome from Crohn's disease, *strictureplasty* is the surgery of choice.

Indication: small bowel strictures, ischemia, small bowel tumors, any small bowel pathology.

Procedure: small bowel *resection* is carried out by isolating and removing the diseased segment. Anastomosis can be achieved by using a stapling technique. The continuity of the small bowel can be reconstructed by a variety of techniques, e.g. end-to-end or side-to-side.

Main blood vessels divided: arteries that supply the segment of bowel.

Postoperative barium appearance: for *end-to-end anastomosis*, some scarring can sometimes be seen to indicate the area of the anastomosis. For *side-to-side anastomosis*, there are often staple lines present and barium may be seen to traverse a chicane.

Strictureplasty (Figure 21.5) is of particular value with benign stricturing patient associated with Crohn's disease, as it preserves small bowel length.

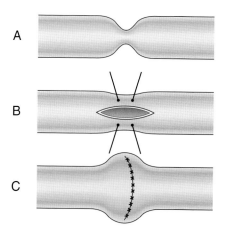

Figure 21.5 Small bowel strictureplasty.

Strictureplasty is a technique whereby a narrowed segment(s) of the small bowel (Figure 21.5A) is individually refashioned to widen the lumen. This is achieved by incising the strictured bowel longitudinally (Figure 21.5B) and then suturing the incision transversely (Figure 21.5C).

Bariatric surgery

Also known as weight loss surgery. There are many types of bariatric surgery. The most common procedure is gastric band. Other procedures that are commonly performed are gastric bypass and sleeve gastrectomy.

Indication: treatment of obesity with body mass index above 35.

Procedure: commonly carried out laparoscopically. *Gastric band insertion* is much like putting a belt round the cardia to create a small gastric pouch of approximately 20 ml size. The tightness of the band is adjusted via a connecting tube to an access port.

Gastric roux-en-Y bypass creates a small 20 ml size gastric pouch with staples. Continuity is reconstructed by roux-en-Y anastomosis. Unlike the standard roux-en-Y, the roux limb is 1–1.5 m in length.

Sleeve gastrectomy involves removing about three quarters of the stomach leaving a narrow gastric tube of about 1–1.5 cm in diameter. The antrum of the stomach is preserved.

Main blood vessels divided: none.

Postoperative barium appearance: in gastric band patients, a band can be seen with barium entering a small pouch before draining into the rest of the stomach. The stomach resembles an uneven hourglass. In gastric bypass, the barium will pass into a small gastric pouch before travelling down the roux limb. The remainder of the stomach is connected to the more distal GI tract via the jejunojejunostomy and therefore likely to be invisible to the barium.

In sleeve gastrectomy, the barium will flow through a narrowed gastric tube before filling the gastric antrum.

Lower gastrointestinal procedures

Regardless of the indication for an operation, whether it is for cancer or inflammatory bowel disease, the surgical principles are the same for colorectal surgery. The pathology needs to be removed with a margin of healthy tissue on each side. The segmental resections of the large bowel are based on the blood supply and lymph node drainage. Even if the area of abnormality is small, a whole segment of colon will be removed depending on which blood vessel has to be divided to aid removal (Figure 21.6). This is because if a blood vessel is divided, the segment of bowel that it supplies will become ischemic unless it is removed completely.

In a cancer operation, the blood vessels will be divided as close to their origin as possible. This is in order to get the maximal lymph node harvest that will allow the pathologist to determine whether any of the lymph nodes contain cancer cells which may have spread from the primary bowel tumor. This is essential for staging the cancer and planning postoperative treatment.

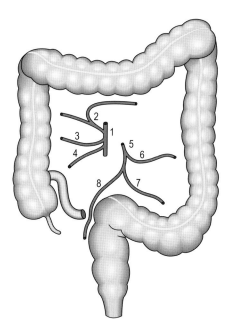

Figure 21.6 Schematic representation of main arteries supplying the colon and rectum. 1. Superior mesenteric artery; 2. middle colic; 3. right colic; 4. ileocolic; 5. inferior mesenteric artery; 6. left colic; 7. sigmoid artery; 8. superior rectal artery.

This section lists the common surgical procedures of the lower gastrointestinal tract, the indications for surgery and the postoperative radiological appearances.

Ileocecectomy

Indication: Crohn's disease or other pathology affecting the distal terminal ileum such as radiation enteritis, benign tumors of the cecal pole, terminal ileum or appendix, conditions which mimic Crohn's disease such as tuberculosis.

Bowel resected: distal ileum (depending on the extent of ileal pathology) and cecal pole.

Main blood vessel divided: ileocecal artery (Figure 21.7).

Postoperative barium appearance: ileum will run straight into colon with no cecal pole and no appendix apparent.

Right hemicolectomy

Indication: colorectal cancer in the right side of the colon, inflammatory bowel disease, diverticulum, cecal volvulus.

Bowel resected: last 5–10 cm terminal ileum, cecum, right colon and hepatic flexure.

Blood vessels divided: ileocolic artery, right colic artery ± right branch of middle colic artery (Figure 21.8).

Postoperative appearance: ileum will run straight into colon with no cecal pole or appendix. Anastomosis will lie anywhere from right side of abdomen to upper midline.

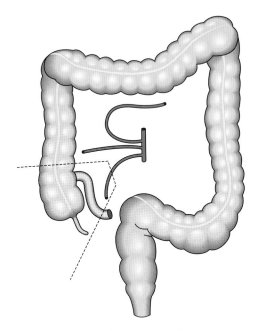

Figure 21.7 Ileocecal resection margins.

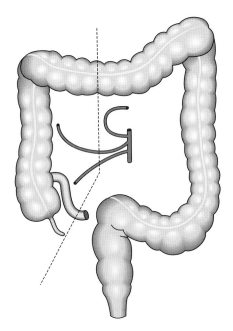

Figure 21.8 Right hemicolectomy margins.

Extended right hemicolectomy

Indication: most commonly a tumor of the mid to distal transverse colon or splenic flexure.

Bowel resected: last 5–10 cm terminal ileum, cecum, hepatic flexure, transverse colon and splenic flexure.

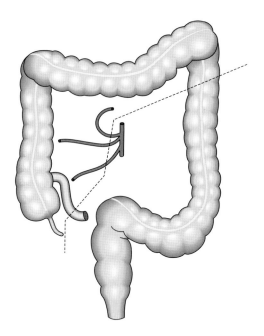

Figure 21.9 Extended right hemicolectomy margins.

Main blood vessels divided: ileocolic artery, right colic artery, middle colic artery (Figure 21.9).

Postoperative appearance: ileum will run straight into colon with no cecal pole or appendix. Anastomosis may lie on left side of abdomen. Only left colon will remain.

Left hemicolectomy

Indication: less common than other resections. It is usually performed for a descending colon tumor. An extended right hemicolectomy is an alternative and will increase lymph node harvest but the left hemicolectomy preserves a greater length of large bowel.

Bowel resected: distal transverse colon, splenic flexure and descending colon.

Main blood vessel divided: left colic artery (Figure 21.10).

Postoperative appearance: shortened colon. The landmarks of the splenic flexure may no longer be apparent.

Sigmoid colectomy

Indication: tumor of sigmoid colon, sigmoid diverticular disease, Crohn's disease or volvulus.

Bowel resected: sigmoid colon.

Main blood vessel divided: sigmoid branch of inferior mesenteric artery (IMA) (Figure 21.11).

Postoperative appearance: this depends on whether the operation was elective or emergency. In the emergency situation, where there may be a lot of fecal

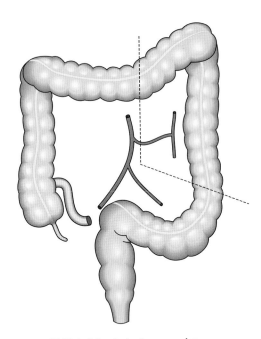

Figure 21.10 Left hemicolectomy margins.

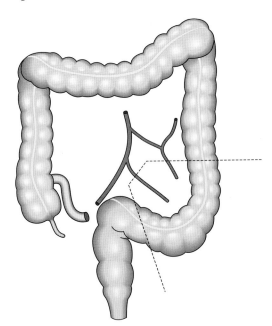

Figure 21.11 Sigmoid colectomy margins.

contamination, e.g. stercoral perforation (a pressure ulcer that can develop in the colon and lead to a perforation), or perforated sigmoid diverticular disease, a *Hartmann's procedure* may be performed. This is where bowel continuity is not restored, the rectal stump is over sewn and the descending colon is brought out as an *end colostomy*. Occasionally, a track might be deliberately formed from the bowel distal to the defunctioning stoma; this track (*a mucus fistula*) leads to a second stoma and produces only mucus.

There is little indication for imaging after this procedure. If the procedure was elective or there was no peritoneal fecal contamination, a primary anastomosis will be performed. In this case, postoperative imaging will show a shortened left colon. The sigmoid colon will no longer be present and the left colon will appear less tortuous.

High and low anterior resections

An anterior resection is a resection of the sigmoid and upper rectum.

High anterior resection

Indication: tumor of distal sigmoid colon or upper rectum or severe sigmoid diverticular disease.

Bowel resected: sigmoid colon and upper rectum.

Main blood vessel divided: inferior mesenteric artery (IMA) at its origin (Figure 21.12).

Postoperative appearance: shortened left colon. The sigmoid colon will no longer be present and the left colon will appear less tortuous. A stapled anastomosis is likely and will be seen in the region of the pelvic brim but may be higher or lower depending on rectal anatomy (Figure 21.12B).

With a high anterior resection, it is not necessary to perform a defunctioning loop ileostomy; however, this may be done if there are doubts about the anastomosis. If this is the case, it is usual to perform water-soluble (Gastrografin) enema postoperatively to check the integrity of the anastomosis prior to closing the ileostomy (Figure 21.12C).

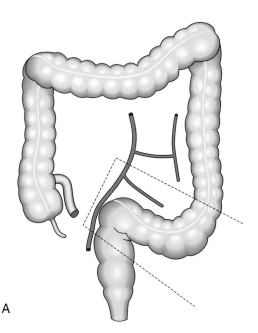

A

Figure 21.12 (A) High anterior resection margins;

(*Continued*)

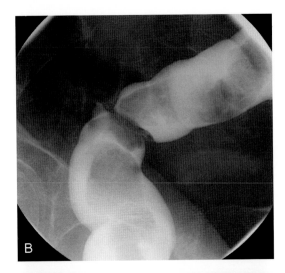

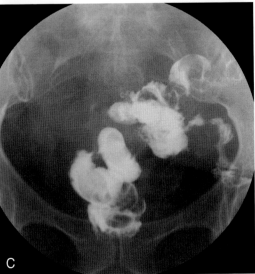

Figure 21.12—cont'd (B) fluoroscopic image of a high anterior resection; (C) leak fistulating from a high anterior resection.

Low anterior resection

Indication: mid to low rectal tumor.

Bowel resected: sigmoid colon and entire rectum down to pelvic floor. This is what is known as a *total mesorectal excision* (TME).

Main blood vessel divided: inferior mesenteric artery (IMA) at its origin (Figure 21.13).

Postoperative appearance: shortened left colon. The sigmoid colon will no longer be present and the left colon will appear less tortuous. A stapled anastomosis is almost certain unless a hand-sewn colo-anal anastomosis has been performed and will be seen just above the pelvic floor (Figures 21.14A, 21.14B).

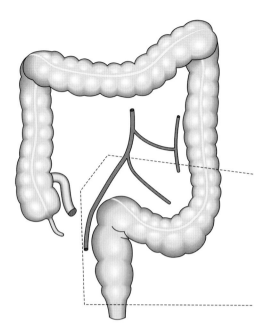

Figure 21.13 Low anterior resection margins.

These operations are almost always defunctioned with a loop ileostomy and again it is usual to perform a water-soluble contrast enema postoperatively to check the integrity of the anastomosis prior to stoma closure.

Subtotal colectomy

Indication: acute fulminant colitis, inflammatory bowel disease (IBD), infective or ischemic colitis, synchronous colorectal tumors, some colorectal cancer syndromes.

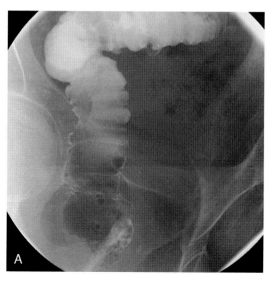

Figure 21.14 (A) Low anterior resection;

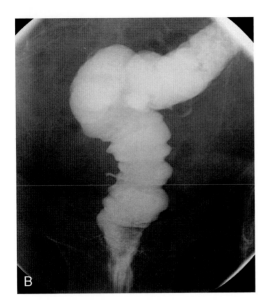

Figure 21.14—cont'd (B) low anterior resection.

Bowel resected: distal 5–10 cm of ileum and entire colon to top of rectum.

Main blood vessels divided: ileocolic, right colic, middle colic, left colic, sigmoid arteries (Figure 21.15).

Postoperative appearance: depends on whether bowel continuity has been restored. In the emergency situation, e.g. acute fulminant colitis, an end ileostomy will be fashioned and the rectal stump will remain in situ. There is little indication for imaging postoperatively unless there is doubt about

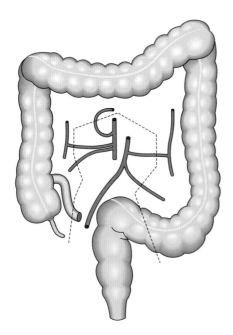

Figure 21.15 Subtotal colectomy margins.

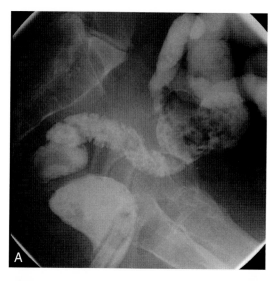

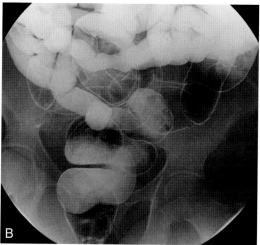

Figure 21.16 (A) Ileorectal anastomosis, lateral view; (B) ileorectal anastomosis, anterior view.

the integrity, health or length of rectal stump. If bowel continuity has been restored, an ileorectal anastomosis will have been performed in which case the ileum will be anastamosed directly to the top of the rectal stump (Figures 21.16A, 21.16B).

Ileoanal pouch

Indication: familial adenomatous polyposis (FAP), ulcerative colitis.

Bowel resected: the entire colon is resected from distal ileum to pelvic floor. In the case of FAP, all colonic mucosa needs to be removed down to the dentate line. In order to restore bowel continuity, the distal ileum is fashioned into a pouch or neo-rectum, which is anastamosed to the top of the anal canal either via a circular stapler or a hand-sewn anastomosis (Figures 21.17, 21.18A, 21.18B and 21.19).

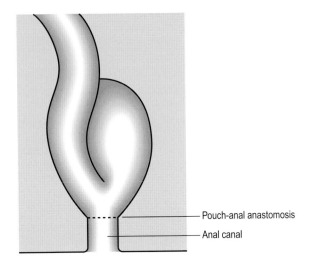

Figure 21.17 **Ileoanal pouch.** A loop of ileum is looped back on itself in a U-shape and sutured or stapled to form a pouch.

Postoperative appearance: a ring of staples may be seen at the top of the anal canal. The appearance of the pouch depends on its configuration. The commonest type is a stapled J pouch, followed by a hand-sewn W.

Abdominoperineal resection (AP resection, APR, APER)

Indication: tumors of the lower rectum/anal canal where there is not enough normal colon distally to restore bowel continuity.

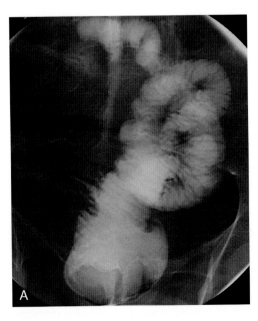

Figure 21.18 (A) Ileoanal pouch;

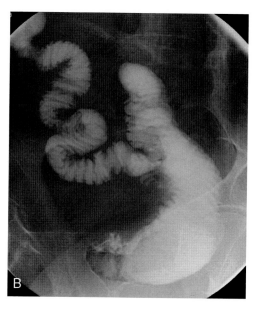

Figure 21.18—cont'd (B) ileoanal pouch.

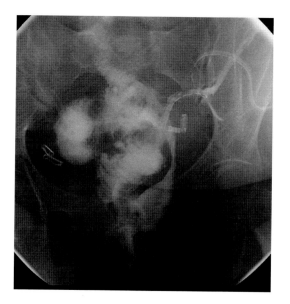

Figure 21.19 Ileoanal pouch; leak from ileoanal anastomosis with drain.

Bowel resected: accessed via the abdomen and from around the anus, the sigmoid, rectum and anal canal are removed and the descending colon is fashioned into an end colostomy.

Type of anastomosis

Anastomoses can be performed using staplers or hand-sewn with sutures. For distal anastomoses of high or low anterior resections, a *circular staple gun* is used which fires a ring of staples that can be clearly seen on x-ray (see

Figures 21.12B, 21.14A). In the pelvis, circular staplers allow anastomoses to be performed that would be impossible or extremely difficult to perform with sutures.

The circular stapled anastomosis can be an end to end or end to side which can cause some confusion in interpreting postoperative images as there is often a 'dog-ear' to the side of the join which may be misinterpreted as a leak.

In other parts of the colon, staples and sutures are interchangeable as it is technically as easy to *hand sew* as it is to staple. The only benefit is that it is arguably quicker to use a stapling device and the join between the two pieces of bowel is usually larger. However, stapling is more expensive. If a hand-sewn anastomosis is performed, this is not visible on x-ray. However, staples are visible and the anastomosis is usually performed in a side-to-side configuration.

Stomas

It is worth mentioning stomas, as the radiographer or radiologist may sometimes be asked for a contrast study via a stoma. Stomas are either ileostomies or colostomies. In general, an *ileostomy* is fashioned in the right iliac fossa (although it could be anywhere on the abdomen) and contains liquid stool in the bag and is spouted.

A *colostomy* is usually in the left iliac fossa, contains more solid stool and is flush with the skin (Figure 21.20).

Stomas are performed for various reasons:

1   It is not anatomically possible to rejoin the bowel, e.g. where an AP resection is performed for a low rectal cancer
2   It is unfavorable to rejoin the bowel. This may be due to the bowel pathology itself, e.g. if there is gross fecal contamination following perforated diverticular disease. Alternatively, this may be due to patient factors, e.g. if a patient is severely malnourished, their protein levels may not support adequate healing
3   To defunction the bowel after surgery or to defunction pathology. For example, an ileostomy is formed after anterior resection. This allows an anastomosis to heal and protects against the consequences of a leak. If a leak develops in the presence of a stoma, the consequence is usually a pelvic abscess, whereas if a stoma is not present, peritonitis will ensue and a second operation may be necessary. A defunctioning

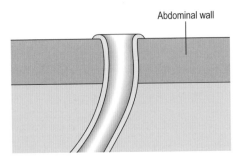

Abdominal wall

Figure 21.20 End colostomy. Colon is sutured flush with abdominal wall.

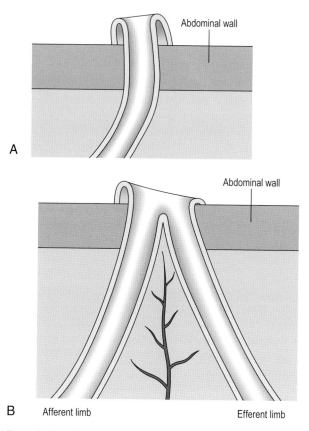

A

B   Afferent limb   Efferent limb

Figure 21.21 (A) End ileostomy. Ileum is spouted onto the abdominal wall to prevent bowel contents excoriating abdominal wall. (B) Loop ileostomy. A loop of bowel is brought up to the abdominal wall. The proximal (afferent) limb is spouted to protect the abdominal wall. The distal (efferent) limb is sutured flush with the abdominal wall.

ileostomy may also be used to defunction distal Crohn's disease or a loop colostomy may be used to defunction a distal tumor

4 For a functional problem (e.g. incontinence) as a last resort.

There are loop or *end stomas* (Figure 21.21A). Temporary defunctioning stomas are almost always *loop stomas*. It is possible to intubate either limb for imaging. In a loop ileostomy, the spouted end will be proximal (Figure 21.21B); in a loop colostomy, the passage of stool usually indicates which end is proximal. Temporary stomas can be closed any time after 6 weeks, but this depends on the fitness of the patient and integrity of the anastomosis on post-operative imaging.

Laparoscopic colorectal surgery

Laparoscopic surgery is minimally invasive surgery where the bulk of the operating is performed using a laparoscope and laparoscopic instruments, inserted through very small incisions. This replaces traditional surgery, which is performed through a midline or transverse incision. The technique was first perfected with laparoscopic cholecystectomy with the benefits of reduced pain and earlier return to normal activities. However, laparoscopic resection has been slower to evolve as a technique for colorectal cancer surgery because it is technically demanding and time consuming, especially when the surgeon is on a learning curve. Early in its evolution there was concern about a high morbidity of up to 21%, which deterred surgeons from adopting the technique (Berends et al., 1994). The incidence of port site metastases led to concern about cancer outcomes and whether laparoscopic surgery was oncologically equivalent to traditional open surgery.

An early British study (the CLASICC trial) reflected the learning curve of surgeons with conversion rates to open surgery of 29%, but there were no differences in mortality, postoperative complications or the number of positive circumferential resection margins (Guillou et al., 2005). Since then, there have been other randomized controlled trials and meta-analyses which have demonstrated short-term benefits from laparoscopic surgery for colon and rectal cancer in terms of reduced blood loss, less pain, earlier return of bowel function and earlier tolerance of a normal diet. Oncologically, the surgery appears to be equivalent in terms of positive circumferential resection margins for rectal cancer, complete resection for colon cancer and numbers of lymph nodes harvested in the specimen (Breunkink et al., 2006; Wexner and Cera, 2006; Aziz et al., 2006).

Reports of longer-term outcomes suggest similar results for both open and laparoscopic surgery for colorectal cancer (Reza et al., 2006), but long-term oncological outcomes in terms of local recurrence, disease-free survival and cancer-related mortality are eagerly awaited by the surgical community. There is also expectation that laparoscopic surgery will reduce the rate of postoperative adhesional obstruction and incisional hernia. After initial scepticism, the National Institute for Clinical Excellence (NICE) has now ruled that laparoscopic resection can be recommended as an alternative to open surgery in England and there is wide uptake of the laparoscopic technique within the confines of supervised training (NICE, 2006).

References

Aziz, O., Constantinides, V., Tekkis, P.P., et al., 2006. Laparoscopic versus open surgery for rectal cancer, a metaanalysis. Ann. Surg. Oncol. 13 (3), 413–424.

Berends, F.J., Kazemier, G., Bonjer, H.J., et al., 1994. Subcutaneous metastases after laparoscopic colectomy. Lancet 344, 58.

Breunkink, S., Pierie, J., Wiggers, T., 2006. Cochrane Database Syst. Rev., issue 4, Art No. CD005400; DOI:10.1002/14651858CD005200.pub2

Guillou, P.J., Quirke, P., Thorpe, H., et al., 2005. Short term endpoints of conventional versus laparoscopically assisted surgery in patients with colorectal cancer (MRC CLASICC trial) multicentre randomised controlled trial. Lancet 365, 1718–1726.

National Institute for Clinical Excellence (NICE), 2006. Technology appraisal guidance 105. Aug 2006. <http://www.nice.org.uk/guidance/index.jsp> Accessed 10.11.08.

Reza, M.M., Blasco, J.A., Andradas, E., 2006. Systematic review of laparoscopic versus open surgery for colorectal cancer. Br. J. Surg. 938, 921–928.

Wexner, S., Cera, S.M., 2006. Laparoscopy for colon cancer. US Gastroenterology Review 1–6.

Further reading

Bauer, J.J., Gorfine, S.R., 1993. Colorectal surgery illustrated: a focused approach. Mosby-Year Book.

Keighley, M.R.B., Fazio, V.W., Pemberton, J.H., 1996. Atlas of colorectal surgery. Churchill Livingstone.

Pearson, F.G., Cooper, J.D., Deslauriers, J., et al., 2002. Esophageal surgery. Second ed. Churchill Livingstone.

Taylor, T.V., Williamson, R.C.N., Watson, A., 1999. Upper digestive surgery, oesophagus, stomach and small intestine. Elsevier Health Sciences.

Lower gastrointestinal procedures

CHAPTER 21

Upper gastrointestinal and colorectal stenting

Robert L. Law, Derrick Martin

Contents

PART 1: UPPER GI TRACT STENTING

Background

Less than 10% of patients with gastro-esophageal cancer survive 5 years (Lee, 2001). Oral intake of nutrition is vital in maintaining quality of life for these patients, particularly when considered by the multidisciplinary team (MDT)

BOX 22.1 Management options to palliate dysphagia resulting from occlusive neoplastic stricturing

- Laser ablation
- Photodynamic therapy
- Argon therapy
- Ethanol injection
- Brachytherapy
- Radiotherapy on its own or chemoradiotherapy
- Self-expanding metal stent (SEMS)

---

to be suitable for palliative treatment only. The development of significant dysphagia to solids and, more particularly, liquids as a result of occlusive neoplastic stricturing requires palliation that is effective and minimally invasive (Box 22.1). In this section, it is intended to review upper gastrointestinal (GI) tract stenting.

History

Historically, palliation of dysphagia resulting from occlusive malignancy has required surgical intervention. Celestin (1959) described a *traction technique* that required endoscopic guidance of an introducer and a mini laparotomy to gain entry high in the stomach; this enabled the tube (Figure 22.1) to be pulled through. Subsequently, the Nottingham introducer precluded the requirement for a laparotomy.

The alternative *pulsion technique* was one where a tube, such as the Atkinson or Soutter tubes, was pushed through the neoplastic stricture, often following bougie dilatation.

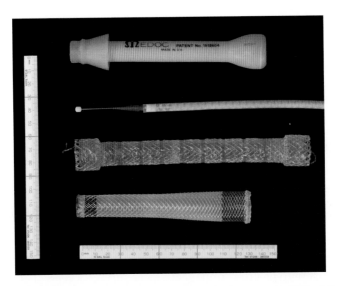

Figure 22.1 Insertion size of the Celestin tube (top) compared with the delivery system for SEMS (underneath), with two SEMS types expanded.

These intubation procedures took less than an hour to perform but required a general anesthetic and hospitalization of between three and ten days (Celestin, 1959; Davis, 1972; Bancewicz, 1979; Unruh and Pagliero, 1985; Kratz et al., 1989; Dunn and Rawlinson, 1992).

Self-expanding metal stent (SEMS) structure

The most common material used to form GI SEMS mesh weave is *Nitinol*, an abbreviation of 'Nickel Titanium Naval Ordinance Laboratory'. Discovered in 1961 by William Buehler, Nitinol is one of the shape memory alloys. It has the property, particularly when warm, of generating a force returning it to a predetermined shape. Nitinol's property and its strength make it an ideal material to be fashioned into the wire that forms SEMS. The membrane of the covered GI stent is most commonly made of silicone or polyurethane:

- *Silicone* is commonly used for the sheath material of covered upper GI SEMS. It is durable and has no effect on the expansile nature of the stent
- *Polyurethane* can biodegrade, particularly in the presence of bile salts, to the extent that holes can appear in the membrane within 8 weeks
- *PTFE* (polytetrafluoroethylene) is most commonly used for vascular stents.

The vast majority of *upper GI SEMS insertions* are associated with neoplastic occlusion or tracheo-esophageal fistula. SEMS have also been used for benign conditions, such as achalasia, where other management options, such as myotomy, balloon dilatation or the injection of botulinum toxin, have failed. In a number of papers, the use of stents is not recommended for benign strictures (De Palma et al., 2001). Ackroyd (2001) suggests that SEMS should be used for benign strictures with caution as they can make matters worse, potentially making a stricture inoperable. The indications for upper GI SEMS insertion are given in Box 22.2.

Removable SEMS

If a temporary stent is being considered, subsequent removal is undertaken endoscopically (Nam et al., 2006; Shin et al., 2008). Removable stents have a

---

BOX 22.2 Indications for upper GI SEMS insertion

- Palliation of malignant occlusion
- Palliation of tumor overgrowth in an in situ stent
- Occlusion of tracheo-esophageal fistula
- Esophageal perforation predominantly as a result of:
  - stricture dilatation
  - iatrogenic endoscopic trauma
  - anastomotic tumor recurrence or leak
  - benign esophageal stricturing
- Stricturing resulting from extrinsic neoplastic compression

lasso woven into their proximal end. Under endoscopic control, forceps are used to grasp the lasso, tension will draw the proximal end of the stent closed and away from the esophageal wall. Maintaining hold of the lasso, the scope and forceps are then drawn out together with the stent.

Approaches to esophageal and gastro-esophageal SEMS insertion

SEMS provide a significant benefit in palliating malignant dysphagia, but there is broad discussion as to the best method to employ for their insertion. The literature suggests a bias towards a *joint endoscopic/fluoroscopic approach* to SEMS insertion. Ramirez et al. (1997) reported that 83% of those members of the American Society of Gastrointestinal Endoscopy (ASGE) who responded to a survey used a combined endoscopic/fluoroscopic approach for the deployment of SEMS. Described by Sarper et al. (2003) and others, the joint approach uses endoscopy to pass the guide wire across the stricture, the subsequent stent deployment being undertaken using fluoroscopic guidance. Singhvi et al. (2000) suggest fluoroscopy is not necessary, advocating the use of a thin gastroscope, possibly in conjunction with a dilator such as the Savrey buginage, to assist with tight strictures. The routine use of general anesthetic for endoscopic SEMS insertion has also been reported (Singhvi et al., 2000; Sarper et al., 2003; Sabharwal et al., 2003; Soussan et al., 2005a, 2005b). The literature, however, also supports the use of *fluoroscopy alone* for deployment (Laasch et al., 2002; Saranovic et al., 2005; Law, 2008). The technical and clinical success rates for the deployment of esophageal SEMS are reported as similar whether using an endoscopic/fluoroscopic technique or fluoroscopic alone (Petruzziello and Costamagna, 2002).

Some units use *endoscopy alone* for the insertion of SEMS, but the advantages of this approach are limited. It can be used where there is limited access to fluoroscopy (Rathore et al., 2006). Singhvi et al. (2000) report using endoscopy alone as being a quick procedure (15 minutes) and resorting to the use of fluoroscopy is not routinely needed.

Points to consider:

- SEMS insertion should be a *minimally invasive* procedure
- *Tumor markers* placed as part of a fluoroscopic SEMS insertion technique can be inaccurate and time consuming (Singhvi et al., 2000)
- Using fluoroscopy only, reduces risk and patient discomfort (Saranovic et al., 2005; Law, 2008)
- Upper GI endoscopy itself carries a significant associated *morbidity* (1:200) and *mortality* (1:2000), little changed over the last ten years (Quine and Bell, 1995; Teague, 2003)
- Endoscopy may have difficulty in differentiating true and false lumen. The guide wire and subsequent SEMS delivery system might be directed through an esophagogastric fistula (Figures 22.2A, 22.2B)
- Endoscopic balloon or bougie dilatation prior to stent insertion has been reported with the attendant risk of perforation (Adam et al., 1997; Sarper et al., 2003; Sabharwal et al., 2003).

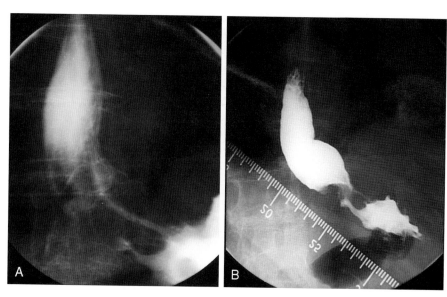

Figure 22.2 (A) Contrast passing through a tumor via an esophagogastric fistula; (B) the strictured true lumen adjacent to the fistulous tract.

- The cost and potential complications associated with general anesthetic (if used), bougie dilatation, endoscopy and endoscopic SEMS insertion should all be taken into account
- Suitably trained advanced practice gastrointestinal radiographers have been demonstrated as safe and cost efficient, able to demonstrate the tumor lumen and transgress it with fine bore tube and guide wire under fluoroscopic control (Law, 2008)
- Fine bore tube and barium contrast enable strictured lumen to be accurately demonstrated and the parameters of the stricture to be identified
- Fluoroscopic SEMS insertion has an overall success rate of 96% which compares well with published literature (Law, 2008).

Fluoroscopically guided SEMS insertion: technique

Fluoroscopy could be considered the optimum approach to esophageal SEMS insertion; it is quick, safe and cost effective. A suggested alternative would be to employ the endoscopic/fluoroscopic approach only in particularly problematic situations and the endoscopy only approach should not be used.

Fine bore intubation is a natural skill progression for GI radiographers or radiologic technologists experienced in demonstrating esophageal pathology. (The techniques and benefits of *technician performed fine bore intubation* are described as a service development in Chapter 11.) In performing complicated fluoroscopically guided naso/orogastric intubation, GI radiographers and radiologic technologists are ideally placed to be involved in a joint approach with a clinician (gastroenterologist, surgeon or radiologist) in performing the first part of SEMS deployment by transgressing the esophageal lumen strictured by tumor (Law, 2008). Suggested protocol inclusions prior to upper GI SEMS insertion are offered in Box 22.3.

BOX 22.3 Pre-upper GI SEMS insertion protocol

- Histological confirmation of a malignancy
- The tumor must be staged
- The patient should have been discussed at the upper GI multidisciplinary team (MDT) meeting and considered suitable for palliation only
- A barium swallow performed to confirm that the degree of dysphagia justifies stenting. (If due to clinical need, stenting is required at short notice, evaluation of the neoplastic stricture with barium can be performed immediately prior to the stent procedure)

Patient preparation

The protocol for upper gastrointestinal SEMS insertion should include:
- Patient commonly admitted overnight but can be as a day case
- Informed consent obtained
- The patient should be nil by mouth for four hours
- The malignancy would already be histologically proven
- Stenting should have been decided upon as the appropriate clinical plan by the MDT.

The barium swallow

- Clinically, the patient considered for esophageal SEMS would demonstrate marked symptoms of *dysphagia to liquids* as well as solids
- The barium swallow is performed to gauge the degree of obstruction to determine if stenting is warranted at that time, demonstrate the location of the lesion and outline and measure the length of the strictured lumen (Figure 22.3)

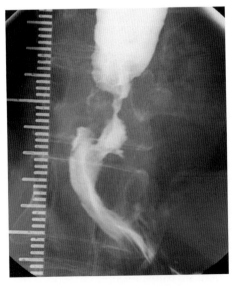

Figure 22.3 Barium outline of neoplastic stricture. A radiopaque rule can help approximate measurement.

- There is not necessarily a need for the barium swallow to be performed in advance of stenting
- As part of a fluoroscopically guided SEMS procedure, barium may be given orally or infused through a fine bore tube sited immediately proximal to the stricture. This is purely to road map the lesion.

Intubation across the stricture

- The patient lies on their side so the pharynx can be easily observed fluoroscopically if there is a problem with tube passage into the esophagus and in case they should aspirate
- The patient may lie on left or right side for esophageal or gastroesophageal stenting. Having the patient lie on their *right side* has the benefit of enabling the practitioner to function from what is traditionally the operational side of the fluoroscopy table. In addition, it also enables gas in the stomach to migrate to and distend the fundus making it easier to pass the fine bore tube and stent delivery system into the gastric body
- *Blood pressure* and *pulse oximetry monitoring* must be available throughout the procedure
- Although *sedation* can be given at this time, it can often be left until after intubation
- Patient cooperation can be of value during intubation. However, constant reassurance may be required
- Prior to intubation, the throat is anesthetized with *xylocaine spray*
- Suction must be available as the procedure carries an inherent risk of reflux and aspiration
- Using a mouth guard, an *8 French gauge tube*, such as the unweighted Coreflo type fine bore tube (E. Merck), is inserted orally
- The tube is manipulated through the strictured lumen into the stomach (Figures 22.4A, 22.4B)
- Adjusting the *guide wire* within the tube alters the rigidity of the distal end of the tube increasing and decreasing its flexibility and assisting in its passage through the tumor
- If a nasogastric fine bore tube is already in situ, the proximal end of the tube can be cut off. Using a tongue depressor, pen torch and long handled forceps, the tube in the oropharynx can be grasped and the trans-nasal aspect of the tube drawn out through the mouth enabling orogastric insertion of a super-stiff guide wire to be introduced without needing to reinsert a tube
- Although the *strictured lumen* tract may be identified, tube passage through the lumen may not be achievable. In these cases, passing the tube tip as far as the proximal margin of the tumor, then a wire such as a straight or curved Jag guide wire or Lunderquist torque controlled wires can often be manipulated through the stricture
- Once the tube is advanced into the stomach, the wire used to site the tube is replaced with one such as the .035 260 cm Amplatz extra (or super) stiff guide wire. It is inserted through the tube exiting into

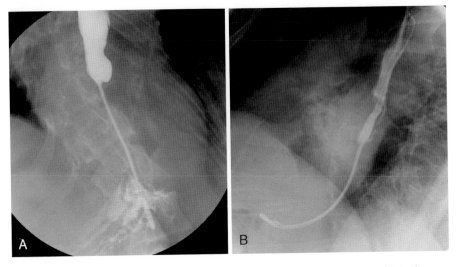

Figure 22.4 (A) Anteroposterior view of the fine bore tube across stricture and into the stomach. (B) Lateral image of tube across lesion and sited in the stomach.

the stomach distal to the lesion (Figure 22.5) and the fine bore tube is withdrawn
- The appropriate type and length of stent is selected
- In the majority of instances, it is of value to sedate the patient for insertion of the delivery system
- Maintaining tension on the guide wire, the *stent delivery system* is inserted over the wire. Advancement of the delivery system is observed fluoroscopically to ensure safe passage through the pharynx and across the stricture

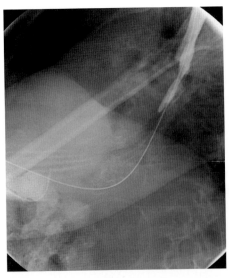

Figure 22.5 A stiff wire sited into the stomach and the tube being withdrawn over the wire.

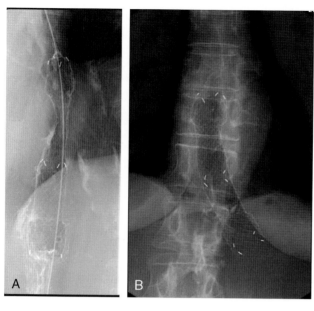

Figure 22.6 (A) SEMS released from delivery system. Proximal, middle and distal markers visible, guidewire in situ. (B) SEMS deployed.

- Identifying the markers of the sheathed stent across the stricture (Figures 22.6A, 22.6B), the stent is deployed maintaining the proximal marker of the stent just above the lesion
- As the delivery sheath is withdrawn, the stent will expand from its distal end
- It is important to maintain close observation of the proximal end of the stent and prevent migration. Once satisfactorily deployed, the wire and delivery system are removed.

High esophageal stricture

Technically, there is nothing to preclude fluoroscopically guided stenting of malignant strictures close to the upper esophageal sphincter. Verschuur et al. (2007), in reporting the safety and effectiveness of stenting high in the esophagus, note that its limitations can include patient intolerance due to pain or globus sensation. Sihoe et al. (2004) reported that, due to the close proximity of the trachea and the upper esophagus, consideration should be given to pre-empt airway stenosis or fistulation by inserting a tracheal stent prior to the insertion of a high esophageal stent. Wyn et al. (2006), although supporting this premise, suggest that airway compression is rare.

Gastric and duodenal SEMS

SEMS insertion can be used to palliate advanced symptomatic malignancy obstructing the stomach or duodenum. It is normally undertaken as a joint endoscopic/fluoroscopic procedure. Symptoms might include vomiting, cachexia and dehydration.

As a precursor to SEMS insertion, location and length of the stricture can be demonstrated fluoroscopically using a water-soluble contrast medium such as Ultravist 240 (Schering Health Care Ltd).

With the patient lying on their *right side*, the contrast pooling (whether in the stomach or duodenum) has the optimum chance of outlining the strictured lumen (Aviv et al., 2002; Lowe et al., 2007; Van Hooft et al., 2007; Hosono et al., 2007).

Technical considerations

- Stenting is normally performed as a joint endoscopic-fluoroscopic procedure.
- The stomach should be empty, if necessary by the prior insertion of a gastric drainage tube
- The use of an endoscope can help direct the guide wire into the proximal origin of the stricture. It can also prevent the wire coiling in the stomach during advancement
- The potential for the stent to abut the normal anatomy at either end of the stricture (such as the duodenal bulb), should be taken into account when deciding SEMS length
- If a duodenal stricture to be stented transgresses the ampulla, it must be confirmed that no further endoscopic intervention of the pancreas or biliary tree is required as the SEMS will obstruct access to the ampulla
- Lowe et al. (2007) reported a 96.6% technical success rate for gastro duodenal SEMS insertion; 75% of patients were able to be supported at home without tube feeding
- The removal of a retrievable stent can be elective or indicated as a result of complications such as pain, migration, new stricture formation, incomplete expansion, airway compression. Care must be taken with removal, as intramural perforation, major bleeding, pneumomediastinum and even death may result (Yoon et al., 2004; Wyn et al., 2006)
- Where the stomach is not over distended and the stricture is outlined by a water-soluble contrast medium, gastric and duodenal SEMS insertion can be performed using fluoroscopy without the aid of endoscopy. The technique is similar to that used in the esophagus. Figures 22.7A–G demonstrate stenting of an incomplete duodenal occlusion from a carcinoma in the head of pancreas

Patient after-care post upper GI SEMS insertion

- Routine 4-hourly pulse and blood pressure observations
- Nil by mouth until sedation and oral anesthesia has worn off
- Overnight admission is normal post SEMS insertion. This is so that analgesia can be given as required. The radial force of the stent can cause focal pain as it stretches open the tumor lumen
- The greatest degree of stent expansion occurs within the first six hours after SEMS deployment. If there is concern about migration, expansion or the efficacy of the stent, a limited barium swallow could be considered at this time

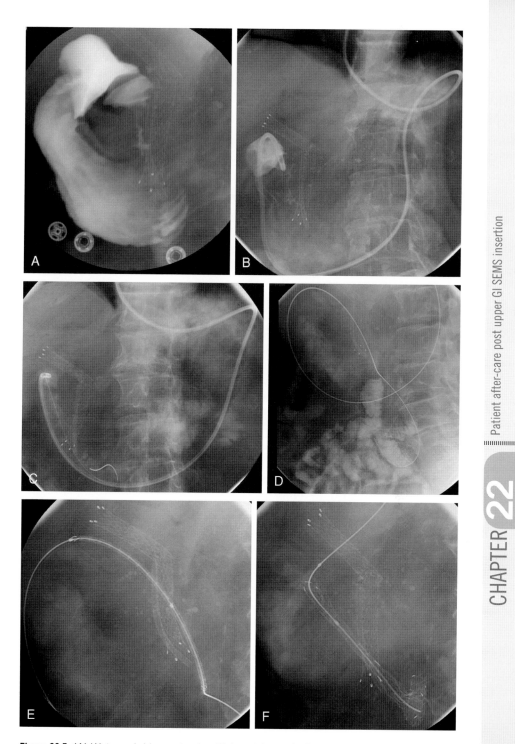

Figure 22.7 (A) Water-soluble contrast outlining stricture in 2nd part of the duodenum. Metal and plastic stent in the common bile duct; (B) 8fg fine bore tube placed at the proximal origin of stricture; (C) guide wire passed across stricture; (D) guide wire passed into jejunum; (E) stent delivery system passed over guide wire; (F) stent deployed;

(Continued)

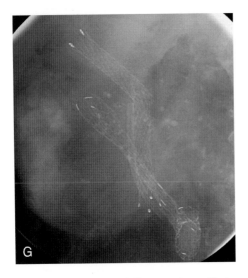

Figure 22.7—cont'd (G) delivery system withdrawn.

BOX 22.4 Gastro-esophageal SEMS complications

- Chest pain often present as the stent expands
- Bleeding, perforation, aspiration, fever, fistula
- Covered stent migration, possibly requiring further stenting
- Esophageal reflux
- Stent impaction
- Tracheal compression

- Fluids only overnight while the stent beds in
- If no overnight complications, start a soft diet and arrange dietetic advice
- Complications directly associated with gastro-esophageal SEMS are given in Box 22.4.

The patient experience

Xylocaine spray to the throat will initially taste unpleasant before making the tongue feel as if it has enlarged. Despite local anesthesia, a degree of *retching* can occur. This can be caused by the initial passage of the tube through the pharynx into the esophagus. With residual fluid collecting above an esophageal occlusion, reflux and possible aspiration is a hazard during the procedure.

The most common experience the patient can expect, particularly in the immediate post SEMS insertion period, is *focal chest pain*. Pain is caused by the radial force of the stent as it opens. Staying in hospital overnight will allow for monitoring and appropriate analgesia to provide pain relief. Complications are not infrequent. Although not related to large patient groups, literature has reported early complication rates of 13% and late complication rate of 20% (Aviv et al., 2002). A complication rate of 44% has been reported for

Table 22.1 SEMS complications

During procedure	Post procedure
Cardiorespiratory distress	Misplacement
Reflux	Perforation
Aspiration	Reflux
Failed deployment	Aspiration
Failed expansion	
Migration	

Delayed complications	Iatrogenic complications
Migration	Aspiration
Tumor overgrowth	Fistula formation
Food impaction	Sepsis
Bleeding	Respiratory failure

SEMS placement for distal esophageal tumor stenoses (Sarper et al., 2003). Major complication rates of 37% have also been reported (Ross et al., 2007). Complications are given in Table 22.1.

PART 2: COLORECTAL SELF-EXPANDING METAL STENTS (SEMS)

Introduction

About 20000 people die in the UK each year from colorectal malignancy (Starkey, 2002; Steele, 2006). Currently, most incidents of colorectal cancer occur in patients in their seventh and eighth decades of life when other comorbidities, such as vascular disease, may limit treatment options. Most patients with colorectal cancer present with colonic symptoms (see Chapter 10), while others may present with disease as a consequence of metastatic spread. A significant number of patients with colorectal cancer present with *acute large bowel obstruction* (Stipa et al., 2008) and it is in this group of patients where colonic stenting is particularly appropriate (Alcantara et al., 2007; Farrell, 2007; Dionigi et al., 2007).

The morbidity and mortality for elective surgery for colorectal cancer is quite low, while urgent surgery for the patient who presents with acute colonic obstruction is significantly higher. Concerns may include:

- Electrolyte imbalance because of nausea and vomiting and a consequent inability to eat or drink
- Pre-renal failure may intervene because of dehydration
- Postoperative chest infection may be a problem because of the pulmonary stasis associated with elevation of the diaphragm from abdominal distension.

Most colorectal cancers which cause intestinal obstruction are on the left side of the colon, where the diameter of the colon is less and the consistency of feces is harder. It has been hypothesized that the relatively *high mortality of urgent surgery* can be avoided by placing a stent across the obstructing tumor and allowing the colon to decompress and the patient to return to a normal physiological state before elective surgery is undertaken. This, it is believed, returns the patient to the risk level for morbidity and mortality associated with elective surgery. Additionally, the use of colorectal stenting in the emergency situation might simplify the type of surgery. In an acutely obstructed patient, it may be necessary to perform colostomy to decompress the colon, closing the distal colonic stump. In some circumstances, it may not even be possible to remove the primary tumor at this time. The patient is then left with a colostomy and probably the need for further surgery at some time in the future when the urgent situation has passed. If a stent is placed and elective surgery is undertaken, then a *primary colocolic anastomosis* may be undertaken and the tumor removed, thereby improving the quality of the patient's existence and reducing the need for second surgery. Under some circumstances, for example, where the patient is not fit even for elective surgery or has extensive metastatic disease, colonic stenting may be *definitive therapy* in the acutely obstructed patient, thereby avoiding the need for potentially futile surgery (Athreya et al., 2006; Soto et al., 2006; Small et al., 2008).

Other indications

While the majority of colorectal stenting is undertaken for the obstructed patient with colonic cancer, other indications exist. *Colonic strictures* from diverticular disease or from Crohn's disease may be treated with stenting when the patient is too unfit for the surgical option. The presence of a *fistula* between the colon and other structures, such as the bladder, small bowel and vagina, can lead to extremely debilitating symptoms for the patient and may be effectively treated by stenting (Laasch et al., 2003; Small et al., 2008).

One of the uncertainties regarding the use of colorectal stenting at present is whether *pre-emptive stenting* in the patient with a left-sided colonic tumor who is unfit for surgery might be of value. It is tempting to try to prevent the onset of colonic obstruction by stenting the patient who appears to have a narrow lumen through the tumor at the time of diagnosis. Opinions here are divided. It is clearly logical to try to avoid an episode of acute large bowel obstruction with its associated morbidity and mortality, but colorectal stenting itself carries a risk and there are no clear predictors that indicate the likelihood of large bowel obstruction in colonic cancer patients. The risk, therefore, is that patients are exposed to the risks of stenting for no clear clinical value. Most intestinal stents have a limited life span eventually becoming obstructed themselves. It may be inappropriate to use a proportion of this lifespan before it is clinically necessary.

Patient preparation

For the patient who presents with acute colonic obstruction, full clinical biochemical, hematological and radiological evaluation is important to reduce risk. *Clinical assessment* is important to determine the presence of comorbidities, particularly cardiac and respiratory disease. *Hematological assessment* is necessary because the patient may be anemic as a consequence of bleeding from the tumor and this may need correcting. *Biochemical abnormality* may be present because of dehydration, vomiting and renal failure. These deficiencies need to be corrected. It is rare that colorectal stenting is required so urgently that the patient cannot be adequately resuscitated from a hematological and biochemical standpoint prior to stenting. While *radiological evaluation* is most commonly undertaken using a *plain film of the abdomen* to determine the presence of obstruction, CT of the abdomen at least is essential. It may be valuable to add a CT of the chest in order to determine the presence of metastatic disease.

Abdominal CT can be carried out without any oral or rectal bowel preparation, but with intravenous contrast medium administration and CT examination carried out during the portal phase of contrast flow.

The CT will demonstrate:

- The degree and level of obstruction, the presence of synchronous tumors
- The normality or otherwise of the large bowel below the level of the obstructing tumor
- The presence of diverticular disease here is particularly important
- Other complications such as fistula formation, tumor perforation and abscess formation can be demonstrated
- The presence of lymph node involvement and metastatic liver disease.

Stent placement technique

Patient management

After a discussion of the results of the evaluations listed above with the patient and the appropriate acquisition of consent, the patient is brought to the radiology department. In all patients, it is helpful to administer a *phosphate enema* in order to clear feces from the distal colon and improve access to the tumor. It is appropriate to use gentle *conscious sedation and analgesia* during the procedure and many will use a combination of fentanyl and midazolam. It is therefore important that the patient is cared for by a nurse who is dedicated to monitoring their status throughout. *Non-invasive monitoring* of oxygen saturation, ECG, blood pressure and pulse rate should normally be undertaken. *Pre-oxygenation* with oxygen administered at 4 litres per minute is universally indicated. The patient is made comfortable lying either on their left side or supine on the fluoroscopy table. It is important to remember that patients can get very cold during prolonged procedures and it is important to make them comfortable and cover them appropriately with blankets.

Colonoscopy or not?

It is generally true to say, with upper GI or lower GI enteral stenting, that the further the lesion from the point of access, the more appropriate it is to use endoscopy. Obstructing tumors in the *rectosigmoid* can usually be traversed and stented using fluoroscopic guidance alone, without colonoscopy (Athreya et al., 2006). However, with more *proximal tumors*, in the descending colon up to the transverse colon, colonoscopy has a definite advantage in that it allows more rapid access to the tumor and therefore reduces radiation dose to the patient, but most importantly to staff (Figures 22.8, 22.9A, 22.9B).

Fluoroscopic stent placement technique

It is appropriate to have a variety of hydrophilic catheters and guide wires to hand. With the patient in the *left lateral position*, a catheter (such as the Headhunter 1, Bernstein or Law 2) loaded with a guide wire is inserted into

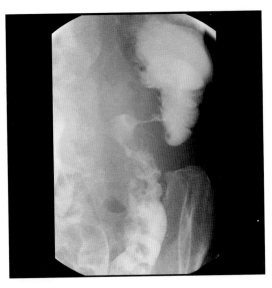

Figure 22.8 Obstructive carcinoma descending colon.

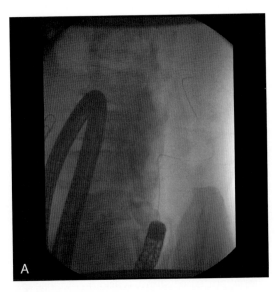

Figure 22.9 (A) Endoscope passed to descending colon;

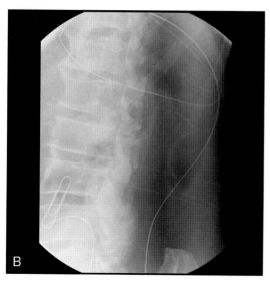

Figure 22.9—cont'd (B) wire passed through stricture.

the rectum and negotiated slowly up to the level of the tumor. This is generally not difficult but can be time consuming. Once arrival at the distal margin of the tumor is achieved, it may be appropriate to inject water-soluble contrast in order to outline the tumor (Figure 22.10).

The *catheter and guide wire* can then be negotiated across the tumor into the dilated colon above (Figures 22.11 and 22.12). This can occasionally be very difficult or impossible and there is a variety of tricks to improve success. Access across the tumor is most easily achieved using a *standard non-stiff, straight tipped, hydrophilic guide wire*. Occasionally, stiff or angled wires may be helpful. A change of catheter should be considered if difficulty is

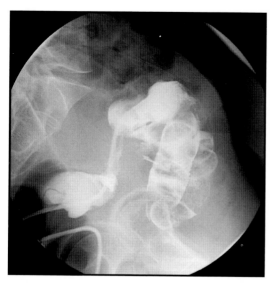

Figure 22.10 Water-soluble contrast infused through catheter to outline tumor.

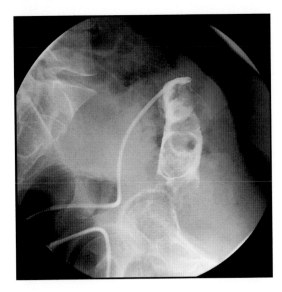

Figure 22.11 Catheter negotiated across tumor lumen.

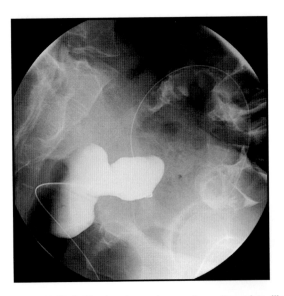

Figure 22.12 Guide wire advanced across tumor lumen into dilated colon.

encountered. The more curved (cobra) or even straight catheters may be successful when the primary choice of catheter fails. Intravenous *Buscopan* to reduce peristalsis may help, as might insufflation of the rectum and distal colon with gas. The placement of a stiffening sheath into the rectum and sigmoid can help to prevent tube looping, but this also removes the effectiveness of the anal sphincter in maintaining continence.

If the proximal margin of the tumor has not been outlined, with the catheter passed through the tumor lumen into dilated colon, the guide wire can be removed and a water-soluble contrast infused. A relatively long, relatively stiff, nitinol plastic coated guide wire should then be passed into the proximal segments of colon. As much wire as possible should be inserted beyond

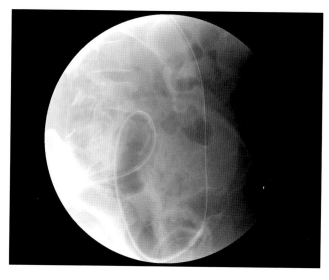

Figure 22.13 Law 2 tube showing guide wire passed into proximal descending colon.

the stricture (Figure 22.13). It may be necessary to allow a soft guide wire to loop its passage through the stricture (Figure 22.14). However, depending on the configuration of the colon, the length of wire passed across the stricture may, by force of circumstances, be short (Figure 22.15).

Short (90 cm) non-endoscopic *stent delivery systems* are available, as well as long (150 cm) delivery systems for endoscopic use. While short systems cannot be used with an endoscope, it is possible to use long (more cumbersome) delivery systems without an endoscope. The well-lubricated and flushed stent system is passed gently over the guide wire under fluoroscopic control, until it lies in an acceptable position.

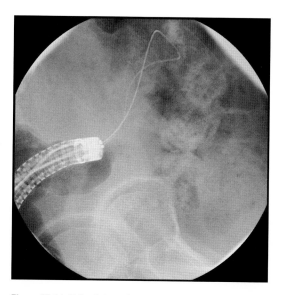

Figure 22.14 Using joint colonoscopic/fluoroscopic guidance a soft wire is allowed to loop to pass across the strictured lumen.

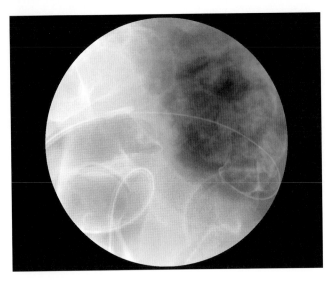

Figure 22.15 Maximum position of guide wire due to a tight loop of bowel immediately proximal to the tumor site.

If the delivery system does not easily pass through the stricture due to the tightness or rigidity of the lumen, pulling the wire to place it under tension can assist in railroading the delivery system into place. If the wire is to be placed under tension, the amount of free wire across the stricture must be very closely monitored as the tension will draw the wire out. Should the amount of wire extracted give concern, stop the advance of the delivery system and reinsert the wire.

With tumors above the rectosigmoid junction, it is probably best to place the middle of the stent in the middle of the tumor, so that there are equal lengths of stent above and below the tumor (Figure 22.16). It is appropriate to use a

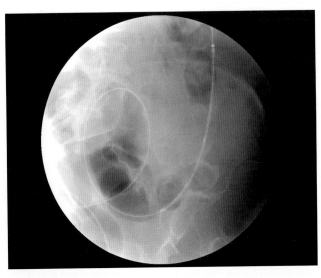

Figure 22.16 Stent delivery system sited across the strictured lumen in the descending colon.

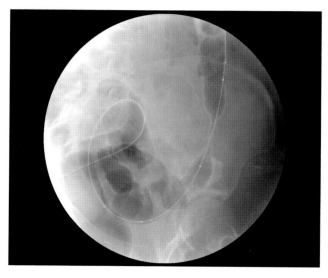

Figure 22.17 Stent deployment (note change in position of delivery system markers from Figure 22.16).

length of stent so that at least 2, preferably 3 or 4 cm, of stent lie above and below the margins of the tumor. This allows for any slippage or movement during placement (Figure 22.17).

Stent types

As described for esophageal stents (see Part 1) *nitinol* or *stainless steel* stents are available. The most appropriate stent in current use has smooth wire ends and no sharp edges. Stents range from 22 to 30 mm in diameter and up to 14 cm in length. Colorectal stents are most commonly *uncovered* because of the better bowel wall grip achieved. Tumor in-growth is of less concern in the colon due to the bowel lumen diameter that can be achieved post stenting. However, *covered stents* may be appropriate in patients with fistula (Laasch et al., 2003; Shin et al., 2008; Small et al., 2008).

Post-procedural management

Generally, the feces at the level of obstruction are liquid and pass readily through the opening stent. A successful procedure is generally indicated by the patient needing a bedpan as they are wheeled out into the recovery area of the interventional suite. Again, it is important to maintain adequate fluid balance for the patient although, once the obstruction is dealt with, *oral intake* can resume quite quickly. In some patients, solid stool is present above the stent and this may make stent dysfunction a problem. *Gentle enemas and orally administered stool softeners*, such as Lactulose, may be helpful in these circumstances. Once the abdominal distension begins to decompress through the stent, oral intake, both liquid and solid, can resume. It may be wise to keep the patient on an orally administered stool softener indefinitely.

Outcomes

Stent placement and technical success is expected in about 90% of cases (Sebastian et al., 2004; Baraza et al., 2008). Failure occurs most commonly because of inability to negotiate either the catheter or colonoscope through the colon up to the level of the tumor. This may be because of tortuosity of the bowel or the presence of diverticular disease or stricture. Failure to negotiate a catheter or guide wire across the stricture may occur because the stricture is very tight (uncommon) or because of an adverse relationship of the lumen of the colon and the lumen of the tumor. Once the guide wire has been placed across the tumor into the proximal colon, failure to place a stent is extremely rare.

Complications

Apart from failure to complete the procedure, complications are few. *Perforation* of the distal colon or perforation of the tumor can occur and, in some series, appear quite common. If the position markers are not held rigidly in place during SEMS deployment, as the stent opens the radial force can migrate the stent into the more proximal colon (Figure 22.18). *Stent migration* appears to be less common in the colon than at the gastro-esophageal junction, perhaps a function of the use of uncovered stents more frequently in the colon. In experienced hands, perforation is uncommon. Failure of a technically well placed stent to function adequately is most likely because of impaction of solid feces into the stent and enemas, together with oral stool softeners, may resolve the situation (Athreya et al., 2006; Pericoli Ridolfini et al., 2007; Shin et al., 2008).

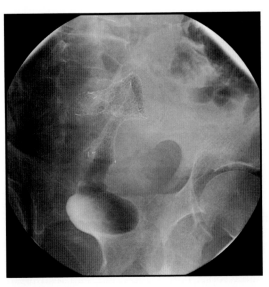

Figure 22.18 Stenting sited around a tight strictured loop, due to stent migration: malignancy not optimally covered.

Late complications

Stent migration can occur late, but is less common than immediate migration. *Stent occlusion* is the most common later sequel and is usually due to tumor through-growth, although fecal impaction may occur. *Late perforation* is reported (Salvi et al., 2004; Pericoli Ridolfini et al., 2007).

Post-stent course

In the majority of patients who undergo colorectal stenting for acute colonic obstruction as a bridge to surgery, further clinical and radiological assessment for the detection of metastatic disease or preliminary treatment with chemotherapy or radiotherapy may be appropriate under certain circumstances. *Elective surgery* can then be undertaken, the stent being removed with the surgical specimen. There does not appear to be any disadvantage to the surgeon caused by the presence of the stent. Some anxieties have been raised about the possibility that the presence of the stent causes dissemination of tumor cells with a possible increased risk of metastatic liver disease (Maruthachalam et al., 2007), but these concerns have yet to be confirmed.

Summary

- Colorectal stenting is a significant advantage in the management of the patient with the acutely obstructed colon
- It is technically a relatively straightforward procedure and not an uncomfortable or distressing procedure for the patient
- It removes the risks of surgery in an acute situation and returns the patient to a more acceptable elective surgical risk
- It allows better assessment of the patient for appropriate colorectal cancer management and is definitive treatment for some not suitable for surgery

References

Ackroyd, R., Watson, D.I., Devitt, P.G., et al., 2001. Expandable metallic stents should not be used in the treatment of benign oesophageal strictures. J. Gastroenterol. Hepatol. 16 (4), 484–487.

Adam, A., Ellul, J., Watkinson, A., et al., 1997. Palliation of inoperable esophageal carcinoma: a prospective randomized trial of laser therapy and stent placement. Radiology 202, 344–348.

Alcantara, M., Serra, X., Bombardó, J., et al., 2007. Colorectal stenting as an effective therapy for preoperative and palliative treatment of large bowel obstruction: 9 years' experience diseases of the colon and rectum. Tech. Coloproctol. 11 (4), 316–322.

Athreya, S., Moss, J., Urquhart, G., 2006. Colorectal stenting for colonic obstruction: the indications, complications, effectiveness and outcome – 5 year review. Eur. J Radiol. 60 (1), 91–94.

Aviv, R.I., Shyamalan, G., Khan, F.H., et al., 2002. Use of stents in the palliative treatment of malignant gastric outlet and duodenal obstruction. Clin. Radiol. 57 (7), 587–592.

Bancewicz, J., 1979. Celestin tubes (letter). Br. Med. J. 2 (6200), 1292.

Baraza, W., Lee, F., Brown, S., et al., 2008. Combination endo-radiological colorectal stenting: a prospective 5-year clinical evaluation. Colorectal Dis. [Epub ahead of print].

Celestin, L.R., 1959. Permanent intubation in inoperable cancer of the oesophagus and cardia: a new tube. Ann. R. Coll. Surg. Engl. 25, 165–170.

Davis, R.S., 1972. Insertion of Celestin tubes (letter). Br. Med. J. 4 (5834), 235.

De Palma, G.D., Iovino, P., Masone, S., Persico, M., et al., 2001. Self-expanding metal stents for endoscopic treatment of esophageal achalasia unresponsive to conventional treatments. Long-term results in eight patients. Endoscopy 33 (12), 1027–1030.

Dionigi, G., Villa, F., Rovera, F., 2007. Colonic stenting for malignant disease: review of literature. Surg. Oncol. 16 (Suppl. 1), S153–S155.

Dunn, D.C., Rawlinson, N., 1992. Surgical diagnosis and management, second ed. Blackwell Scientific Publications.

Farrell, J.J., 2007. Preoperative colonic stenting: how when why? Curr. Opin. Gastroenterol. 23 (5), 544–549.

Hosono, S., Ohtani, H., Arimoto, Y., et al., 2007. Endoscopic stenting versus surgical gastroenterostomy for palliation of malignant obstruction: a meta-analysis. J. Gastroenterol. 42 (4), 283–290.

Kratz, J.M., Reed, C.E., Crawford, F.A., et al., 1989. A comparison of endoesophageal tubes: improved results with Atkinson tube. J. Thorac. Cardiovas. Surg. 97 (1), 19–23.

Laasch, H., Marriott, A., Wilbraham, L., et al., 2002. Effectiveness of open versus antireflux stents for palliation of distal esophageal carcinoma and prevention of symptomatic gastrointestinal reflux. Radiology 225 (2), 359–365.

Laasch, H.U., Wilbraham, L., Marriott, A., Martin, D.F., 2003. Treatment of colovaginal fistula with coaxial placement of covered and uncovered stents. Endoscopy 35 (12), 1081.

Law, R.L., 2008. Radiographer involvement with stent insertion to palliate symptomatic dysphagia resulting from neoplastic obstruction. Radiography 14, 39–44.

Lee, S.H., 2001. The role of oesophageal stenting in the non surgical management of oesophageal strictures. Br. J. Radiol. 74 (886), 891–900.

Lowe, A.S., Bechett, C.G., Jowett, S., et al., 2007. Self-expandable metal stent placement for the palliation of malignant gastroduodenal obstruction: experience in a large UK centre. Clin. Radiol. 62 (8), 738–744.

Maruthachalam, K., Lash, G.E., Shenton, B.K., et al., 2007. Tumour cell dissemination following endoscopic stent insertion. Br. J. Surg. 94 (9), 1151–1154.

Nam, D.H., Shin, J.H., Song, H.Y., et al., 2006. Malignant esophageal-tracheobronchial strictures: parallel placement of covered retrievable expandable nitinol stents. Acta Radiologica 47 (1), 3–9.

Pericoli Ridolfini, M., Sofo, L., Di Giorgio, A., et al., 2007. Late complication after colon self-expandable metal stent placement: a case report. Minerva Chirurgie 62 (1), 69–72.

Petruzziello, L., Costamagna, G., 2002. Stenting in oesophageal strictures. Dig. Dis. 20, 154–166.

Quine, M.A., Bell, G.D., 1995. Prospective audit of upper gastrointestinal endoscopy in two regions of England: safety, staffing, and sedation methods. Gut 36, 462–467.

Ramirez, F.C., Dennert, B., Zierer, S.T., et al., 1997. Esophageal self expanding metal stents – indications, practice, technique and complications; results of a national survey. Gastrointest. Endosc. 45 (5), 360–364.

Rathore, O.I., Cross, A., Patchett, S.E., et al., 2006. Direct-vision stenting: the way forward for malignant oesophageal obstruction. Endoscopy 38 (4), 382–384.

Ross, W.A., Alkassab, F., Lynch, P.M., et al., 2007. Evolving role of self-expanding metal stents in the treatment of malignant dysphagia and fistulas. Gastrointest. Endosc. 65 (1), 70–76.

Sabharwal, T., Hamady, M.S., Chui, S., et al., 2003. A randomized prospective comparison of the Flamingo wall stent and Ultraflex stent for the palliation of dysphagia associated with lower third oesophageal carcinoma. Gut 52, 922–926.

Salvi, P.F., Leone, G., Corona, F., et al., 2004. Colonic perforations after self-expandable metallic stenting: two cases. G. Chir. 25 (6–7), 211–216.

Saranovic, D.J., Djuric-Stefanovic, A., Ivanovic, A., et al., 2005. Fluoroscopically guided insertion of self expanding metal esophageal stents for palliative treatment of patients with malignant stenosis of esophagus and cardia: comparison of covered and uncovered stent types. Dis. Esoph. 18 (4), 230–238.

Sarper, A., Oz, N., Cihangir, C., et al., 2003. The efficacy of self expanding metal stents for palliation of malignant esophageal strictures and fistulas. Eur. J. Cardio-thorac. Surg. 23, 794–798.

Sebastian, S., Johnston, S., Geoghegan, T., et al., 2004. Pooled analysis of the efficacy and safety of self-expanding metal stenting in malignant colorectal obstruction. Am. J. Gastroenterol. 99 (10), 2051–2057.

Shin, S.J., Kim, T.I., Kim, B.C., et al., 2008. Clinical application of self-expandable metallic stent for treatment of colorectal obstruction caused by extrinsic invasive tumors. Dis. Colon. Rectum. 51 (5), 578–583.

Sihoe, A.D.L., Wan, I.Y.P., Yin, A.P., et al., 2004. Airway stenting for irresectable esophageal cancer. Surg. Oncol. 13 (1), 17–25.

Singhvi, R., Abbasakoor, F., Manson, J.M., et al., 2000. Insertion of self-expanding metal stents for malignant dysphagia: assessment of a simple endoscopic method. Ann. R. Coll. Surg. Engl. 82 (4), 243–248.

Small, A.J., Young-Fadok, T.M., Baron, T.H., 2008. Expandable metal stent placement for benign colorectal obstruction: outcomes for 23 cases. Surg. Endosc. 22 (2), 454–462.

Soussan, E.B., Antonietti, M., Lecleire, S., et al., 2005a. Palliative esophageal stent placement using endoscopic guidance without fluoroscopy. Gastroenterol. Clin. Biol. 29 (8–9).

Soussan, E.B., Antonietti, M., LeCleire, S., 2005b. Palliative oesophageal stent. Gastroenterol. Clin. Biol. 29 (8–9), 785–788.

Soto, S., López-Rosés, L., González-Ramírez, A., 2006. Endoscopic treatment of acute colorectal obstruction with self-expandable metallic stents: experience in a community hospital . Surg. Endosc. 20 (7), 1072–1076.

Starkey, B.J., 2002. Screening for colorectal cancer. Ann. Clin. Biochem. 39 (4), 351–365.

Steele, R.J., 2006. Modern challenges in colorectal cancer. Surgeon 4 (5), 285–291.

Stipa, F., Pigazzi, A., Bascone, B., et al., 2008. Management of obstructive colorectal cancer with endoscopic stenting followed by single-stage surgery: open or laparoscopic resection? Surg. Endosc. 22 (6), 1477–1481.

Teague, R., 2003. Clinical practice guidelines update: safety and sedation during endoscopic procedures. British Society of Gastroenterology. <http://www.bsg.org.uk>

Unruh, H.W., Pagliero, K.M., 1985. Pulsion intubation versus traction intubation for obstructing carcinomas of the esophagus. Ann. Thorac. Surg. 40 (4), 337–342.

Van Hooft, J., Mutignani, M., Repici, A., 2007. First data on the palliative treatment of patients with malignant gastric outlet obstruction using the Wall-flex enteral stent: a retrospective multicenter study. Endoscopy 39 (5), 434–439.

Verschuur, S.M., Kuipers, E.J., Siersema, P.D., 2007. Esophageal stents for malignant strictures close to the upper esophageal sphincter. Gastrointest. Endosc. 66 (6), 1082–1090.

Wyn, D., Shah, R., Talwar, A., 2006. Left main stem airway obstruction after esophageal stent placement for metastatic mediastinal mass. J. Bronchol. 13 (2), 72–73.

Yoon, C.J., Shin, J.H., Song, H.Y., et al., 2004. Removal of retrievable esophageal and gastrointestinal stents: experience in 113 patients. Am. J. Roentgenol. 183 (5), 1437–1444.

Radiotherapy and chemotherapy of GI tract malignancy

Neil Bayman, Mark P. Saunders

Contents ||||||||||||||||||||||||||||||||||||||||||||||||||||||||||||||||||||||||||||

Introduction

Chemotherapy and radiotherapy can be used as separate treatment modalities or together as combination chemoradiotherapy (CRT). *Chemotherapy* is a systemic treatment used to treat established tumors and micrometastatic disease. The anticancer drugs effective in gastrointestinal (GI) tract malignancies are either injected intravenously or ingested orally. In contrast, *radiotherapy* is a localized treatment using megavoltage photons or electrons targeted to a specific volume (usually the primary tumor).

GI malignancies are a heterogeneous group and chemotherapy/radiotherapy has a role as *definitive radical treatment* (e.g. esophageal cancer, anal cancer), as *adjuvant treatment* to definitive surgery (e.g. colorectal cancer) and as *palliative treatment* to reduce tumor burden, prolong survival and control symptoms in advanced disease.

Chemotherapy and radiotherapy both have a significant *toxicity profile*. Patients with GI malignancies are often unwell with symptoms of their disease and thus the potential benefit of treatment must be measured against the potential risks and side effects, which can be life threatening. *Chemotherapy toxicity* is dependent on the drug regimen employed, but most chemotherapy drugs used to treat GI malignancies can cause lethargy, nausea, vomiting, diarrhea and, most importantly, myelosuppression with the subsequent risk of anemia, thrombocytopenia and neutropenic sepsis. *Radiotherapy toxicity* is dependent on the specific site of irradiation. Irradiation of the upper GI tract causes problems such as esophagitis, gastritis, nausea and vomiting. Irradiation of the lower GI tract can lead to severe diarrhea and proctitis.

Table 23.1 Definitions of outcome parameters used to measure efficacy of a treatment regimen

Outcome parameter	Definition
Median survival[1]	The time from either diagnosis or start of treatment at which half of the patients with a given disease are found to be, or expected to be, still alive
5 year survival	Proportion of patients still alive 5 years after diagnosis or start of treatment
Cancer specific survival	Can be used as median survival or 5 year survival but includes patients who are still alive and those who died of causes not related to their cancer
Progression-free survival[1]	The length of time from either diagnosis or start of treatment in which a patient is living with a disease that does not get worse
Time to progression[1]	A measure of time after a disease is diagnosed (or treated) until the disease starts to get worse
Response rate[1]	The percentage of patients whose cancer shrinks or disappears after treatment

[1] Definitions adapted from the National Cancer Institute, www.cancer.gov [accessed 4 June 2008]

There are several different parameters used to measure 'benefit' from chemotherapy or radiotherapy (Table 23.1). These terms are often used as endpoints in clinical trials assessing the efficacy of a treatment regimen.

This chapter provides an overview of the role of chemotherapy and radiotherapy in GI malignancies and presents the current evidence-base for accepted treatments.

Colorectal cancer (CRC)

Radiotherapy

The risk of local recurrence of rectal cancer following surgery correlates with the presence of microscopic tumor cells within 1 mm of the *circumferential resection margin* (CRM) (Quirke et al., 1986; Nagtegaal et al., 2002). *External beam megavoltage radiotherapy* can be administered to sterilize the surgical field and has therefore established a role in the treatment of rectal cancer as an adjunct to definitive surgery. There is no established role for adjuvant radiotherapy in the treatment of colon cancer.

The three adjuvant radiotherapy regimens in common practice are:

1 short course preoperative radiation
2 long course preoperative CRT
3 long course postoperative CRT.

If a rectal cancer is considered operable at the outset, then a short course of radiotherapy may be given prior to surgery to reduce the risk of local recurrence. If a rectal cancer is considered to be inoperable or only potentially operable, then a long course of rectal radiotherapy, with or without chemo-therapy, is given to downsize the tumor and increase the chance of a clear resection margin.

The 'operability' of a rectal cancer is determined by a pelvic magnetic resonance imaging (MRI) scan. A large European multicenter prospective study (MERCURY study) has demonstrated that MRI scans can accurately measure the depth of extramural tumor spread to within 0.5 mm (MERCURY, 2007). It is essential that each patient has a pelvic MRI scan which is discussed at a multidisciplinary meeting prior to commencing treatment to determine the optimal sequencing of the multimodality treatment. Patients are selected for *long course preoperative radiotherapy* (with or without chemotherapy) if there is felt to be a high chance that the surgeon will not be able to perform a curative (R0) resection based on the following findings on the pelvic MRI scan:

1 primary tumor involving or extending beyond the mesorectal fascia
2 primary tumor within 2 mm of the mesorectal fascia
3 involved regional lymph nodes outside of the mesorectal fascia.

Should the primary tumor be contained at least 2 mm from the mesorectal fascia, a *short course preoperative radiotherapy* can be considered.

Short course preoperative radiotherapy

The principal aim of short course preoperative radiotherapy is to sterilize any microscopic spread from an operable primary tumor that appears well contained within the mesorectum on MRI scan, thereby reducing the risk of local recurrence.

The Northwest Cancer Group published a randomized study evaluating a short course of preoperative radiotherapy for patients with tethered or fixed tumors (Marsh et al., 1994). A recurrence rate of 36.5% with surgery alone was significantly reduced to 12.8% by the addition of 20 Gy in 4 fractions ($P = 0.0001$). A survival advantage was demonstrated in the radiotherapy arm for patients that had a curative resection (53.3% versus 44.9% at 8 years, $P = 0.033$).

The well-quoted 'Swedish' study randomized 1168 patients planned for surgery to a short course preoperative radiotherapy regimen of 25 Gy in 5 fractions or surgery alone (Anonymous, 1997). An improvement in local recurrence rate (11% versus 27%; $P < 0.001$) and a 10% absolute improvement in 5-year survival (48% versus 58%; $P = 0.004$) was demonstrated.

The practice of *total mesorectal excision* (TME) has also led to improved local recurrence rates. The 'Dutch' study compared the benefits of TME with or without preoperative radiotherapy (Kapiteijn et al., 2001). A total of 1861 operable patients were randomized to receive preoperative radiotherapy (25 Gy in 5 fractions) followed by TME or TME alone. The local recurrence at 2 years was significantly lower in the radiotherapy arm (2.8% versus 8.2%; $P < 0.001$) but overall survival was the same (82% for both groups).

The MRC CR07 trial randomly assigned 1350 patients with operable rectal cancer stage I to III to preoperative short-course radiotherapy (25 Gy in 5 fractions over 1 week) or surgery alone (Sebag-Montefiore et al., 2006). Patients in the surgery alone arm underwent postoperative chemoradiotherapy (45 Gy in 25 fractions with concomitant infusional 5-fluorouracil (5-FU)) if the resected specimen had positive circumferential margins. Compared to selective postoperative radiotherapy, preoperative radiotherapy reduced local recurrence from 11% to 5%. As expected, local recurrence rates were lower in the 596 patients who underwent optimal surgery with a total mesorectal excision (TME). In this group, local recurrence reduced from 6% with selective postoperative radiotherapy to 1% with preoperative radiotherapy. There was no difference in overall survival.

The benefits in local control demonstrated by these studies must be balanced against long-term toxicity from this *hypofractionated regimen* in the large numbers of patients with operable, good prognosis rectal cancer. Both the Dutch and Swedish studies have demonstrated increased incidence of bowel dysfunction in the irradiated group compared with surgery alone (Peeters et al., 2005; Birgisson et al., 2005). The Swedish group have also shown an increased incidence of second malignancies in the irradiated group (Birgisson et al., 2005). The early Northwest Cancer Group study demonstrated the benefit of using a lower dose regimen of 20 Gy in 4 fractions preoperatively (Marsh et al., 1994). A more recent retrospective audit from the Northwest group has suggested that delivering the lower dose regimen preoperatively to a smaller treatment volume than adopted in the Swedish and Dutch trials provides comparable local recurrence rates in patients with operable rectal cancer (Saunders et al., 2006).

Long-course radiotherapy

The rationale behind long-course radiotherapy is to downsize the primary tumor that breaches the CRM on MRI scan to increase the chance of a R0 resection and thus reduce the risk of local recurrence in inoperable or potentially operable cancers. In contrast to short-course preoperative radiotherapy where the surgery usually takes place within 10 days of the final fraction, a longer gap is required after long-course radiotherapy to allow for maximal shrinkage of the tumor.

The MRC CR02 trial showed a 10% reduction in local recurrence when surgery was preceded by radiotherapy (40 Gy in 20 fractions) in potentially operable rectal cancers (5 year local recurrence 36% versus 46%, $P = 0.04$) (MRCRCWP, 1996). A more recent Cochrane meta-analysis assessing the role of preoperative radiotherapy in rectal cancer confirmed an improvement in local control with greater benefits in patients treated with a *biologically equivalent dose* (BED) of >30 Gy (Wong et al., 2007). The addition of chemotherapy to long-course radiotherapy has been shown to improve locoregional control. This was first demonstrated in the NSABP-02 trial randomizing patients with Dukes B or Dukes C rectal cancer to postoperative chemotherapy alone or concomitant long course postoperative CRT (Wolmark et al., 2000). A reduction in locoregional relapse from 13% in the chemotherapy arm to 8% in the CRT arm led to postoperative CRT becoming the standard adjuvant treatment of rectal cancer in North America (NIH, 1990). The EORTC 22921 trial randomly assigned patients with clinical stage T3 or T4 resectable rectal cancer to receive one of four regimens:

- Preoperative radiotherapy
- Preoperative chemoradiotherapy
- Preoperative radiotherapy and postoperative chemotherapy
- Preoperative chemoradiotherapy and postoperative chemotherapy.

Radiotherapy consisted of 45 Gy in 5 weeks. Two courses of chemotherapy (5-FU 350 mg/m^2 per day and leucovorin 20 mg/m^2 per day for 5 days) were combined with preoperative radiotherapy and four courses were used for adjuvant postoperative chemotherapy. With a median follow-up of 5.4 years, overall survival was comparable in all four groups. The 5-year cumulative incidence rates for local recurrences were 8.7%, 9.6% and 7.6% in the groups that received chemotherapy preoperatively, postoperatively, or both, respectively, and 17.1% in the group that did not receive chemotherapy ($P = 0.002$) (Bosset et al., 2006).

The German Rectal Cancer Study Group directly compared preoperative long-course chemoradiotherapy to postoperative chemoradiotherapy. *Preoperative chemoradiotherapy* resulted in reduced 5-year local recurrence (6% versus 13%, $P = 0.006$) and fewer grade 3 or 4 acute toxicities (27% versus 40%, $P = 0.001$) and late toxicities (14% versus 24%, $P = 0.01$) compared to *postoperative chemoradiotherapy* (Sauer et al., 2004).

Chemotherapy

Meta-analyses have shown that chemotherapy for advanced CRC can slow progression and prolong disease survival compared with best supportive care (Simmonds, 2000, Anonymous, 2000). For nearly 50 years, *5-fluorouracil (5-FU)* has been the mainstay of chemotherapy treatment for CRC and fluoropyrimidine-based chemotherapy remains a key component of the treatment algorithm for advanced disease. Indeed, until 10 years ago, 5-FU was the only chemotherapy option available to patients. 5-FU administered as a continuous infusion has superior efficacy when compared with 5-FU administered as an intravenous (IV) bolus (RR 22% versus 14%) (Anonymous, 1998a) and is associated with fewer World Health Organization grade 3 and 4 toxicities (Anonymous, 1998b).

Oral fluoropyrimidines, such as capecitabine and tegafur/uracil (UFT) are converted to 5-FU through various enzymatic conversions. Randomized trials (Hoff et al., 2001; Douillard et al., 2002; Carmichael et al., 2002; Van Cutsem et al., 2004a) have shown equivalence to bolus 5-FU/folinic acid (FA) but have not compared oral fluoropyrimidines to infusional 5-FU. Oral fluoropyrimidines now offer the patient a more convenient form of chemotherapy compared to single-agent infusional or bolus 5-FU.

Optimal 5-FU-based therapy for the treatment of advanced CRC lies in its combination with newer agents with non-overlapping toxicity profiles, such as the topoisomerase I inhibitor *irinotecan* and the third-generation platinum compound *oxaliplatin*.

The addition of irinotecan to 5-FU/FA, irrespective of regimen, conferred a significant clinical benefit, in terms of *response rate* (RR), *progression-free survival* (PFS) and *overall survival* (14.8 versus 12.6, 20.1 versus 16.9, 17.4 versus 14.1 months) compared with the corresponding 5-FU/FA regimen alone (respectively for Saltz et al., 2000; Douillard et al., 2000; Kohne et al., 2005), although it was associated with a higher incidence of grade 3 diarrhea.

Oxaliplatin is also effective first-line in the treatment of advanced CRC when combined with 5-FU (Giacchetti et al., 2000; de Gramont et al., 2007). RRs and median PFS times were longer in the oxaliplatin/5-FU/FA arms compared to the 5-FU/FA alone arms. However, median overall survival was not increased in the oxaliplatin arms. This may be attributable to cross-over from the 5-FU/FA to the oxaliplatin/5-FU/FA arms. The principal *dose-limiting toxicities* are neurotoxicity (which may be acute or chronic) and neutropenia (Grothey and Goldberg, 2004).

The relative efficacy of these two regimens was directly compared in the randomized Tournigand trial (Tournigand et al., 2004). Patients were randomized to one of two treatment arms. Those in arm A received FOLFIRI (irinotecan 180 mg/m^2 and FA 200 mg/m^2 on day 1, followed by bolus 5-FU 400 mg/m^2 and continuous 5-FU, 2400–3000 mg/m^2, by 46-hour infusion) until disease progression or unacceptable toxicity, at which time they crossed over to receive oxaliplatin (100 mg/m^2 on day 1) in combination with the same modified de Gramont 5-FU/FA regimen (FOLFOX6). Conversely, the patients assigned to arm B received FOLFOX6 until disease progression, at which time they crossed over to receive FOLFIRI. The median overall survival was 21.5 months in arm A (FOLFIRI followed by FOLFOX6) and 20.6 months for patients assigned to arm B (FOLFOX6 followed by FOLFIRI), leading to the conclusion that the two regimens were essentially indistinguishable in terms of efficacy. However, it was noted that a significantly higher number of patients in arm B had their metastatic disease rendered resectable ($P = 0.02$). The most important observation from the Tournigand study was therefore that median survival was in excess of 20 months for both arms when the two combinations were used sequentially (i.e. the use of three active drugs during the course of the patient's treatment).

The UK MRC CR08 FOCUS trial was designed to assess the role of irinotecan or oxaliplatin combined with the modified de Gramont (MdG) infusional 5-FU/FA regimen, in the first- and second-line treatment of patients with advanced CRC. Patients with good performance status were randomly allocated to receive either *single agent chemotherapy* first line followed by *combination chemotherapy* at failure or combination chemotherapy upfront. Nonsignificant increases in overall survival were seen with each combination therapy over the staged single-agent arm (Seymour, 2005). This suggests that staged combination therapy may provide an alternative treatment strategy for those patients unable to tolerate first-line combinations. The optimum duration of treatment was assessed in the CR06 study (Maughan et al., 2003). After 12 weeks (6 cycles) of chemotherapy, patients with evidence of response or stable disease were randomized to stopping treatment, restarting with the same regimen on progression or continuing chemotherapy until progression. The study showed no benefit in continuing chemotherapy indefinitely and patients in the intermittent group had significantly fewer toxicities and adverse events.

Targeted agents

As our knowledge of tumor biology and genetics matures, a range of agents that interact with novel disease-associated targets are emerging into the clinical setting. Two drugs already approved for the treatment of CRC are the monoclonal antibodies cetuximab (Erbitux®), which binds to and inhibits activation of the epidermal growth factor receptor (EGFR) (Li et al., 2005), and bevacizumab (Avastin®), which binds vascular endothelial growth factor (VEGF-A) thereby interfering with signaling through the VEGF-1 and -2 receptors and inhibiting angiogenesis (Hicklin and Ellis, 2005).

Cetuximab has been approved in both Europe and the USA for use in combination with irinotecan, as second-line therapy in CRC patients who have failed prior irinotecan treatment. In the pivotal study, Cunningham and colleagues (Cunningham et al., 2004) randomized previously-treated patients who had progressed during or immediately following irinotecan-based therapy into two groups which received either cetuximab plus irinotecan or cetuximab alone. They demonstrated a higher RR (22.9% versus 10.8%) and an increase in the median time to progression (4.1 versus 1.5 months) for the combination-therapy group compared to the monotherapy group. More recently, single agent cetuximab has been shown to improve overall survival compared to best supportive care in patients with advanced colorectal cancer who had previously been treated with a fluoropyrimidine, irinotecan and oxaliplatin or had contraindications to treatment with these drugs (hazard ratio for death, 0.77; 95% confidence interval [CI], 0.64 to 0.92; $P = 0.005$) (Jonker et al., 2007). The importance of determining the K-ras status of CRC prior to treatment with cetuximab has been demonstrated. Recent studies showed that patients with a colorectal tumor bearing mutated K-ras did not benefit from cetuximab, whereas patients with a tumor bearing wild-type K-ras did benefit (Karapetis et al., 2008; Van Cutsem et al., 2009).

Cetuximab does not appear to increase the intensity or frequency of the characteristic *side effects of cytotoxic chemotherapy*. The most common cetuximab related adverse event reported is the development of an acne-like rash. This class effect of EGFR inhibitors is generally manageable (Segaert et al., 2005) and may be indicative of a response to cetuximab (Van Cutsem et al., 2004b).

Bevacizumab in combination with irinotecan/bolus 5-FU/FA has been approved for the first-line therapy of patients with advanced CRC based on the data from the Hurwitz trial (Hurwitz et al., 2004). Adding bevacizumab to a bolus irinotecan/5-FU regimen resulted in an improved median duration of survival (20.3 versus 15.6 months), an increased RR (44.8% versus 34.8%) and a longer median progression free survival (10.6 versus 6.2 months). Similarly, the second-line use of bevacizumab in combination with oxaliplatin/5-FU (FOLFOX) has shown a statistically significant survival advantage versus FOLFOX alone (12.5 versus 10.7 months) (Giantonio et al., 2005).

The use of bevacizumab has been associated with a low level of gastrointestinal perforation events (Kozloff et al., 2006) and some concern has been expressed as to whether anti-VEGF therapy might inhibit wound healing (Scappaticci et al., 2005). This concern led to the recommendation that a patient should not undergo elective hepatic resection during or within 8 weeks of bevacizumab treatment (Ellis et al., 2005).

Adjuvant treatment

Adjuvant treatment is aimed at preventing disease recurrence or increasing the time to relapse after a patient has undergone a curative resection of their tumor. Randomized trials from North America and Europe have demonstrated a 6–10% absolute improvement in overall survival for patients receiving adjuvant 5-FU based chemotherapy with Dukes C disease and a 2–5% benefit in Dukes B disease (Wolmark et al., 1988, 1993; Moertel et al., 1995; IMPACT, 1995; O'Connell et al., 1997; Gray et al., 2007). Common practice is to offer adjuvant chemotherapy postoperatively to all patients with Dukes C disease and 'high-risk' Dukes B disease (Dukes B tumors with evidence of tumor perforation, serosal involvement and/or vascular invasion, and patients who underwent non-elective emergency surgery).

Until recently, the standard therapy most widely used in the UK was a weekly bolus 5-FU/FA regimen, as pioneered in the QUASAR trial (Gray et al., 2007). The X-ACT study comparing capecitabine to bolus 5-FU/FA in patients with resected stage III CRC (Twelves et al., 2005) showed equivalent disease-free survival. The MOSAIC study aimed to show that the addition of oxaliplatin to a conventional 5-FU/FA regimen was beneficial to patients in the adjuvant setting (Andre et al., 2004). Patients who had undergone curative resection for stage II or III CRC were randomized to an infusional 5-FU/FA regimen with or without oxaliplatin (FOLFOX). The DFS at three years was 78.2% in the oxaliplatin group, compared to 72.9% for 5-FU/FA group ($P = 0.002$). A recent update has shown a significant benefit in overall survival (OS) for stage III patients at 6 years (hazard ratio for death, 0.80; 95% confidence interval [CI], 0.66 to 0.98) (de Gramont et al., 2007). However, there was not OS benefit for patients with stage II disease. A recent phase III study showed no advantage of adding bevacizumab to adjuvant FOLFOX chemotherapy in stage II or III CRC (3 year DFS 75.5% for FOLFOX vs 77.4% for FOLFOX and bevacizumab, hazard ratio, 0.89; 95% CI, 0.76–1.04) (Wolmark et al., 2009).

The convenience of *adjuvant oral capecitabine chemotherapy* has led to a phasing out of the previously standard weekly 5-FU regimen. The improved efficacy of the combination FOLFOX regimen provides another option for the clinician and patient at the cost of increased toxicity in the adjuvant setting.

Anal cancer

The treatment of anal carcinoma with CRT has evolved dramatically over the last 20 years with a drift from surgical resection (abdominoperineal resection (APR)) to a combination of radiotherapy and chemotherapy.

In 1987, a multicenter anal cancer trial (ACT I) was set up by the UK Coordinating Committee on Cancer Research (UKCCR) to compare the most promising regimens of radiotherapy alone with combined modality therapy. Five hundred and eighty-five patients were randomized to receive either 45 Gy radiotherapy (RT) over 4–5 weeks (n = 290) or the same RT combined with *mitomycin* (MMC)/5-FU. Patients who had a good response after 6 weeks underwent a further radiotherapy boost; patients who had not responded after 6 weeks underwent salvage surgery. *Combined chemoradiotherapy* showed a 46% reduction in local failure after a median survival of 42 months, although there was increased early morbidity and no survival advantage (58% with RT versus 65% with chemoradiotherapy after 3 years, $P = 0.25$) (UKCCCR, 1996). The EORTC conducted a similar trial also demonstrating a significant increase in locoregional control (18% improvement at 5 years) and colostomy free survival (32% improvement at 5 years) with chemoradiotherapy compared to radiotherapy alone (Bartelink et al., 1997).

The ACT II trial randomized patients to RT totalling 50.4 Gy in 28 fractions together with either 5-FU/MMC or 5-FU/cisplatin during the first and fifth weeks of RT. Patients are also further randomized to two courses of chemotherapy or just follow up after CMT. There was no difference in the complete response rate between concurrent 5-FU/MMC or 5-FU/cisplatin

(94% vs 95%, $P = 0.53$) and no difference in recurrence free survival (HR 0.89, 95% CI 0.68 to 1.18; $P = 0.42$) or overall survival (HR 0.79, 95% CI 0.56 to 1.12; $P = 0.19$) with the addition of maintenance chemotherapy (James et al., 2009).

The recently published RTOG 98-11 study has questioned the efficacy of RT and 5-FU/CDDP in the treatment of anal cancer (Ajani et al., 2008). This multicenter phase III study randomized patients to either 5-FU ($1000\,mg/m^2$ on days 1–4 and 29–32) plus MMC ($10\,mg/m^2$ on days 1 and 29) and RT (45–59 Gy starting on day 1) or 5-FU ($1000\,mg/m^2$ on days 1–4, 29–32, 57–60 and 85–88) plus cisplatin ($75\,mg/m^2$ on days 1, 29, 57 and 85) and RT (45–59 Gy starting on day 57). There was no difference between the two arms in disease-free survival, overall survival, locoregional control and distant metastasis rates. The cumulative rate of colostomy was significantly better for mitomycin-based than cisplatin-based treatment (10% versus 19%; $P=0.02$). However, this was not a direct comparison of mitomycin/5-FU versus cisplatin/5-FU as the cisplatin arm incorporated two cycles of induction chemotherapy prior to starting RT. Induction chemotherapy may have resulted in accelerated repopulation and an increase in the number of clonogens at the onset of radiation in the cisplatin arm. The ACT II study does not incorporate induction chemotherapy in either arm and the results of ACT II should help clarify the optimum chemo-RT regimen for anal carcinomas.

Upper GI malignancy

Esophageal cancer

Carcinoma of the esophagus can be treated with definitive surgery, CRT or radiotherapy alone. For patients with *operable tumors*, standard practice in the UK is to offer two cycles of *neoadjuvant cisplatin/5-FU chemotherapy* based on the OE02 trial. Eight hundred and two patients with operable esophageal cancer were randomly assigned to resection alone or resection preceded by two courses of cisplatin ($80\,mg/m^2$ on day 1) and 5-FU ($1000\,mg/m^2$ by continuous infusion days 1 to 4) given three weeks apart. *Preoperative chemotherapy* was associated with significantly greater overall survival (hazard ratio for mortality 0.79, 95% confidence interval, 0.67 to 0.93), two-year survival (43% versus 34% percent) and median survival (16.8 versus 13.3 months) (OE02, 2002). The current MRC OE05 phase III study is comparing four cycles of neoadjuvant epirubicin, cisplatin and capecitabine to the standard OE02 regimen preoperatively. In the United States Intergroup trial 0113, 467 patients with potentially resectable esophageal or gastro-esophageal (GOJ) junction cancer were randomly assigned to surgery alone or three cycles of preoperative cisplatin/5-FU chemotherapy followed by surgery (Kelsen et al., 1998). There was no difference between the groups in survival at one, two or three years (59%, 35% and 23% versus 60%, 37% and 26% percent, respectively). The OE02 and Intergroup trials had populations with very similar pretreatment characteristics. The different outcomes may partly be explained by the difference in dose intensities and time to definitive surgery between the studies. The Intergroup trial used three cycles of cisplatin/5-FU compared to two cycles in the OE02 study. In using a less demanding regimen than the Intergroup trial, more patients completed the full course of preoperative chemotherapy in the

OE02 study (80% versus 71%) and the time to surgery after completion of the chemotherapy was shorter (median 63 days versus 93 days).

There is evidence to suggest that a *concurrent trimodality approach* (concomitant CRT followed by surgery) provides a survival benefit compared to surgery alone. An Irish trial randomly assigned patients with esophageal or GOJ adenocarcinoma to surgery alone or preceded by CRT (Walsh et al., 1996). Preoperative treatment consisted of radiotherapy (40 Gy in 15 fractions over three weeks) and two courses of cisplatin/5-FU starting on day one of the radiotherapy regimen. CRT was associated with significantly longer median survival (16 versus 11 months, $P = 0.01$) and three-year survival (32% versus 6%, $P = 0.01$). These results were criticized because of the lower than expected survival with surgery alone.

The only trial directly to compare induction chemoradiotherapy to chemotherapy alone was the multicenter German POET (Preoperative chemotherapy or radiochemotherapy in esophagogastric adenocarcinoma trial), which focused exclusively on GOJ adenocarcinomas. Patients were randomly assigned to 16 weeks of cisplatin/5-FU chemotherapy alone or 12 weeks of the same chemotherapy regimen followed by radiotherapy (30 Gy over three weeks) concurrent with cisplatin (50 mg/m^2 on days 2 and 8) and etoposide (80 mg/m^2 on days 3 to 5) (Stahl et al., 2007). The trial was closed early because of poor accrual. In a preliminary report with a median follow-up of 46 months, patients undergoing CRT had better median survival (33 versus 21 months) and three-year survival (47% versus 28%, $P = 0.07$), but these potentially clinically meaningful differences were not statistically significant.

For *bulky and borderline unresectable tumors*, chemotherapy alone may not achieve sufficient downstaging. Definitive radiotherapy alone has been reported to give 5-year survivals of less than 10% and median survivals ranging from 6 to 12 months (Sun, 1989; Okawa et al., 1989; Araujo et al., 1991; Wan et al., 1991; Sykes et al., 1998). The Radiation Therapy Oncology Group (RTOG) 85-01 trial was the landmark trial that established the superiority of chemoradiation over radiation alone (Herskovic et al., 1992). Patients were randomized to receive either CRT with 50 Gy in 25 fractions, 5 days per week and concurrent adjuvant cisplatin/5-FU or 64 Gy in 32 fractions of radiotherapy without chemotherapy. The 5-year survival rate was 27% in the combined therapy arm compared with 0% in the control arm ($P < 0.0001$). In the Intergroup Study 0123, all 236 patients received concurrent chemotherapy with cisplatin and 5-FU (as in RTOG 85-01), but they were randomly assigned to one of two different RT doses: 50.4 Gy (28 fractions of 1.8 Gy each, 5 fractions per week) or 64.8 Gy (36 fractions of 1.8 Gy each, 5 fractions per week). Higher radiotherapy doses were not associated with a higher median survival (13 months [95% confidence interval, 10.5 to 19.1 months] versus 18 months [95% confidence interval, 15.4 to 23.1 months]). High-dose radiotherapy was associated with significantly more toxicity (Minsky et al., 2002). The UK SCOPE trial is currently recruiting patients to determine the role of the EGFR inhibitor cetuximab in combination with definitive, RTOG 85-01 type CRT for inoperable esophageal cancer.

Stomach cancer

Surgery remains the definitive treatment for gastric cancer. The standard adjuvant approaches vary between Europe and North America. Practice in the UK has been influenced by the MAGIC trial. Five hundred and three patients with potentially resectable gastric, distal esophageal or GOJ adeno-carcinomas were randomly assigned to surgery alone or surgery plus peri-operative chemotherapy (three preoperative and three postoperative cycles of epirubicin, cisplatin and infusional 5-fluorouracil (ECF)). Only 42% of patients were able to complete protocol treatment, including surgery and all three cycles of the postoperative chemotherapy. Nevertheless, with median four-year follow-up, progression-free survival was significantly worse in the surgery alone group (hazard ratio [HR] for progression 0.66, 95 percent confidence interval, 0.53 to 0.81; $P < 0.001$) as was overall survival (HR for death 0.75, 95% confidence interval, 0.60 to 0.93, $P = 0.009$). The 25% reduction in the risk of death favoring chemotherapy translated into an improvement in five-year survival from 23% to 36% ($P = 0.009$) (Cunningham et al., 2006). The US Intergroup study INT-0116 randomly assigned 556 patients follow-ing potentially curative resection of gastric cancer to observation alone or adjuvant combined CRT (Macdonald et al., 2001). Treatment consisted of one cycle of 5-FU and leucovorin daily for five days, followed one month later by 45 Gy (1.8 Gy/day) radiotherapy given with 5-FU and leucovorin on days 1 to 4 and on the last three days of radiotherapy. Two more five-day cycles of che-motherapy were given at monthly intervals beginning one month after com-pletion of radiotherapy. Three-year disease-free (48% versus 31%, $P < 0.001$) and overall survival rates (50% versus 41%) were significantly better with combined modality therapy and median survival was significantly longer (36 versus 27 months, $P = 0.005$). Grade 3 and 4 toxic effects occurred in 41% and 32% of the CRT group, respectively, while three patients (1%) died from treatment-related toxic effects. These results changed the standard of care in the USA following potentially curative resection of gastric cancer from obser-vation alone to surgery followed by adjuvant combined CRT.

A criticism of the American Intergroup trial was the limited extent of the surgical procedure in most cases. Although D2 lymph node dissection (removal of nodes along the hepatic, left gastric, celiac and splenic arteries as well as those in the splenic hilum) was recommended in the protocol, it was only performed in 10% of the patients and 54% did not have clearance of the D1 (perigastric) nodal regions. As a significant proportion of patients did not receive optimal surgery, the CRT may have been simply compensating for poor surgical resection. However, the study was randomized and the surgi-cal limitations would have influenced both arms equally.

In the USA, the on-going Cancer and Leukemia Group B phase III study (80101) is comparing pre- and post-radiotherapy bolus 5-FU to ECF chemo-therapy, both arms having radiotherapy (45 Gy) with infusional 5-FU. In the UK, the MAGIC 2 trial is comparing pre- and postoperative epirubicin, cispl-atin and capecitabine chemotherapy (ECX) with and without bevacizumab.

Palliative chemotherapy improves survival in advanced gastric cancers (Murad et al., 1993; Pyrhonen et al., 1995; Glimelius et al., 1997). Two random-ized studies and a meta-analysis support the use of the epirubicin, cisplatin and infusional 5-FU regimen (ECF) often used first line for advanced gas-tric cancer (Webb et al., 1997; Ross et al., 2002; Wagner et al., 2006). A recent study has shown a regimen using epirubicin, oxaliplatin and oral capecit-abine (EOX) is as effective as ECF (Cunningham et al., 2008). The authors suggest that EOX is a more convenient regimen for the patient as the oral capecitabine is at least as effective as the infusional 5-FU and the oxaliplatin (which does not require hydration) is at least as effective as cisplatin (which does require hydration).

Pancreatic cancer

Systemic chemotherapy, RT or a combination of chemotherapy and RT have all been applied following surgery in an effort to improve outcome in patients undergoing potentially curative (R0) resection of exocrine pancreatic cancers. The European Study Group for Pancreatic Cancer 1 Trial (ESPAC 1) was a 2×2 factorial design trial with four groups: adjuvant CRT, adjuvant chemotherapy, adjuvant CRT followed by chemotherapy, or surgery alone. Chemoradiotherapy consisted of 20 Gy radiotherapy plus three days of concomitant 5-FU, repeated after a planned break of two weeks. *Adjuvant chemotherapy* consisted of bolus leucovorin-modulated 5-FU (leucovorin 20 mg/m^2, 5-FU 425 mg/m^2), administered daily for five days, every 28 days, for six months. Adjuvant chemotherapy demonstrated a survival benefit compared to surgery alone (5-year survival 21% versus 8%, $P = 0.009$). *Postoperative CRT* was found to be detrimental with an estimated five-year survival rate of 10% among patients assigned to receive CRT and 20% among patients who did not receive CRT ($P = 0.05$) (Neoptolemos et al., 2004). The ESPAC 3 trial is currently randomizing patients to surgery alone or surgery followed by gemcitabine chemotherapy or surgery followed by 5-FU chemotherapy. Results are awaited.

The guidelines on 'good practice' in the UK from the NHS Executive recommends that chemoradiotherapy and not radiation alone may be considered for 'fit' patients *with inoperable locally advanced pancreatic cancer* (Department of Health, 2001). The evidence of benefit for CRT over radiation alone in the treatment of locally advanced pancreatic cancer was provided by the gastrointestinal tumor study group (GITSG.) They demonstrated a small advantage in survival of 3–4 months with chemoradiotherapy compared to radiotherapy alone. One-year survival was 40% with CRT and 10% with RT alone (Moertel et al., 1981). Current practice is to use radiotherapy in combination with 5-FU or capecitabine. Several phase II trials recruiting in the UK are assessing the role of targeted agents in combination with radiotherapy for treating inoperable pancreatic cancer.

Palliative chemotherapy is the treatment of choice for metastatic pancreatic cancers. This approach is also used for locally advanced disease not suitable for CRT. Single agent *gemcitabine* (1000 mg/m^2 weekly for seven weeks followed by a week of rest, then weekly for three out of every four weeks) has shown improved 1-year survival over 5-FU (600 mg/m^2 weekly) (18% versus 2%) (Burris et al., 1997). A multinational phase III trial comparing gemcitabine alone to gemcitabine and capecitabine showed no significant benefit in overall survival (7.2 versus 8.4 months, $P = 0.234$). Unplanned subgroup analysis did show a significant benefit in overall survival (10.1 versus 7.4, $P = 0.014$) with gemcitabine/capecitabine versus gemcitabine alone in patients with a good performance score (Karnofsky performance score 90 to 100) (Herrmann et al., 2007). In contrast, gemcitabine in combination with cisplatin has been shown to improve overall survival in advanced or metastatic biliary tract cancer (ABC) compared to gemcitabine alone (median OS 11.7 vs 8.2 months, $P = 0.002$) (Valle et al., 2009).

Future directions

The future treatment of GI malignancies will be influenced by further developments in *targeted molecular therapies*. As an alternative to cytotoxic chemotherapy, the novel agents have a different and often less severe toxicity profile. When combined with conventional cytotoxic chemotherapy and/or radiotherapy, there is often only limited increase in the overall toxicity of a treatment. The targeted therapies are currently being investigated in large, phase III multicenter studies for both upper and lower GI malignancies.

With the advent of *intensity modulated radiotherapy* (IMRT) allowing for more conformal shaping of a treatment volume and *image guided radiotherapy* (IGRT) resulting in more accurate treatment delivery, toxicity from radiotherapy dose to normal tissues should be reduced. Future studies in dose escalation in upper and lower GI malignancies should incorporate IMRT and IGRT to ensure acute and late toxicities are kept to a minimum.

Conclusions

Chemotherapy and radiotherapy are integral to the multimodality approach essential for the effective treatment of GI malignancies. A multidisciplinary team approach is critical, not only to ensure the patient receives the optimum treatment for their disease but also the appropriate support in dealing with the physical and psychological impact of both the disease and its treatment with chemotherapy and radiotherapy.

References

Anonymous, 1997. Improved survival with preoperative radiotherapy in resectable rectal cancer. Swedish Rectal Cancer Trial. N. Engl. J. Med. 336, 980–987.

Anonymous, 1998a. Efficacy of intravenous continuous infusion of fluorouracil compared with bolus administration in advanced colorectal cancer. Meta-analysis Group In Cancer. J. Clin. Oncol. 16, 301–308.

Anonymous, 1998b. Toxicity of fluorouracil in patients with advanced colorectal cancer: effect of administration schedule and prognostic factors. Meta-Analysis Group In Cancer. J. Clin. Oncol. 16, 3537–3541.

Anonymous, 2000. Palliative chemotherapy for advanced or metastatic colorectal cancer. Colorectal Meta-analysis Collaboration. Cochrane Database Syst. Rev. CD001545.

Ajani, J.A., Winter, K.A., Gunderson, L.L., et al., 2008. Fluorouracil, mitomycin, and radiotherapy vs fluorouracil, cisplatin, and radiotherapy for carcinoma of the anal canal: a randomized controlled trial. J. Am. Med. Assoc. 299, 1914–1921.

Andre, T., Boni, C., Mounedji-Boudiaf, L., et al., 2004. Oxaliplatin, fluorouracil, and leucovorin as adjuvant treatment for colon cancer. N. Engl. J. Med. 350, 2343–2351.

Araujo, C.M., Souhami, L., Gil, R.A., et al., 1991. A randomized trial comparing radiation therapy versus concomitant radiation therapy and chemotherapy in carcinoma of the thoracic esophagus. Cancer 67, 2258–2261.

Bartelink, H., Roelofsen, F., Eschwege, F., et al., 1997. Concomitant radiotherapy and chemotherapy is superior to radiotherapy alone in the treatment of locally advanced anal cancer: results of a phase III randomized trial of the European Organization for Research and Treatment of Cancer Radiotherapy and Gastrointestinal Cooperative Groups. J. Clin. Oncol. 15, 2040–2049.

Birgisson, H., Pahlman, L., Gunnarsson, U., et al., 2005. Adverse effects of preoperative radiation therapy for rectal cancer: long-term follow-up of the Swedish Rectal Cancer Trial. J. Clin. Oncol. 23, 8697–8705.

Bosset, J.F., Collette, L., Calais, G., et al., 2006. Chemotherapy with preoperative radiotherapy in rectal cancer. N. Engl. J. Med. 355, 1114–1123.

Burris, H.A. 3rd, Moore, M.J., Andersen, J., et al., 1997. Improvements in survival and clinical benefit with gemcitabine as first-line therapy for patients with advanced pancreas cancer: a randomized trial. J. Clin. Oncol. 15, 2403–2413.

Carmichael, J., Popiela, T., Radstone, D., et al., 2002. Randomized comparative study of tegafur/uracil and oral leucovorin versus parenteral fluorouracil and leucovorin in patients with previously untreated metastatic colorectal cancer. J. Clin. Oncol. 20, 3617–3627.

Cunningham, D., Allum, W.H., Stenning, S.P., et al., 2006. Perioperative chemotherapy versus surgery alone for resectable gastroesophageal cancer. N. Engl. J. Med. 355, 11–20.

Cunningham, D., Humblet, Y., Siena, S., et al., 2004. Cetuximab monotherapy and cetuximab plus irinotecan in irinotecan-refractory metastatic colorectal cancer. N. Engl. J. Med. 351, 337–345.

Cunningham, D., Starling, N., Rao, S., et al., 2008. Capecitabine and oxaliplatin for advanced esophagogastric cancer. N. Engl. J. Med. 358, 36–46.

de Gramont, A., Boni, C., Navarro, M., et al., 2007. Oxaliplatin/5FU/LV in adjuvant colon cancer: updated efficacy results of the MOSAIC trial, including survival, with a median follow-up of six years. J. Clin. Oncol., 2007 ASCO Annual Meeting Proceedings Part I 25, 4007.

Department of Health, 2001. Improving outcomes in upper gastro-intestinal cancers. National Executive, London.

Douillard, J.Y., Cunningham, D., Roth, A.D., et al., 2000. Irinotecan combined with fluorouracil compared with fluorouracil alone as first-line treatment for metastatic colorectal cancer: a multicentre randomised trial. Lancet 355, 1041–1047.

Douillard, J.Y., Hoff, P.M., Skillings, J.R., et al., 2002. Multicenter phase III study of uracil/tegafur and oral leucovorin versus fluorouracil and leucovorin in patients with previously untreated metastatic colorectal cancer. J. Clin. Oncol. 20, 3605–3616.

Ellis, L.M., Curley, S.A., Grothey, A., 2005. Surgical resection after downsizing of colorectal liver metastasis in the era of bevacizumab. J. Clin. Oncol. 23, 4853–4855.

Giacchetti, S., Perpoint, B., Zidani, R., et al., 2000. Phase III multicenter randomized trial of oxaliplatin added to chronomodulated fluorouracil-leucovorin as first-line treatment of metastatic colorectal cancer. J. Clin. Oncol. 18, 136–147.

Giantonio, B.J., Catalano, P.J., Meropol, N.J., et al., 2005. High-dose bevacizumab improves survival when combined with FOLFOX4 in previously treated advanced colorectal cancer: results from the Eastern Cooperative Oncology Group (ECOG) study E3200. J. Clin. Oncol. 23, 2.

Glimelius, B., Ekstrom, K., Hoffman, K., et al., 1997. Randomized comparison between chemotherapy plus best supportive care with best supportive care in advanced gastric cancer. Ann. Oncol. 8, 163–168.

Gray, R., Barnwell, J., McConkey, C., et al., 2007. Adjuvant chemotherapy versus observation in patients with colorectal cancer: a randomised study. Lancet 370, 2020–2029.

Grothey, A., Goldberg, R.M., 2004. A review of oxaliplatin and its clinical use in colorectal cancer. Expert Opin. Pharmacother. 5, 2159–2170.

Herrmann, R., Bodoky, G., Ruhstaller, T., et al., 2007. Gemcitabine plus capecitabine compared with gemcitabine alone in advanced pancreatic cancer: a randomized, multicenter, phase III trial of the Swiss Group for Clinical Cancer Research and the Central European Cooperative Oncology Group. J. Clin. Oncol. 25, 2212–2217.

Herskovic, A., Martz, K., al-Sarraf, M., et al., 1992. Combined chemotherapy and radiotherapy compared with radiotherapy alone in patients with cancer of the esophagus. N. Engl. J. Med. 326, 1593–1598.

Hicklin, D.J., Ellis, L.M., 2005. Role of the vascular endothelial growth factor pathway in tumor growth and angiogenesis. J. Clin. Oncol. 23, 1011–1027.

Hoff, P.M., Ansari, R., Batist, G., et al., 2001. Comparison of oral capecitabine versus intravenous fluorouracil plus leucovorin as first-line treatment in 605 patients with metastatic colorectal cancer: results of a randomized phase III study. J. Clin. Oncol. 19, 2282–2292.

Hurwitz, H., Fehrenbacher, L., Novotny, W., et al., 2004. Bevacizumab plus irinotecan, fluorouracil, and leucovorin for metastatic colorectal cancer. N. Engl. J. Med. 350, 2335–2342.

IMPACT, 1995. Efficacy of adjuvant fluorouracil and folinic acid in colon cancer. International Multicentre Pooled Analysis of Colon Cancer Trials (IMPACT) investigators. Lancet 345, 939–944.

James, R., Wan, S., Glynne-Jones, R., et al., 2009. A randomized trial of chemoradiation using mitomycin or cisplatin, with or without maintenance cisplatin/5FU in squamous cell carcinoma of the anus (ACT II). J. Clin. Oncol. 27, 18s (suppl; abstr LBA4009).

Jonker, D.J., O'Callaghan, C.J., Karapetis, C.S., et al., 2007. Cetuximab for the treatment of colorectal cancer. N. Engl. J. Med. 357, 2040–2048.

Kapiteijn, E., Marijnen, C.A., Nagtegaal, I.D., et al., 2001. Preoperative radiotherapy combined with total mesorectal excision for resectable rectal cancer. N. Engl. J. Med. 345, 638–646.

Karapetis, C.S., Khambata-Ford, S., Jonker, D.J., 2008. K-ras mutations and benefit from cetuximab in advanced colorectal cancer. N. Engl. J. Med. 359, 1757–1765.

Kelsen, D.P., Ginsberg, R., Pajak, T.F., et al., 1998. Chemotherapy followed by surgery compared with surgery alone for localized esophageal cancer. N. Engl. J. Med. 339, 1979–1984.

Kohne, C.H., van Cutsem, E., Wils, J., et al., 2005. Phase III study of weekly high-dose infusional fluorouracil plus folinic acid with or without irinotecan in patients with metastatic colorectal cancer: European Organisation for Research and Treatment of Cancer Gastrointestinal Group Study 40986. J. Clin. Oncol. 23, 4856–4865.

Kozloff, M., Cohn, A., Christiansen, N., et al., 2006. Safety of bevacizumab (BV) among patients (pts) receiving first-line chemotherapy for metastatic colorectal cancer: updated results from a large observational study in the US (BRITE). ASCO Gastrointestinal Cancer Symposium abstract 247.

Li, S., Schmitz, K.R., Jeffrey, P.D., et al., 2005. Structural basis for inhibition of the epidermal growth factor receptor by cetuximab. Cancer Cell 7, 301–311.

Macdonald, J.S., Smalley, S.R., Benedetti, J., et al., 2001. Chemoradiotherapy after surgery compared with surgery alone for adenocarcinoma of the stomach or gastroesophageal junction. N. Engl. J. Med. 345, 725–730.

Marsh, P.J., James, R.D., Schofield, P.F., 1994. Adjuvant preoperative radiotherapy for locally advanced rectal carcinoma. Results of a prospective, randomized trial. Dis. Colon Rectum 37, 1205–1214.

Maughan, T.S., James, R.D., Kerr, D.J., et al., 2003. Comparison of intermittent and continuous palliative chemotherapy for advanced colorectal cancer: a multicentre randomised trial. Lancet 361, 457–464.

MERCURY, 2007. Extramural depth of tumor invasion at thin-section MR in patients with rectal cancer: results of the MERCURY study. Radiology 243, 132–139.

Minsky, B.D., Pajak, T.F., Ginsberg, R.J., et al., 2002. INT 0123 (Radiation Therapy Oncology Group 94–05) phase III trial of combined-modality therapy for esophageal cancer: high-dose versus standard-dose radiation therapy. J. Clin. Oncol. 20, 1167–1174.

Moertel, C.G., Fleming, T.R., Macdonald, J.S., et al., 1995. Intergroup study of fluorouracil plus levamisole as adjuvant therapy for stage II/Dukes' B2 colon cancer. J. Clin. Oncol. 13, 2936–2943.

Moertel, C.G., Frytak, S., Hahn, R.G., et al., 1981. Therapy of locally unresectable pancreatic carcinoma: a randomized comparison of high dose (6000 rads) radiation alone, moderate dose radiation (4000 rads + 5-fluorouracil), and high dose radiation + 5-fluorouracil: The Gastrointestinal Tumor Study Group. Cancer 48, 1705–1710.

MRCRCWP, 1996. Randomised trial of surgery alone versus radiotherapy followed by surgery for potentially operable locally advanced rectal cancer. Medical Research Council Rectal Cancer Working Party. Lancet 348, 1605–1610.

Murad, A.M., Santiago, F.F., Petroianu, A., et al., 1993. Modified therapy with 5-fluorouracil, doxorubicin, and methotrexate in advanced gastric cancer. Cancer 72, 37–41.

Nagtegaal, I.D., Marijnen, C.A., Kranenbarg, E.K., et al., 2002. Circumferential margin involvement is still an important predictor of local recurrence in rectal carcinoma: not one millimeter but two millimeters is the limit. Am. J. Surg. Pathol. 26, 350–357.

Neoptolemos, J.P., Stocken, D.D., Friess, H., et al., 2004. A randomized trial of chemoradiotherapy and chemotherapy after resection of pancreatic cancer. N. Engl. J. Med. 350, 1200–1210.

NIH, 1990. NIH consensus conference. Adjuvant therapy for patients with colon and rectal cancer. J. Am. Med. Assoc. 264, 1444–1450.

O'Connell, M.J., Mailliard, J.A., Kahn, M.J., et al., 1997. Controlled trial of fluorouracil and low-dose leucovorin given for 6 months as postoperative adjuvant therapy for colon cancer. J. Clin. Oncol. 15, 246–250.

OE02, 2002. Surgical resection with or without preoperative chemotherapy in oesophageal cancer: a randomised controlled trial. Lancet 359, 1727–1733.

Okawa, T., Kita, M., Tanaka, M., et al., 1989. Results of radiotherapy for inoperable locally advanced esophageal cancer. Int. J. Radiat. Oncol. Biol. Phys. 17, 49–54.

Peeters, K.C., van de Velde, C.J., Leer, J.W., et al., 2005. Late side effects of short-course preoperative radiotherapy combined with total mesorectal excision for rectal cancer: increased bowel dysfunction in irradiated patients – a Dutch colorectal cancer group study. J. Clin. Oncol. 23, 6199–6206.

Pyrhonen, S., Kuitunen, T., Nyandoto, P., et al., 1995. Randomised comparison of fluorouracil, epidoxorubicin and methotrexate (FEMTX) plus supportive care with supportive care alone in patients with non-resectable gastric cancer. Br. J. Cancer 71, 587–591.

Quirke, P., Durdey, P., Dixon, M.F., et al., 1986. Local recurrence of rectal adenocarcinoma due to inadequate surgical resection. Histopathological study of lateral tumour spread and surgical excision. Lancet 2, 996–999.

Ross, P., Nicolson, M., Cunningham, D., et al., 2002. Prospective randomized trial comparing mitomycin, cisplatin, and protracted venous-infusion fluorouracil (PVI 5-FU) With epirubicin, cisplatin, and PVI 5-FU in advanced esophagogastric cancer. J. Clin. Oncol. 20, 1996–2004.

Saltz, L.B., Cox, J.V., Blanke, C., et al., 2000. Irinotecan plus fluorouracil and leucovorin for metastatic colorectal cancer. Irinotecan Study Group. N. Engl. J. Med. 343, 905–914.

Sauer, R., Becker, H., Hohenberger, W., et al., 2004. Preoperative versus postoperative chemoradiotherapy for rectal cancer. N. Engl. J. Med. 351, 1731–1740.

Saunders, M.P., Alderson, H., Chittalia, A., et al., 2006. Preoperative radiotherapy for operable rectal cancer – is a lower dose to a reduced volume acceptable? Clin. Oncol. (Royal College of Radiologists) 18, 594–599.

Scappaticci, F.A., Fehrenbacher, L., Cartwright, T., et al., 2005. Surgical wound healing complications in metastatic colorectal cancer patients treated with bevacizumab. J. Surg. Oncol. 91, 173–180.

Sebag-Montefiore, D., Steele, R., Quirke, P., et al., 2006. Routine short course pre-op radiotherapy or selective post-op chemoradiotherapy for resectable rectal cancer? Preliminary results of the MRC CR07 randomised trial. J. Clin. Oncol., ASCO Annual Meeting Proceedings Part I 24, 3511.

Segaert, S., Tabernero, J., Chosidow, O., et al., 2005. The management of skin reactions in cancer patients receiving epidermal growth factor receptor targeted therapies. J. Dtsch. Dermatol. Ges. 3, 599–606.

Seymour, M.T., 2005. Fluorouracil, oxaliplatin and CPT-11 (irinotecan), use and sequencing (MRC FOCUS): a 2135-patient randomized trial in advanced colorectal cancer (ACRC). J. Clin. Oncol., 2005 ASCO Annual Meeting Proceedings Part I 23, 3518.

Simmonds, P.C., 2000. Palliative chemotherapy for advanced colorectal cancer: systematic review and meta-analysis. Colorectal Cancer Collaborative Group. Br. Med. J. 321, 531–535.

Stahl, M., Walz, M.K., Stuschke, M., et al., 2007. Preoperative chemotherapy (CTX) versus preoperative chemoradiotherapy (CRTX) in locally advanced esophagogastric adenocarcinomas: first results of a randomized phase III trial. J. Clin. Oncol., 2007 ASCO Annual Meeting Proceedings Part I 25, 4511.

Sun, D.R., 1989. Ten-year follow-up of esophageal cancer treated by radical radiation therapy: analysis of 869 patients. Int. J. Radiat. Oncol. Biol. Phys. 16, 329–334.

Sykes, A.J., Burt, P.A., Slevin, N.J., et al., 1998. Radical radiotherapy for carcinoma of the oesophagus: an effective alternative to surgery. Radiother. Oncol. 48, 15–21.

Tournigand, C., Andre, T., Achille, E., et al., 2004. FOLFIRI followed by FOLFOX6 or the reverse sequence in advanced colorectal cancer: a randomised GERCOR study. J. Clin. Oncol. 22, 229–237.

Twelves, C., Wong, A., Nowacki, M.P., et al., 2005. Capecitabine as adjuvant treatment for stage III colon cancer. N. Engl. J. Med. 352, 2696–2704.

UKCCCR, 1996. Epidermoid anal cancer: results from the UKCCCR randomised trial of radiotherapy alone versus radiotherapy, 5-fluorouracil, and mitomycin. UKCCCR Anal Cancer Trial Working Party. UK Coordinating Committee on Cancer Research. Lancet 348, 1049–1054.

Valle, J.W., Wasan, H.S., Palmer, D.D., et al., 2009. Gemcitabine with or without cisplatin in patients (pts) with advanced or metastatic biliary tract cancer (ABC): Results of a multicenter, randomized phase III trial (the UK ABC-02 trial). J. Clin. Oncol. 27, 15s (suppl; abstr 4503).

CHAPTER 23

Van Cutsem, E., Hoff, P.M., Harper, P., et al., 2004a. Oral capecitabine vs intravenous 5-fluorouracil and leucovorin: integrated efficacy data and novel analyses from two large, randomised, phase III trials. Br. J. Cancer 90, 1190–1197.

Van Cutsem, E., Mayer, R.J., Gold, P., et al., 2004b. Correlation of acne rash and tumor response with cetuximab monotherapy in patients with colorectal cancer refractory to both irinotecan and oxaliplatin. EORTC-NCI-AACR Symposium: Abstract 279.

Van Cutsem, E., Kohne, C.-H., Hitre, E., et al., 2009. Cetuximab and chemotherapy as initial treatment for metastatic colorectal cancer. N. Engl. J. Med. 360, 1408–1417.

Wagner, A.D., Grothe, W., Haerting, J., et al., 2006. Chemotherapy in advanced gastric cancer: a systematic review and meta-analysis based on aggregate data. J. Clin. Oncol. 24, 2903–2909.

Walsh, T.N., Noonan, N., Hollywood, D., et al., 1996. A comparison of multimodal therapy and surgery for esophageal adenocarcinoma. N. Engl. J. Med. 335, 462–467.

Wan, J., Guo, B.Z., Gao, S.Z., 1991. Accelerated hyperfractionation radiotherapy in esophageal cancer. An analysis of 172 cases. Chin. Med. J. (Engl.) 104, 228–229.

Webb, A., Cunningham, D., Scarffe, J.H., et al., 1997. Randomized trial comparing epirubicin, cisplatin, and fluorouracil versus fluorouracil, doxorubicin, and methotrexate in advanced esophagogastric cancer. J. Clin. Oncol. 15, 261–267.

Wolmark, N., Fisher, B., Rockette, H., et al., 1988. Postoperative adjuvant chemotherapy or BCG for colon cancer: results from NSABP protocol C-01. J. Natl. Cancer Inst. 80, 30–36.

Wolmark, N., Rockette, H., Fisher, B., et al., 1993. The benefit of leucovorin-modulated fluorouracil as postoperative adjuvant therapy for primary colon cancer: results from National Surgical Adjuvant Breast and Bowel Project protocol C-03. J. Clin. Oncol. 11, 1879–1887.

Wolmark, N., Wieand, H.S., Hyams, D.M., et al., 2000. Randomized trial of postoperative adjuvant chemotherapy with or without radiotherapy for carcinoma of the rectum: National Surgical Adjuvant Breast and Bowel Project Protocol R-02. J. Natl. Cancer Inst. 92, 388–396.

Wolmark, N., Yothers, G., O'Connell, M.J., et al., 2009. A phase III trial comparing mFOLFOX6 to mFOLFOX6 plus bevacizumab in stage II or III carcinoma of the colon: Results of NSABP Protocol C-08. J. Clin. Oncol. 27, 18s (suppl; abstr LBA4).

Wong, R.K., Tandan, V., De Silva, S., et al., 2007. Pre-operative radiotherapy and curative surgery for the management of localized rectal carcinoma. Cochrane Database Syst. Rev. CD002102.

Index

Notes: Page references followed by 'b', 'f' and 't' refer to boxed material, figures and tables respectively. Abbreviations used in subentries are defined in the main body of the index. Please also note that all entries refer to gastrointestinal imaging unless otherwise stated.

Index